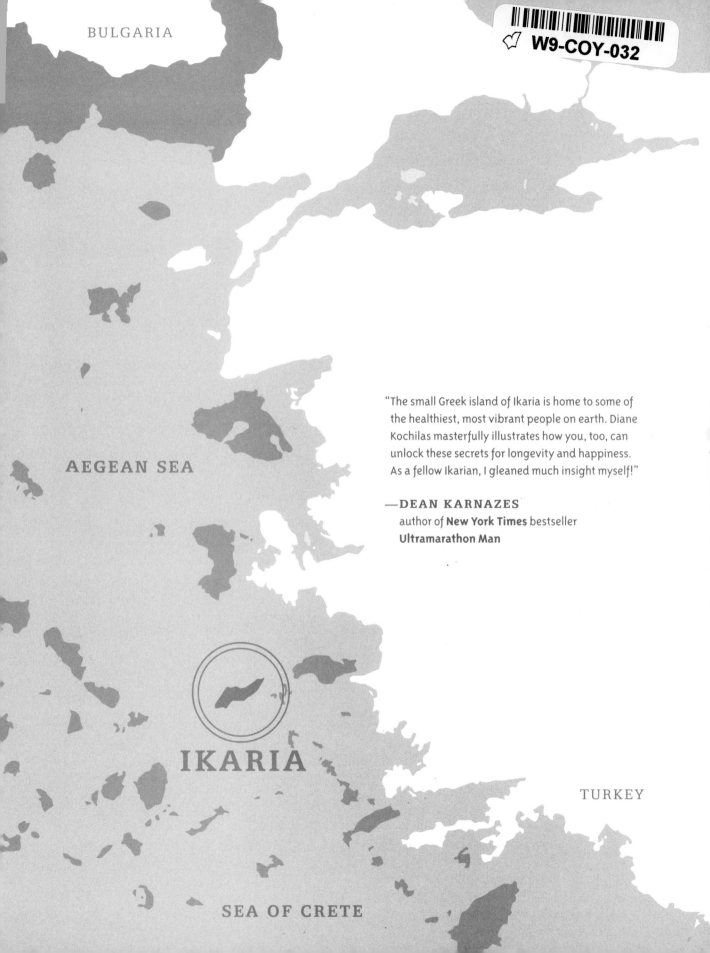

BULGARIA

AEGEAN SEA

"The small Greek island of Ikaria is home to some of
the healthiest, most vibrant people on earth. Diane
Kochilas masterfully illustrates how you, too, can
unlock these secrets for longevity and happiness.
As a fellow Ikarian, I gleaned much insight myself!"

—**DEAN KARNAZES**
author of **New York Times** bestseller
Ultramarathon Man

IKARIA

TURKEY

SEA OF CRETE

IKARIA

Lessons on Food, Life, and
Longevity from the Greek Island
Where People Forget to Die

Diane Kochilas

photography by VASSILIS STENOS

RODALE

In memory of my parents, Tom Kochilas and Zoe Picos Kochilas.

To Vassili, Kyveli, Yiorgo, Athinoula, Koko, Uncle Pauli, Trif, Kris,
Katharine, George, and Tom, for all the reasons families love each other.

© 2014 by Diane Kochilas
Photographs by Vassilis Stenos

Rodale books may be purchased for business or promotional use or for special sales. For information, please write to:
Special Markets Department, Rodale Inc., 733 Third Avenue, New York, NY 10017

Printed in the United States of America
Rodale Inc. makes every effort to use acid-free ∞, recycled paper ♻.

Book design by Kara Plikaitis
Food stylists: Despina Velonia and Ilias Demertzgiou
Kitchen director: Lizana Mitropoulou

Library of Congress Cataloging-in-Publication Data is on file with the publisher.
ISBN 978–1–62336–295–9

Distributed to the trade by Macmillan

2   4   6   8   10   9   7   5   3   1   hardcover

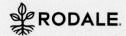

We inspire and enable people to improve their lives and the world around them.
rodalebooks.com

CONTENTS

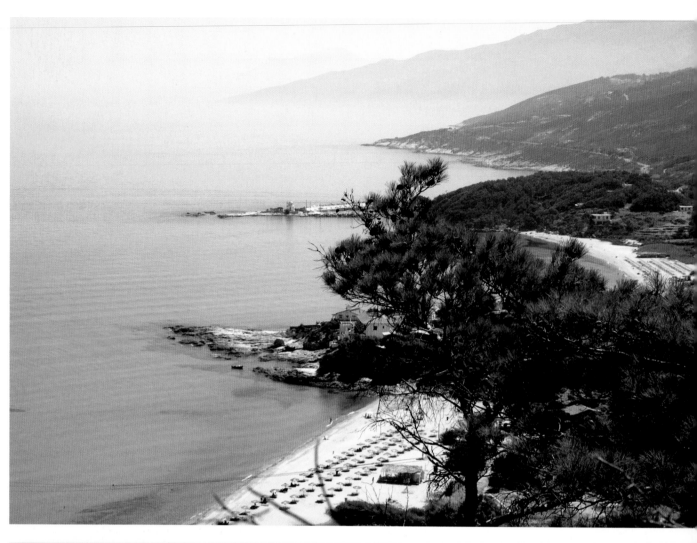

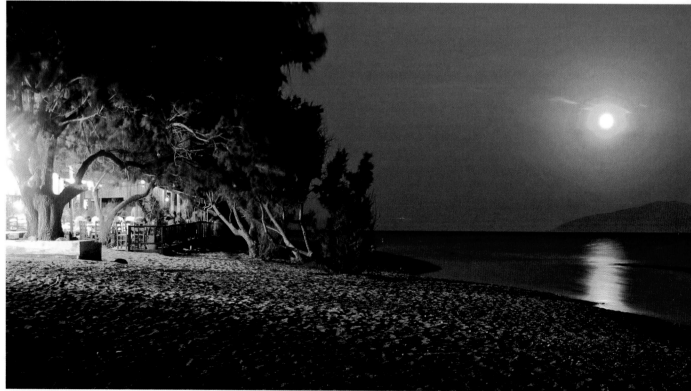

INTRODUCTION

Ikaria feeds the soul.

I first touched foot on the island in 1972 as a 12-year-old New York City kid inured to sticky urban summers, insipid American food, and strict curfews. My Greek was nonexistent, but somehow it didn't matter. I felt at home, as though Ikaria was in my bones. It was, I guess. I grew up with it all around, the child of Ikarian immigrants. My father left his village, Raches, in 1937 and never was able to make it back, settling instead, right after the war, in New York City. Despite our physical distance from it, Ikaria was woven into the texture of our lives. We lived in an Ikarian enclave in Jackson Heights, Queens, and all my parents' friends were from the island; by default and design, we kids were also friends. Now, so are our own children. Bonds among islanders from Ikaria cross oceans and generations. We never thought these ties and our roots to the island to be anything but the norm, even in a society as mobile as America.

Historically, Ikaria has always been isolated and poor, a speck of rock 99 miles long in the middle and roughest part of the Aegean, where political undesirables were exiled from the Byzantine era to the 1960s. But in remoteness and want, islanders learned to be self-reliant, independent of thought, and close-knit, to disdain the pursuit of material acquisition and live simply and essentially, to pay little heed to the zeitgeist of the times, indeed, to pay no heed to time at all. Ikaria is known as the island where people do not live by the clock, where punctuality is not necessarily a virtue, where the time of day is always "late thirty," a kind of running joke. Yet, they outlive most clocks, for the island is home to some of the longest-living people on earth, a demographic and statistical anomaly that has catapulted Ikaria and its people to unexpected fame in the last few years.

Ikaria is one of the Blue Zones,® a term coined by the Belgian demographer Dr. Michel Poulain, who together with Dr. Gianni Pes of the University of Sassari in Italy and Dan Buettner, author of the book *The Blue Zones,* have been studying the planet's pockets of longevity since 2003, under the aegis of the National Geographic Foundation and, in the case of Ikaria, the AARP as well as a series of other corporate funders. Poulain, blue pen in hand, literally drew circles (in blue) on the map one day around places such as Ikaria, Okinawa, Sardinia, Costa Rica, and a community of Seventh Day Adventists in Loma Linda, California, where people seem to live an inordinately long time. His blue-circled zones gave birth to the term that has become synonymous with longevity, but the trademark is owned by Buettner.

What sets Ikarians apart, even from other nonagenarians around the world, is that they live well—with little cancer, cardiovascular disease, dementia, or other age-related ailments—drinking wine, enjoying sex, walking, gardening, and socializing, in other words, being very much alive, in their veritable, modern-day Shangri-La. Since 2008, a battery of scientists, journalists, demographers, and others has been trying to figure out the secrets to this seeming paradise. Food, lifestyle, and such a deep-rooted disregard for living by the clock that there is really no stress have all, somehow, played a role in giving Ikarians good, long lives.

In this book, a tribute to the place and to our countless friends there, both of which have given me and my family more than words can ever express, I set out not to codify Ikaria's diet or lifeways in hopes of uncovering some key, but, rather, to honor them and shine a loving, and, I hope, knowing, light on this once-forgotten piece of rock, that looks like a wing and is named for the Icarus of Greek myth. I hope that anyone who picks up this book might glean a few lessons for how to live more essentially and less anxiously, by cooking and eating simple, real food that is largely plant-based, by ignoring the clock's reign, if even for a bit, and by forging relationships that defy generations and are both meaningful and long-lasting. Those are the things Ikaria has given me and that I hope to share with others.

> THEY LIVE WELL—WITH LITTLE CANCER, CARDIO-VASCULAR DISEASE, DEMENTIA, OR OTHER AGE-RELATED AILMENTS—DRINKING WINE, ENJOYING SEX, WALKING, GARDENING, AND SOCIALIZING, IN OTHER WORDS, BEING VERY MUCH ALIVE, IN THEIR VERITABLE, MODERN-DAY SHANGRI-LA.

IKARIA'S "LONGEVITY" DIET

In researching the diet and foods that people who are now well into old age ate while growing up, I consulted Dan Buettner's book (*The Blue Zones*), read through the Ikaria study (which was compiled by a group of international scientists), and asked a lot of my own questions of the 80-plus set on the island. What I discovered was that it wasn't so much what people ate a generation or two ago on Ikaria, but it was more the fact that they simply did not eat very much at all. Food was not nearly as plentiful then as it is today, so if anything, the dearth, rather than the type, of food defined their diet.

Equally important, of course, was and still is the quality of food. On Ikaria, to this day, people eat very little processed food. Sure, fast food has made some inroads, mainly in the form of souvlaki joints, pizzerias, and a few places selling handheld phyllo pies, most of which are slathered with hydrogenated oils. Chips, candy, and the kind of ice cream so filled with stabilizers that it doesn't melt even under an August sun (an experience I had with my own daughter a few years ago on the island) are all now, unfortunately, part of the dietary vernacular. But so are the wild greens and tomatoes and fruits picked in season, fish just minutes out of the sea, the pigs raised in the family barn and fed leftovers from the table and acorns from the forest, the goats that are grazed or fed on clover and bramble, and the chickens that also eat scraps left over from dinner.

Olive oil flows in copious amounts and mostly everyone produces their own. The local variety is not the Koroneiki olive, which produces some of the finest, fruitiest oils in Greece, but a larger variety called Hondroelia, or "fat olive," which makes more rustic-flavored oils. It is all extra virgin, of course, and almost all of it, like most of the food produced on Ikaria, is organic. Dr. Antonia Trichopoulou, professor emeritus at the Athens School of Pubic Health, who helped administer the surveys that shaped the present picture of Ikaria and its long-lived people, noted that the unprocessed nature of the islanders' diet means that they eat far fewer pesticides and many more nutrients. The purity of the foods they consume might indeed yield up to 4 more years of life expectancy compared with the typical American diet.

Breakfast

Breakfast for the people who are now in their golden years was almost always liquid! Goat's milk, loaded with antioxidants and much easier to digest than cow's milk, was and still is available for about half the year, during periods when the goats are not nursing. It remains one of the bedrock breakfast treats. But so was *krasopsihia*, bread dipped in wine (also loaded with antioxidants), even for children (the wine might have been diluted), a combination that has nursed Greek hunger for eons. "Sometimes we had sage tea with Nounou," said my friend Popi, close to 80, from the town of Manganitis, on the south side of the island. Nounou, for anyone not familiar with it, is nothing more than the brand name of a popular canned condensed milk. Three generations of Greeks have grown up on this.

HERBAL TEAS, HONEY, AND A CLOVE OF GARLIC WORK WELL AS ANTIBIOTICS.

Herbal teas played an important part on the breakfast table, with sage and pennyroyal the most common. "If we were sick, my mother would give us pennyroyal tea with honey and a clove of garlic inside. It was our antibiotic," says Yiorgos Stenos, 83, and active as a beekeeper and merchant.

Sage tea sweetened either with honey or *petimezi* (grape molasses, page 293), a few olives, maybe a rusk or two were also common foods on the breakfast table. That and *koumara*, or arbutus berries, which grow all over Ikaria and provide fodder not only for breakfast but for the still, too, as they are processed into liquor. Koumara blossoms also nourish bees, whose bittersweet arbutus honey is thought to be especially therapeutic.

Wild and Foraged Foods

Ikarians a generation or two ago were lucky, for even in poverty they lived (and still do) in a rich natural environment that provided many foods, available in every season, literally just for the picking: several kinds of berries; fruits from both wild and cultivated trees, among them pears, apples, cherries, sour cherries, figs, and prickly pears; dozens of different wild mushrooms and perhaps hundreds of wild greens, certainly more than I could count and codify for this book. Nuts were and still are part of the diet, and as a kid I recall the awe, city-kid awe, when I first discovered what the snapping sound was on the hottest summer days: pinecones bursting open! We used to spend hours in the forests meticulously fishing for the pine nuts inside the warm, rough cones.

Fish and game, of course, have always been available if one were so inclined to catch them. The two main game animals on Ikaria are partridges and hares. Snails, periwinkles, sea urchins are still accessible treats, too, but less so, as pollution has done its job, diminishing their numbers and quality. I talk about fish in a later chapter (page 207).

What I surmised in countless conversations with people over 80 is that the diet in their formative years comprised a few basics, with foraged foods, especially greens, providing a solid foundation. Breakfast, mentioned on page vii, was almost always either goat's milk or herbal tea; lunch, the main meal of the day, consisted of a lot of beans and pulses. "We ate beans 6 days a week, split peas, broad beans, white beans, fresh beans, you name it. And maybe some boiled greens," says Popi. For the poorest families, dishes such as pies and fritters with foraged greens were a mainstay.

WHAT I SURMISED IN COUNTLESS CONVERSATIONS WITH PEOPLE OVER 80 IS THAT THE DIET IN THEIR FORMATIVE YEARS COMPRISED A FEW BASICS, WITH FORAGED FOODS, ESPECIALLY GREENS, PROVIDING A SOLID FOUNDATION.

Accounts of dinner surprised me, for almost everyone I spoke with recounted it as being mainly starch-based: *matsi*, a kind of noodle; *trahana*, the fermented yogurt- or milk-based pebbly wheat product (page 96); or either fried potatoes or potatoes cooked in tomato sauce. "If we had a pig and it was pork season, we added a little to the beans or potatoes," says Popi. Indeed, pork has always been very important as a protein source and more. The best childhood treat for the over-80 crowd was a piece of bread spread with lard and *petimezi* (grape molasses) or honey. Everyone who mentioned this to me recalls it as being a special treat, one woven into the maternal fabric of the family, something delicious that a grandmother or mother would slip to a child with an extra helping of TLC.

But the type of grains they ate also came as a surprise. Wheat, so closely associated with the Mediterranean diet, was less prevalent on Ikaria proper than barley and rye. Most wheat was cultivated by Ikarians on land they owned across the sea in Asia Minor (Turkey), and wheat flour was either mixed with rye or barley to make bread or used alone in holiday breads or to make pasta and trahana. Corn was also a vital part of the diet, in soups, stuffings, and as flour. So were carob and even acorns, both nutritionally dense and both milled into flour for use in fritters and even as porridge.

As Dan Buettner wrote in a pivotal *New York Times Magazine* article in 2012, ". . . every one of the Ikarians' dietary tendencies had been linked to increased life spans: low intake of saturated fats from meat and dairy was associated with lower risk of heart disease; olive oil—especially unheated—reduced bad cholesterol and raised good cholesterol. Goat's milk contained serotonin-boosting tryptophan and was easily digestible for older people. Some wild greens had 10 times as many antioxidants as red wine. Wine—in moderation—had been shown to be good for you if consumed as part of a Mediterranean diet, because it prompts the body to absorb more flavonoids, a type of antioxidant. And coffee, once said to stunt growth, was now associated with lower rates of diabetes, heart disease, and, for some, Parkinson's. Local sourdough bread might actually reduce a meal's glycemic load. You could even argue that potatoes contributed heart-healthy potassium, vitamin B_6, and fiber to the Ikarian diet. Another health factor at work might be the unprocessed nature of the food they consume."

Essentially, Ikaria's longevity diet is the Mediterranean diet of half a century ago, tailored to what was available locally and defined more by the struggle to procure food than by any contemporary sense of abundance.

LONG LIVES, GOOD LIVES: BLUE ZONES AND THE IKARIA STUDY

The Blue Zones is a large demographic and anthropologic study of various long-living peoples from different parts of the world, different nationalities, and different cultures. And yet they share certain behavioral characteristics, such as closely knit family relations, avoidance of smoking (not necessarily the case among Ikarians), plant-based diets, moderate daily physical activity, and community engagement among people of all ages with little discrimination.

Ikaria's renown as a place where people live exceptionally long—and good—lives was born by accident in 2008, when a Greek researcher involved in the Blue Zones project realized that Ikaria is inhabited by some of the oldest people on the planet. The sleuthing got under way to discover more about the remote, but intriguing, island.

As the team gathered data, cross-referencing birth, baptism, and military service records, they realized that people on Ikaria were, in fact, reaching the age of 90 at more than twice the rate that Americans do. Ikarian men in particular are four times more likely to reach 90 and be in good physical and mental health than their American counterparts. Other characteristics set them apart, even from other long-livers, such as the virtual nonexistence of dementia.

The story of Ikaria began to gain traction. Then, in 2009, a group of seven Greek physicians and medical researchers associated with the University of Athens Medical School, among them the cardiologist Dr. Christodoulos Stefanadis (of Ikarian descent), assessed the socio-demographic, clinical, psychological, and lifestyle characteristics of 1,420 people from the island, a large proportion of whom were over the age of 80, in what has become known as the Ikaria study. The study concluded that indeed Ikaria could and should be considered a candidate for the Blue Zones.

The Athens Medical School team looked at lifestyle, diet, and income levels. They assessed dietary patterns, using quantitative questionnaires that looked at the consumption

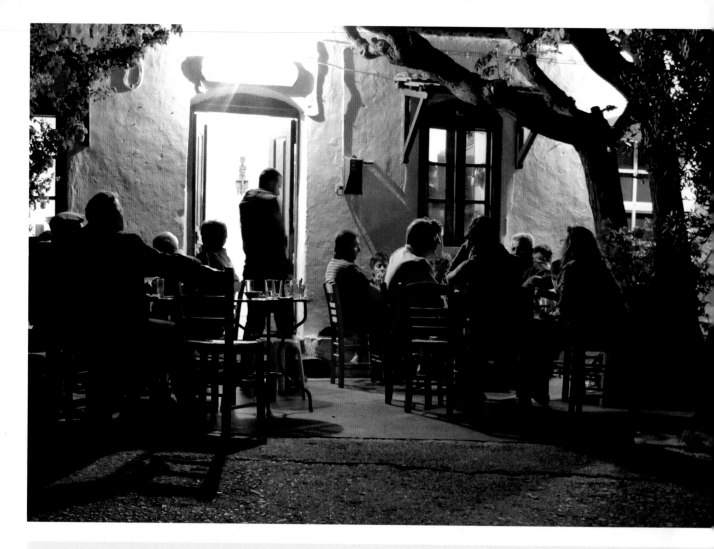

frequency of all the major food and beverage groups and devised a score sheet to gauge the adherence to the Mediterranean diet (the higher the score, the better the diet).

Many of their discoveries were startling. For example, the average life expectancy in Greece is 79.78 years and the number of people over the age of 80 makes up just 5% of the population. Globally, the over-80 set accounts for just 1% of the world's population. On Ikaria, 13% of the study's total sample was over the life expectancy age of 80. (In North America and Europe only 3% of the population reaches past 80.) In addition, 1.6% of the men and 1.1% of women participants in the Ikaria study were over the age of 90, which means that Ikarians were 10 times more likely to reach their ninth, and maybe even tenth decade than either Americans or Western Europeans, and to do so while maintaining a healthy, active life.

Another interesting discovery was the ratio of men to women over 80, which in the West is roughly 1:2; on Ikaria, men and women seem to reach their sunset years together, in a ratio of about 1.1:1. But that said, the majority of men over 80 were married, whereas the majority of women over 80 were widowed.

Income levels were fascinating, and in other parts of this book I mention that Ikarians are not particularly money-driven. A "good" income, for example, on Ikaria is anywhere between 9,600 and 18,000 euros per year, far below what one would ever consider a decent wage in the United States. Half of the people over 80 on the island reported incomes that were below their needs, meaning less than 6,000 euros per year. And yet, these people are neither poor nor damned to misery, as they would be, say, in an urban environment in the West, since for the most part they live with their children and are taken care of with love and a sense of inclusion. In addition, 3.3% of the oldest men and 4.1% of the oldest women still worked, either in their own small businesses or as farmers.

THERE WAS VIRTUALLY NO DEPRESSION AND NO DEMENTIA, WHEREAS ALMOST HALF OF AMERICANS OVER THE AGE OF 85 SHOW SIGNS OF ALZHEIMER'S.

A majority (69%) of the participants in the Ikaria study were found to adhere to a traditional Mediterranean diet, with one difference being their higher rates of potato consumption.

Almost all of them napped regularly, a practice that reduces stress and may lower a person's chances of heart disease. Very few reported any signs of depression, perhaps because of the strong sense of community on the island and the fact that most did not actually live alone.

Older Ikarians are not just mentally and emotionally healthier than their counterparts in other parts of both Greece and the world, they also seem to be physically healthier. The people of Ikaria had 20% less cancer than and half the rate of cardiovascular disease of Americans; not only that but if and when they did get sick from either cancer or heart disease, it was often 8 to 10 years later in life than Americans did. There was virtually no depression and no dementia, whereas almost half of Americans over the age of 85 show signs of Alzheimer's.

Time for Life

My husband and I got married on the island in 1984 and I was 2 hours late for my own wedding. I finally arrived only to learn that the priest had not gotten there yet either! It honestly wasn't a big deal. People were enjoying themselves, the groom was testing the wine, the goats were on a spit, and after the ceremony took place the actual festivities went on for almost 2 days. Imagine that happening in New York City!

Signs here and there in shops around the island read "Clocks, Anxiety and Stress Have No Place on Ikaria." A running joke, when you ask someone what time it is, is to answer *argamisi*, or "late-thirty."

On the northern side of the island, the villages in Raches are renowned for their odd shop schedule. In the summer, for example, when we live on the island, you can buy everything from a glass of wine to clothes, shoes, and groceries until 2 and 3 in the morning. You can't do the same at 10 a.m. though, because the village is mostly still asleep. There's actually a historical reason for the late-night mentality, dating to the era half a millennium ago, when pirates were a constant threat. Ikaria's villages are unlike the villages on most Greek islands. Houses are spread apart and surrounded by land, not clustered together. People lived inland because the coast was too dangerous, and they moved about cautiously at night, after their farm and household chores were done, so as not to be seen from afar. The custom of shopping, socializing, whatever, into the wee hours has remained to this day.

The quirky schedule (if I dare even use that word in the context of Ikaria) and the embrace of serendipity both key into Ikarians' unique, and arguably nonexistent, relationship to time. Read that to mean that they are untouched by the stress that comes with living a programmed, by-the-clock life. You don't need to call a friend to visit him or her; dropping by is just fine and visitors are always welcome (and fed). You don't need to explain yourself if things change midway through a plan. In fact, when you do try to make real, solid plans with someone, the answer is often an uncommitted "we'll see," not because people hedge their bets waiting for something better to come along, but because they know that the adage "man plans, God laughs" is really how life is.

But being tuned in to life's ephemeral truths means being open to chance. It means being sent for coffee to the general store by your mother, as our friend Christos Kourdos once was, and coming back 3 months later, after having met a group of buddies on their way to a *panygyri* (local festival), hooking up with them, cavorting all night, heading with them all the way to Athens, landing a temporary job, and, finally, returning home, coffee, of course, long forgotten. At some point early on, he probably called home.

Is this reason for a misunderstanding? Absolutely not! Quite the contrary, it's reason to savor the unexpected. Does it mean that appointments, promises, and other bound-by-time commitments are never met? No. It just means there is always a little wiggle room in every social interaction, enough to keep people limber and flexible, unhardened by the stress of a ticking clock. Open to life.

No talk of Ikaria and its legendary longevity could ever be complete without mention of the island's ways, the abhorrence of rigidity and rules, and the generally pervasive philosophy of "live and let live."

To this day, a relative disinterest in material wealth, a penchant for last-minute planning, if any at all, and a deep-rooted recognition of the fleeting quality of life still pervade and define the Ikarian mind-set. Most of the values that define and constrict the West are anathema in Ikaria; of course, no one could ever quantify this, but these, together with what was once a lean, almost exclusively plant-based diet, are the values that account for the islanders' legendary longevity.

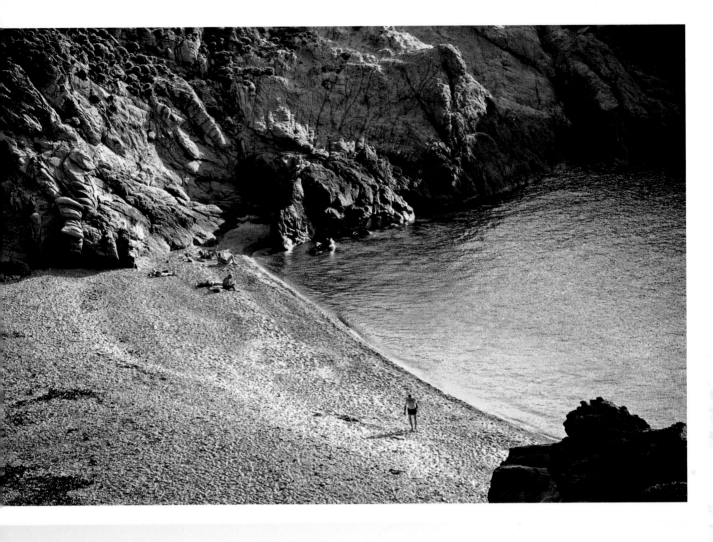

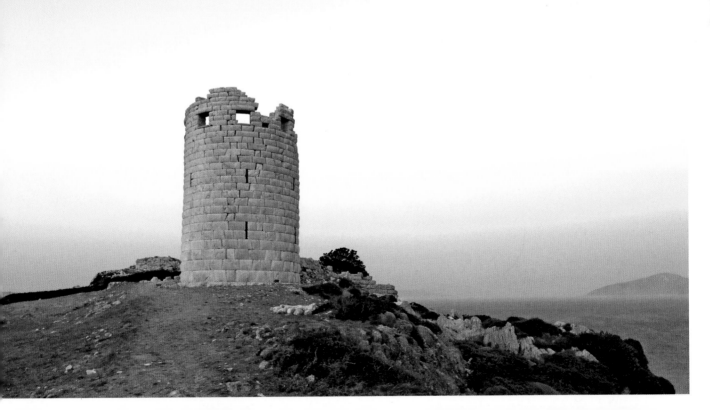

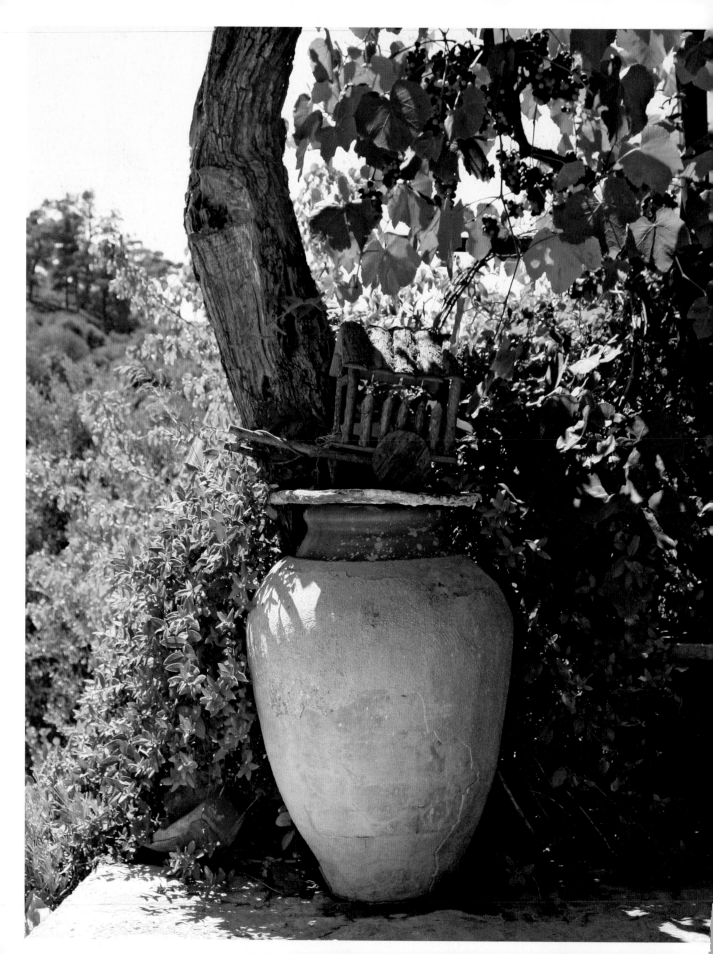

MEZEDES

SMALL BITES
OF BIG
HOSPITALITY

TO UNDERSTAND THE IDEA OF SHARED FOOD—

small bites or *mezedes*—on Ikaria is to understand the sense of community, camaraderie, and generosity that permeates just about every aspect of life on the island. Every table, literally, is an open invitation; plans to meet up with friends don't really exist, they just take shape on the spur of the moment, or people just come around. When they do, which is often, i.e., daily, you always put a little something out, starting with wine and then with whatever else you've either cooked that day or prepared as a preserve, including bread, olives, pickled vegetables, and cheese.

Most of the permanent residents on the island are fairly self-sufficient: They produce their own wine, milk their own goats and make cheese; pick their own *volvoi* (bulbs) to pickle; go foraging for greens, wild asparagus, mushrooms; they fish, and some even hunt. Almost all keep a large garden and other farm animals, like chickens.

So the literal cost of so much open-ended hospitality is one's own labor, but the rewards cannot be monetized because in every single bite offered to someone there is the whole experience of either having gathered or made it, and there is immense pride at having done so. This is all fodder for a conversation, too, which is, in turn, a show of appreciation for what's been offered. Greeks love to sit around the table and talk about the food they're eating! So, even if you've just popped by a friend's and been served something as simple as boiled eggs with olive oil and oregano, the flavors are inimitable—eggs with yolks as yellow as marigolds, oregano whose smell reaches you at the dining room table from the jar just opened in the kitchen, olive oil that is pressed from the olives that grew on the tree outside the front door.

In cities anywhere, you just can't replicate these things—neither the quality and freshness of the food, nor the kind of unregimented life that enables you to visit a friend unannounced (which is different from uninvited), and find him or her at the ready with wine, food, and time to spare.

But that's not to say that the tradition of serving *mezedes*—small communal plates of savory and varied foods—is exclusive to Ikaria. It is not, of course; the need to share our experiences is universal and human. That Greeks do so with the backdrop of tangy dishes—and Ikarians in an environment that is uber-relaxed, clockless, and in tune to the rhythms and bounty of nature—just makes their meze table all the more enviable!

HOMEMADE IKARIAN GOAT'S MILK CHEESE

Kathoura

Kathoura, the local Ikarian cheese, is always made with goat's milk and yet is surprisingly mild, especially in comparison to the strong caprine aromas of American goat cheeses. It almost tastes like mozzarella and has a similar consistency, although it is not steeped in hot whey and kneaded, the way mozzarella and other cheeses in the *pasta filata* family are. You can eat it fresh, as in hours' old or a day or two old; you can salt it and dry it so that it dehydrates and hardens, and you can take it at that stage and preserve it either in olive oil or a 10% salt brine.

MAKES ABOUT 1 POUND

3 quarts unpasteurized goat's milk

¼ teaspoon powdered animal rennet

Coarse salt, preferably sea salt

SPECIAL TOOLS: 10- or 12-quart stainless steel pot, a dairy thermometer, and fine-weave cheesecloth

Measure out ¼ cup of the milk and set aside. Pour the remaining milk into a 10- to 12-quart stainless steel pot and bring to a boil. As soon as the milk boils, turn off the heat. Cover the pot with a clean kitchen towel and let the milk cool to tepid, about 98°F (37°C).

Dissolve the rennet in the reserved ¼ cup milk. Pour it into the tepid milk and stir with a clean, stainless steel spoon. Season with 1 tablespoon salt.

Cover the pot again with a clean cloth and let it stand until the rennet coagulates the milk, anywhere from 1 to 4 hours, depending on the outside temperature. The cheese mass will look a little like Greek yogurt.

Remove the cloth. Cut the cheese mass into small curds using a sharp, clean knife. Resalt to taste. Heat it over low flame until the whey separates from the mass.

Line a large fine-mesh sieve with a double layer of cheesecloth. Using a slotted spoon, transfer the separated curds to the cheesecloth. Gather up the corners of the cheesecloth, joining two and two on each side, almost like folding a sheet. Tie the corners together to form a double knot. The end result should look like a beggar's purse. Hang this over a bowl in the sink, bathtub, or outdoors overnight, to drain. Discard the whey.

The next day, unwrap the cheese and rub it with a little salt. Let it sit for 1 hour in the refrigerator before serving. The cheese will keep for up to 1 week in the refrigerator. If the exterior gets a little wet, rub it with coarse salt.

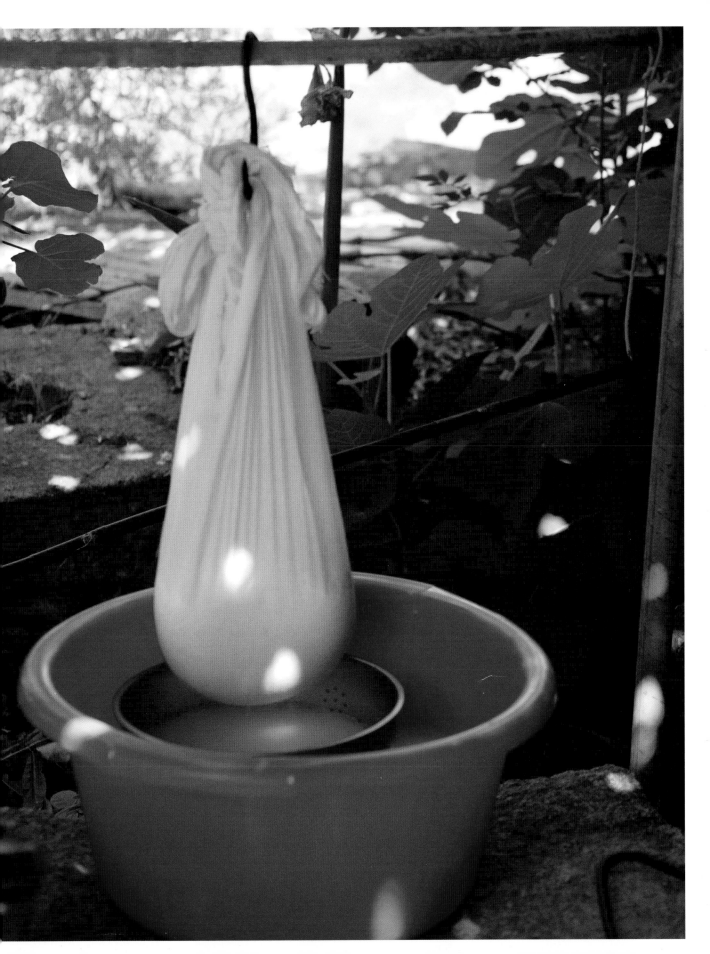

A FEW DIPS AND SPREADS

MARY SAFOS'S IKARIAN-STYLE NEW YORK KOPANISTI

Kariotiki Kopanisti stin Nea Yorki

Kopanisti, a soft, sharp cheese, is to an Ikarian home what a bag of peanuts or chips is to an American kitchen cupboard: something that's almost always on hand, and offered freely to anyone who comes to visit, ad lib or planned.

Such is the case with our friend Basil's mom, Mary, whose American-born recipe speaks tomes about the way Ikarians in the wider immigrant community across the globe maintain and transform traditions, adapting to what's available. "Every summer, I have to pick *throumbi* for my mother," Basil explains when I ask him what his mom's recipe is. *Throumbi* is the herb called savory and it's one of the foremost wild herbs on the island, so peppery and earthy and very much beloved in all sorts of dishes. So, with a bag full of savory, which Basil manages to dry out before leaving the island in August, Mary makes her *kopanisti*, which is a mixture of feta cheese, blue cheese, a little cottage cheese, *throumbi*, and a most unexpected ingredient, at least to this culinary scribe, chile oil. Her mission, for sure, when first attempting to reproduce this spicy local cheese in a New York City home was to create a close approximation of the original, which is peppery because it "fires up" as they say on the island, over the months of fermenting.

MAKES ABOUT 3 CUPS

- 2 cups crumbled Greek feta cheese
- ½ cup crumbled Roquefort or other good-quality blue cheese
- ½ cup cottage or ricotta cheese
- ⅓ cup Greek extra virgin olive oil
- 3 tablespoons dried savory, Greek oregano, or thyme
- Several drops of chile oil or hot sauce
- Freshly ground black pepper

In a food processor, combine the cheeses, olive oil, herb, and chile oil or hot sauce and black pepper to taste and pulse until smooth. Keep in a sealed container for up to 2 weeks, refrigerated. Over the course of a few days, the *kopanisti* will acquire a more peppery flavor.

WHIPPED FETA KOPANISTI

Kopanisti me Feta

Here's another facsimile of the traditional Ikarian *kopanisti*, but made easily with feta (more accessible to American cooks), olive oil, and herbs. It can be made in a flash. With a bowl of kopanisti, a little bread or rusks, and a glass or two of wine on the table, you've got the makings of an ad hoc get-together.

MAKES ABOUT 3 CUPS

3 cups crumbled Greek feta or kalathaki Limnou (see Note)

1 tablespoon dried savory or 2 teaspoons dried Greek oregano

⅔ cup Greek extra virgin olive oil, plus more for storing

In a food processor, combine the cheese and savory (or oregano) and pulse on and off, drizzling in the olive oil, until the mixture is creamy.

Transfer to a sealed container or glass canning jar. Pour ¼ inch (1 cm) olive oil over the surface to cover the cheese and store in the refrigerator for 3 to 5 days before consuming.

NOTE: Kalathaki Limnou *is a brine cheese, like feta, made with 100% goat's milk.*

KOPANISTI: IKARIA'S SOFT CHEESE

Kopanisti, which means "beaten" or "whipped," is actually the name given to various soft, sharp cheeses throughout Greece, mainly in the islands.

To make the Ikarian *kopanisti*, you need authentic Ikarian *kathoura* cheese (or an American homemade version, page 4). Take the fresh cheese, crumble it, and mix it with 3 tablespoons of dried savory or oregano, 1 heaping teaspoon salt, and about ½ cup olive oil. Pack it into a glass jar and pour enough olive oil over the surface to seal it. Store it in the refrigerator. In a few days' time it will sour and ferment. The longer you keep it, the more pungent it will be. Stir it up every few days. You can keep replenishing it with additional fresh, crumbled *kathoura* and herbs and salt. It will keep for up to several weeks, refrigerated.

You can also make *ersatz*, which are delicious versions of this creamy spread shown on these two pages, with ingredients readily available in American supermarkets.

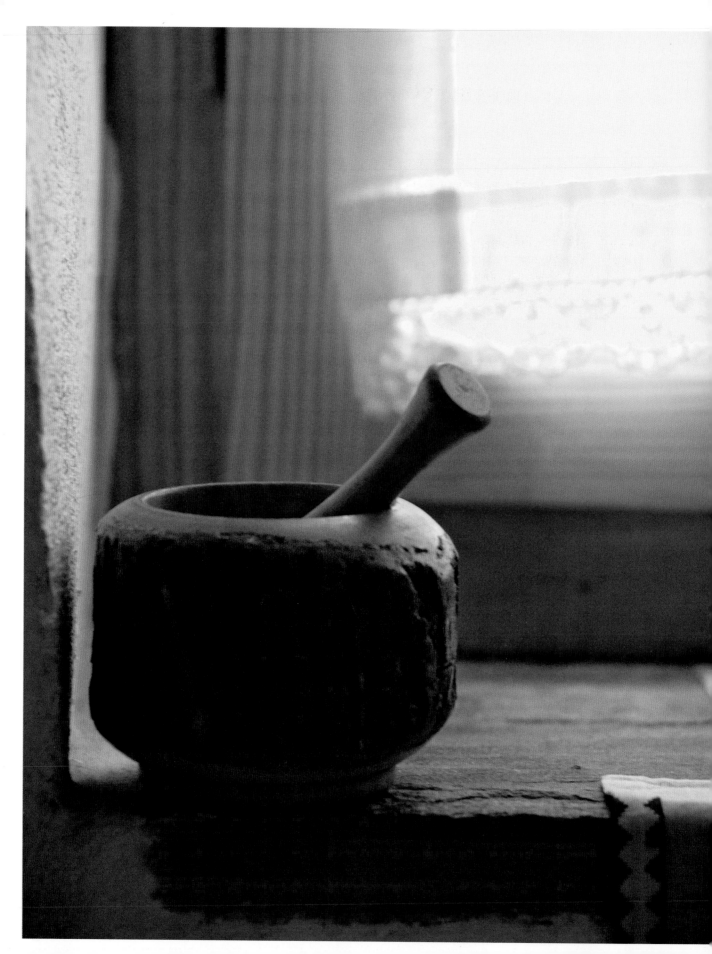

TARO ROOT SKORDALIA

Skordalia

Skordalia, the garlicky dip made with either a bread, potato, or nut base elsewhere in Greece, was traditionally made with taro root on Ikaria. That's not to say that the other versions don't exist—they do—especially the bread-based version. But the taro root–garlic puree below is purely Ikarian; I haven't come across this dish anywhere else in Greece. Its flavor is unique, too. Taro imparts a starchy neutrality to the base, much more so than either potatoes, which are sweeter, or bread, which can get gummy.

This garlicky dip goes beautifully with beet salad, fried or grilled fish, boiled greens, crispy fried or baked pumpkin, and vegetable patties.

MAKES 4 TO 6 SERVINGS

1 large taro root about 1 pound (450 g)

Salt

5 to 7 garlic cloves, chopped (to taste)

½ to 1 cup Greek extra virgin olive oil (to taste)

2 to 4 tablespoons red wine vinegar (to taste)

Using a sharp knife or vegetable peeler, remove the crusty hard peel of the taro root. Rinse well under cold water.

Cut the taro into chunks and place in a medium pot with cold water and a little salt. Bring to a boil over medium heat, reduce to low, and simmer the taro root until fork-tender, 20 to 30 minutes.

Drain and transfer to a food processor. Add the garlic and pulse on and off, drizzling in the olive oil and vinegar in alternating doses, until the mixture is creamy and smooth and reaches desired acidity. Season to taste with salt. Store in the refrigerator.

CLASSIC SKORDALIA WITH BREAD

Klassiko Skordalia me Vasi to Psomi

There are a handful of regional *skordalia* recipes throughout Greece, some made with a potato base, others with a bread base, others still with almonds or walnuts or a combination of starch and nuts. The most common version of *skordalia* on Ikaria is made with a bread base, as in the recipe below. There is another, older recipe for *skordalia* made with taro root, too (page 9). When you make this with leftover, really good sourdough bread, the dip is rustic and pleasantly sharp. It's the perfect foil to many of the island's crispy fried vegetables and a real favorite with fried pumpkin (page 20).

MAKES 6 SERVINGS

4 thick slices (2-inch [5 cm]) stale country bread, preferably sourdough

5 to 6 garlic cloves (to taste)

Sea salt

¾ to 1 cup Greek extra virgin olive oil (as needed and to taste)

4 to 6 tablespoons red wine vinegar (to taste)

Run the bread under the flowing tap water to dampen, then squeeze dry and crumble. (You can remove the crusts, if desired, before dampening.)

Place the garlic in a large mortar and, using the pestle, pound with 2 pinches of salt to form a paste. Slowly add the bread, olive oil, and vinegar, alternating between each and seasoning to taste with salt as you continue to pound. The end result should take about 10 minutes and should be dense and spreadable.

VARIATION

Old-Fashioned Skordalia with Purslane (*Skordalia me Glistrida*): Purslane *skordalia* was the traditional summer accompaniment to boiled potato salads, fried small fish, and boiled beets. Add to the above recipe 2 cups of trimmed purslane. Stir it into the *skordalia*.

VASSILI'S TARAMOSALATA

Taramosalata is a whipped dip with a base of fish roe (*tarama*) and either potatoes, bread, or a combination of either of those and nuts. On Ikaria, there is no one specific recipe; most people make the classic stale-bread version. My husband makes a mean *taramosalata*, which is exceedingly creamy thanks to the unabashed use of olive oil. He spikes it with refreshing dill and pink peppercorns, definitely not traditional but delicious nevertheless.

MAKES ABOUT 2 CUPS (8 TO 12 SERVINGS)

2 medium potatoes, about ½ pound (225 g), peeled and cubed

2 heaping tablespoons *tarama* (fish roe)

Juice of 2 lemons

2 cups Greek extra virgin olive oil, or more if necessary

½ cup snipped fresh dill

1 tablespoon pink peppercorns, crushed

Place the potatoes in a saucepan with enough water to cover and bring to a boil. Reduce to a simmer and cook until tender, about 20 minutes.

Reserving the potato cooking liquid in the pan, use a slotted spoon to transfer the hot potatoes to a food processor. Add the *tarama* and lemon juice. Pulse on and off continuously until the mixture is pureed. Then add ½ cup of the hot potato cooking liquid and pulse a few more times.

Then, pulsing all the while, add the olive oil, slowly drizzling it into the mixture, for about 4 minutes total. Taste and if the mixture is too sour because of the lemon juice, add more olive oil. If the mixture is too dense, add a few more drops of the hot cooking liquid and pulse on and off again. Transfer to a bowl and mix in the dill and peppercorns.

NUTRIENT-DENSE TARAMA

Tarama, the tiny beads of fish roe from cod or carp, is so nutrient dense that it could easily be labeled a superfood. The roe provides a boost of cancer-fighting vitamin D and brain-supporting omega-3 fatty acids. The high content of vitamins A and K_2 work synergistically to prevent toxicity and overcalcification of the bones, heart, and kidneys, explains nutritionist Maria Byron Panayidou. When combined with bread or potatoes to make *taramosalata*, the dish becomes a great source of protein, complex carbohydrates, monounsaturated fat (the good fat from olive oil), vitamin E, vitamin B_{12}, potassium, selenium, phosphorus, and copper. The fact that *taramosalata* is a seminal part of the traditional fasting menu is not accidental at all.

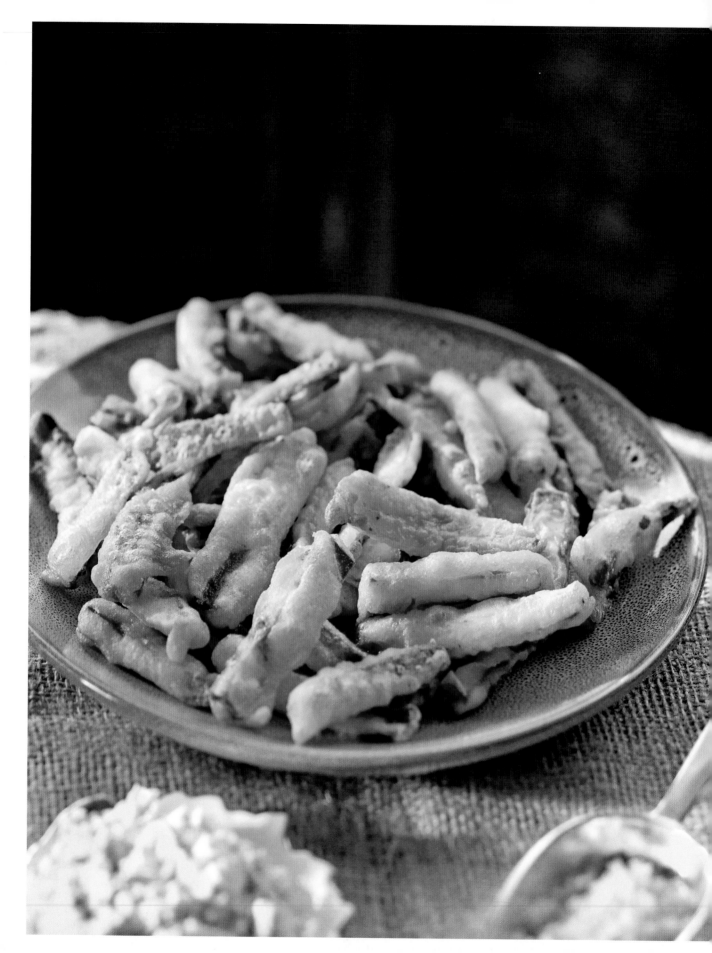

NIKOS POLITIS' ZUCCHINI STICKS

Maridaki Kariotiko

Father and son Theodosis and Nikos Politis run several restaurants on the north side of Ikaria, all of which serve up a combination of traditional fare and contemporary Ikarian-inspired food. The zucchini sticks are whimsically called *maridaki* (the Greek word for smelts), because smelts, long and slim, are typically floured and fried just like these little sticks. They're great.

One caveat: It's really hard to replicate the texture and flavor of Greek garden vegetables in the United States and elsewhere because farming techniques are different and so is the common attitude toward seasonal foods. In Greece, most people still tailor their diets to what really is in season. Summers are dry, sunny, and hot, and vegetables are not overwatered. Greek zucchini, eaten almost always and only in the summer, is crisper, smaller, and more intensely flavored than what I typically find in an American supermarket. So, please, cook this in season, try to find zucchini from a farm that's nearby, and tweak the frying time as needed if the zucchini is waterlogged.

MAKES 4 TO 6 SERVINGS

1 pound (450 g) medium summer zucchini

Salt

Olive oil, for frying

All-purpose flour, for dredging

3 tablespoons grated Greek *kefalotyri* cheese

2 teaspoons dried mint or 1 tablespoon chopped fresh mint

Rinse and pat dry the zucchini. Cut each one into sticks about 2½ inches (6 cm) long and ¼ inch (75 mm) wide. Layer in a colander, sprinkling each layer with salt. Place a plate and a weight over the zucchini and let drain for at least 1 hour. Dry with a clean kitchen towel.

In a large, heavy-bottomed pot, heat 2 inches (5 cm) of oil over medium heat. Test for temperature by tossing a piece of bread into the pot. If it crisps up and turns golden within about 10 seconds, the oil is ready.

Toss the zucchini in flour, shaking off the excess. Using a slotted spoon or spider, slip a small handful of zucchini into the hot oil and fry without moving around too much, until crisp and golden. Remove with the slotted spoon and drain on paper towels. Continue with remaining zucchini sticks, clearing out any burnt clumps of flour that might accumulate in the hot oil.

Once the zucchini are cooked, toss in a serving bowl with the grated cheese and mint. They are great with any of the *kopanisti* and/or *skordalia* recipes (pages 6 to 10).

FRIED AND/OR STUFFED ZUCCHINI FLOWERS

Tiganitoi Kolokythoanthoi

Zucchini flowers are a gardener's delicacy on Ikaria, as they are, really, throughout the Greek countryside. A few island cooks I know have a way with them—a light touch when it comes to batter-frying them or a good hand at placing them as space-fillers in a tray full of other stuffed vegetables, including the zucchini itself, but also tomatoes, peppers, and eggplants.

Popi Manoli, who runs a little snack-bar-cum-taverna in Manganitis, on the south side of Ikaria, is one of those cooks who knows how to fry the flowers so that they are crisp on the outside and delicate within. Sometimes she stuffs them with a little *kathoura*, Ikaria's local cheese.

Ikaria's home cooks also use the flowers in fillings for their summer *pitarakia*, the small, long, slim handheld phyllo pastries that are a local specialty (the contents of the filling change somewhat with each season). Flowers, cleared of pistils and/or stamens, are chopped up as an additional treat in the local zucchini fritter, too, and a few more adventurous local cooks add them here and there to salads.

Pick fresh zucchini flowers early in the morning, when they are open wide. You can use the male and female flowers interchangeably: The male flowers grow on the stems of the zucchini plant

FRYING IN THE GREEK DIET

It always strikes me as ironic that in Ikaria, as well as throughout the Greek islands, where the Mediterranean diet is still alive and well, the number of fried dishes eaten on a regular basis is astonishingly vast. Fried foods do not a healthy diet make, so their prevalence seems counterintuitive—unless we see them in context.

Frying prevails all over the Greek islands because electric ovens are a relatively new phenomenon, and fuel, i.e., wood, for outdoor ovens, was used sparingly, and also because frying is easy and fast. So, there is a whole range of fried foods all over Greece, but mainly on the islands: vegetable, mushroom, and other fritters, bean patties, fried fish, even desserts that are made in a skillet.

The trick is to know which fat to use for frying and how to use it. Olive oil, canola oil, and peanut oil are best. Ikarians fry almost exclusively in olive oil. "We all need fat in our diet. In fact, 25% to 30% of our total caloric intake should come from fat. We have to keep the very important fat-soluble vitamins (A, D, and E) happy!" says Maria Byron Panayidou, who contributed the nutrition notes in this book. "The pleasures of fried food are not forbidden for the health-conscious," says Maria.

and are a little smaller. They contain pistils, which most people remove. The female flowers grow on the end of the vegetable itself, are a little larger, and contain the stamens.

To store (they keep for a few days), place one flower inside the other, to keep them from closing. Place on a tray lined with paper towels, and place a dry paper towel over them and a dampened one on top. Cover with plastic wrap.

Like the zucchini, the flowers are a good source of folate, potassium, manganese, and vitamin A.

MAKES 6 SERVINGS

18 zucchini flowers, preferably organic

2 cups all-purpose flour

Salt and freshly ground black pepper

1 cup milk, water, seltzer, or beer

2 eggs, lightly beaten

CHEESE STUFFING (OPTIONAL)

1/4 cup crumbled Greek Manouri cheese or ricotta salata

1/2 cup crumbled Greek feta cheese

1/3 cup finely chopped fresh mint

1 teaspoon grated lemon zest

Salt and freshly ground black pepper

Olive oil, for frying

Carefully remove the stamens or pistils from the zucchini flowers, and any insects that might be on the inside of the flowers.

Place the flour in a large bowl and season with salt and pepper. Make a well in the center. Add the liquid and the beaten eggs. Whisk until smooth.

For the cheese stuffing (if using): In a bowl, thoroughly combine the cheeses, mint, lemon peel, and salt and pepper to taste. Fill each flower with about 2 teaspoons of the mixture and twist the tips to close.

In a large, heavy-bottomed pot, heat about 4 inches (10 cm) oil until just before the smoke point. To test the oil, drop in a small piece of bread. If it sizzles up and turns golden in about 5 seconds, the oil is ready.

Dip the stuffed or unstuffed zucchini flowers in the batter and hold up over the bowl to drain off excess batter. Carefully drop a few flowers at a time in the hot oil, frying until lightly golden and crisp, about 45 seconds. Remove with a slotted spoon or spider and drain on paper towels. Continue with remaining flowers until done. Serve hot.

TSIFIA: DRYING SUMMER'S BOUNTY FOR WINTER

Food drying is actually one of the oldest methods of preserving food. The process removes the moisture to prevent bacteria, yeast, and mold from spoiling the food. Drying also slows down the action of enzymes without inactivating them. Thus, the veggies get to retain their natural nutritional value with the exception of vitamin C, which is volatile, meaning it's heat and light sensitive.

Ikarians call dried fruits and vegetables *tsifia* and to this day a good portion of the summer garden ends up sliced, salted, and dried to be used later in the year as a meze to go with *ouzo* or *tsipouro* and as an addition to bean dishes and other vegetable stews.

My neighbor Titika salts and air-dries potatoes, zucchini, peppers, tomatoes, and eggplants as well as local summer pears, apricots, and peaches. Figs, a staple in Greece, are also sun-dried but not considered *tsifia*. They are in their own separate category, arguably because they are so packed with nutrition and flavor. Figs saw Ikarians through the long period of Lent, when the larder thinned.

Beguiled by the notion of savoring our own garden vegetables in the winter, I went to Titika for advice.

Apparently, there are several methods to make *tsifia*, among them stringing cut vegetables like a necklace and leaving them to hang until crisp. But following her lead, I simplified the task as outlined below, then oven-baked them in the Final Step as a safety precaution, as per her instructions.

For Zucchini and Eggplants

Slice the vegetables into thin rounds, about ⅛ inch thick.

Place in a framed screen or other surface where air can circulate. Sprinkle generously with salt (preferably sea salt) on one side. Leave them to dry for 1 day in indirect sunlight. Bring them indoors at night because the evening's moisture will spoil them. The next day, turn and salt on the other side and leave outdoors in indirect sunlight, returning them indoors at night. Keep them outside in the daytime for several days, turning every few hours but not adding additional salt unless necessary, until dehydrated and flaky.

For Potatoes

There are several ways to sun-dry potatoes, according to the various islanders I asked. The simplest is to do as above, opting to peel the potatoes or not, first. The second, according to Stefanos Tsantiris, one of the best farmers and gardeners in Raches, is to boil them whole first, with skins, then peel, slice into thin rounds, and sun-dry, all in one day. You have to work fast and start early and the day has to be sunny and hot. If the potatoes take several days to dry, they darken, according to Stefanos.

For Tomatoes

This process is the same, too, but seed the tomatoes and remove the pulp. Salt and turn over several days, as you do with eggplant, covering them with cheesecloth, and remember to bring indoors at night.

For Pears

Slice the pears lengthwise and leave to dry on a screen, turning, for several days. The pears will oxidize and turn deep dark amber.

Final Step

The fruits and vegetables need to be oven-dried at a low temperature to kill any impurities or potential bugs. Preheat the oven to 250°F (130°C). Place them on a baking sheet in a single layer and bake until completely dried and a little chewy, anywhere between 20 minutes and 1 hour. Baking times will vary depending on the water content inherent in each vegetable.

How to Use Dried Vegetables

The rule of thumb when cooking them depends on the recipe. If you want to fry the dried vegetable slices, then you have to rehydrate them in water for a few hours until soft, then either dip them in a simple batter or in flour before frying. They are great with *skordalia* (pages 9 and 10). You can also add them to stews and braised dishes, such as *tourlou* (page 135) or *mageirio* (page 131). If adding to a stew, they don't need to be reconstituted.

Sun-dried fruits and vegetables are rich in concentrated amounts of nutrients, so these old-timers knew something!

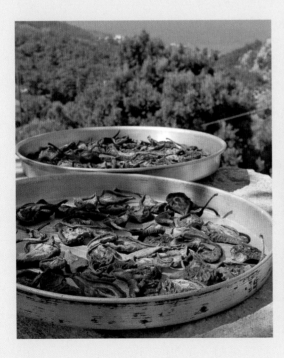

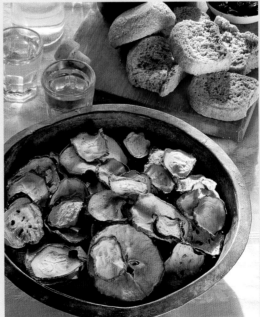

FRIED OR BAKED ZUCCHINI FRITTERS WITH OREGANO AND MINT

Kolokythokeftedes sto Tigani y sto Fourno

Everywhere you look on Ikaria between July and September, whether in local tavernas or in homes, these fritters are there! Zucchini grows like crazy in Ikarian summer gardens and these are a meze that people never tire of. In the last few years, I've taken to baking, rather than frying them, a trick I learned from my good friend Eleni Karimali (see Note below).

MAKES 6 SERVINGS

2 pounds (900 g) zucchini,* grated

2 teaspoons salt

²/₃ cup crumbled feta cheese

2 large eggs, lightly beaten

5 scallions, white and tender green parts, finely chopped

¹/₃ cup finely chopped fresh mint

¹/₄ cup finely chopped fresh oregano

1 to 1¹/₂ cups all-purpose flour, plus more for dredging

Salt and freshly ground black pepper

Olive oil or other oil, for frying

Put the grated zucchini in a colander, sprinkle with the salt, and rub between your palms until wilted, wringing out as much liquid as possible from the vegetable. For the best result, you can even leave the grated zucchini overnight, pressed down in a colander with a plate and several cans as weights.

Transfer the zucchini to a bowl and add the feta, eggs, scallions, and herbs. Add half the flour and stir. Add additional flour a few tablespoons at a time, until the mixture is a very thick batter. The amount of flour may vary depending on the consistency and water content of the zucchini. Season with salt, if needed, and pepper to taste. Refrigerate the mixture, covered, for 1 hour.

In a large, heavy skillet, heat 2 inches (5 cm) olive oil over medium heat. Put about 1 cup flour in a shallow bowl. Using a tablespoon, take a little of the mixture at a time and shape into patties. Dredge the patties lightly in flour, shaking off any excess, and fry a few at a time in the hot oil. Turn carefully with a spatula to fry on both sides. Remove with a slotted spoon and drain on paper towels. Repeat with remaining mixture. Serve hot.

*Grated fresh pumpkin can be used in place of zucchini.

NOTE: *Nowadays, many home cooks, myself included, opt to bake, not fry, the patties. To do so, follow the directions for shaping the fritter patties (no need to dredge them). Preheat the oven to 375°F (190°C). Line a shallow baking pan with parchment paper and bake the patties, in batches if necessary, until golden and crisp, 15 to 20 minutes, turning once.*

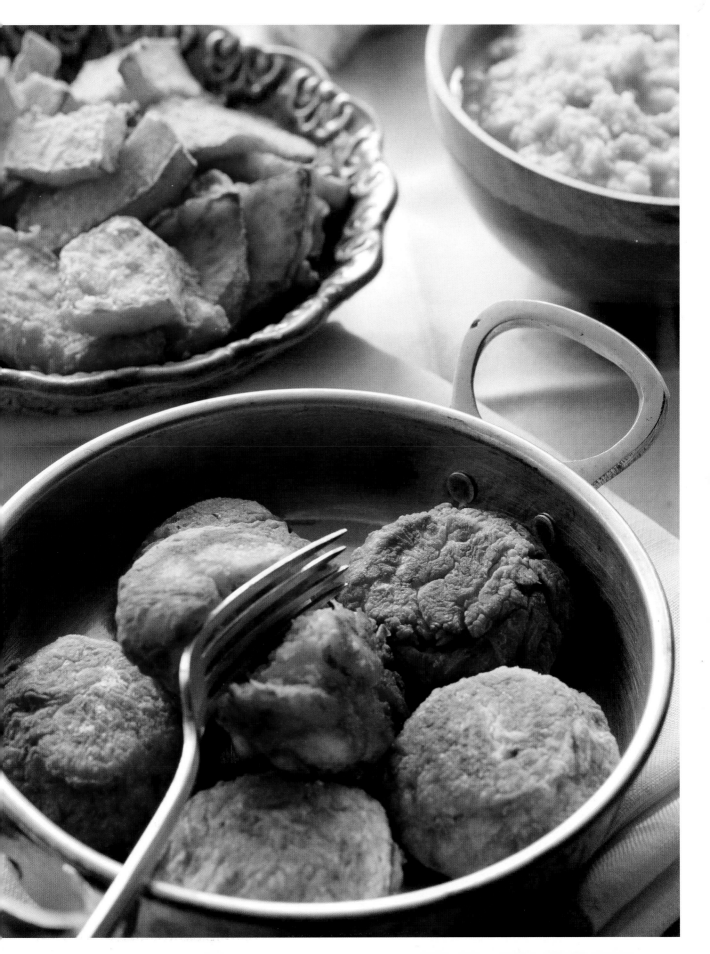

PUMPKIN WEDGES PAN-FRIED IN OLIVE OIL

Tiganiti Kolokytha

Pumpkins dangle from the vine in Ikarian gardens and start to ripen under the end-of-August sun. They provide a winter staple and sometimes last well into the late spring, kept cool in sheds and cellars, next to baskets of potatoes, onions, garlic, and all the other staples of an Ikarian larder. Fried pumpkin and *skordalia* (pages 9 and 10) are a classic Ikarian meze.

MAKES 6 SERVINGS

1 pound (450 g) pumpkin, peeled, seeded, and cut into wedges ¼ inch (75 mm) thick

Sea salt

All-purpose flour, for dredging

Freshly ground black pepper

Olive oil or a combination of corn oil and olive oil, for frying

Place the pumpkin slices in a colander, layering and seasoning lightly with salt. Press down with a plate weighted down with cans, and let the pumpkin sit to drain for at least 1 hour. Pat dry very well with paper towels.

Place some flour in a large bowl and season with salt (taste the pumpkin for saltiness and season accordingly) and a little pepper, too. Set up a large bowl of cold water.

In a nonstick skillet, heat 1 inch (2.5 cm) oil. Dip a few pumpkin wedges at a time in the flour, dip them quickly into the water, then flour them again. Immediately slip a few at a time into the hot oil. Fry, turning once, until crisp and golden brown on both sides, a few minutes. Remove and drain on paper towels. Repeat with remaining slices and flour. Serve hot.

WHOLE ROASTED ONIONS
WITH VINEGAR AND OLIVE OIL
Kremmydia Ofta kai Xidata

I couldn't possibly replicate the real McCoy of this dish in an American kitchen unless I had a working, wood-burning hearth and plenty of hot embers with which to roast everything from onions to potatoes. So many of the most delicious foods that evolved in Ikarian kitchens of yore are foods so humble they seem almost banal. But that's hardly the case when you consider the pungency of a homegrown onions that've been perfectly charred, smoked, and softened in embers, then dressed with peppery olive oil and aromatic local wine vinegar. This was the kind of poor man's food that made for a poor man's feast. Perfect food for guests, both expected and not.

All you need are onions, coarse sea salt, good Greek olive oil, and a strong red wine vinegar. You can do this in a fireplace that burns real wood, on an outdoor grill, or in the oven in your kitchen.

1 ONION PER PORTION

As many large whole, unpeeled onions as you want to roast

Greek extra virgin olive oil (about 1 teaspoon per onion), plus more for dressing

Coarse sea salt

Good aged red wine vinegar

Preheat the oven to 450°F (200°C). (If using a fireplace, wait until the fire dies down and the embers are red-hot. If using a grill, it should be hot, but do not place onions over direct flame.)

Rub each of the onions with about 1 teaspoon olive oil and place in a baking pan. Roast, uncovered, until the skins are deep golden brown and the onions very soft, about 1 hour. (If roasting under embers, don't rub the onions with olive oil. Place whole—wrapped in foil if desired, but this is not necessary—under the hot ash and roast until tender, about 45 minutes. If doing this on the grill, place the whole onions on the side, over indirect heat, cover with the lid, and roast for about 1 hour.)

Remove, cool slightly, and peel. Dress to taste with sea salt, olive oil, and vinegar. Serve hot.

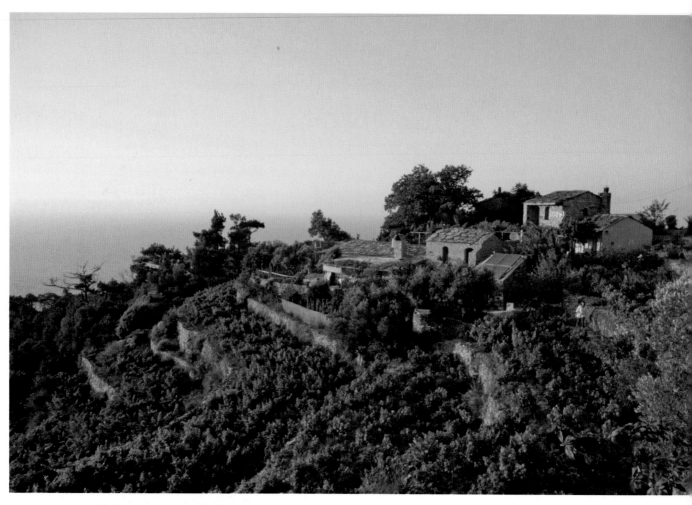

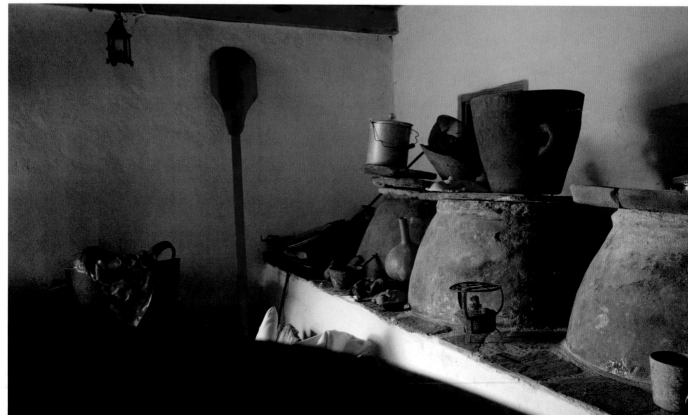

IKARIA'S POTENT WINE

Mezedes are the ultimate convivial food, meant to be shared and enjoyed over a glass or two of wine or spirits. On Ikaria, the local wine is as unique as just about everything else.

The island has been known since antiquity for its wine, which was known as Pramnios Oinos in antiquity. (Pramnos is the name of a mountain peak on the island.) In Hellenistic and Roman times, the entire mountain range was a continuous vineyard and the wine was so prized that most of it was exported to Rome.

What set it apart was its strength. Pramnios oinos, which was produced from sun-dried grapes, was about 18% alcohol.

Today in Ikaria almost every family produces its own wine and they do so the ancient, traditional way: They let the grapes ripen on the vine and then lay them in the sun for about a week so that the sugar levels rise even more. Their juice is pressed in traditional stone presses and in many cases it is still stored the ancient way, in clay amphorae that are buried in the ground. Each clay vessel holds about 250 liters.

Even now, the wine in Ikaria is very strong, between 16% and 18% alcohol. In most wine-making regions, it is impossible to produce wines so strong in alcohol because normally the wine yeasts die when the alcohol level rises above 16%. But modern oenologists on Ikaria isolated a natural, indigenous yeast that can continue the fermentation process even when the alcohol content of the must rises above 16% alcohol. To this day, Ikarians still drink their strong wine the way the ancients did, by watering it down.

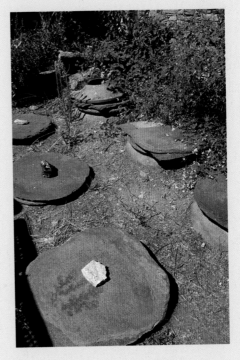

The main grape varieties on the island are the Begleri, a white variety; Fokiano, a red variety that was imported from Asia Minor about two centuries ago and flourishes on the island because the climatic conditions are similar; and, finally, the Koundouro, which is similar to a variety found all over the Aegean called Mandilaria. This grape is prized for its deep red color and is usually mixed with the more aromatic Fokiano. Muscat grapes, a few minor local varieties, and several international varieties have also been planted. There are three commercial vineyards: the Afianes estate, Tsantiris, and the Karimalis estate. Afianes exports his wines and I have seen them on menus as far away as New York City.

POTATO-CHEESE CROQUETTES

Patatokeftedes

This is a popular meze and snack during the 3 weeks of Carnival, right before the 48 days of Lent begin. The croquettes are soft, light, and easy to eat in quantity. The herbs help foil some of the pungency of the feta. These make an excellent accompaniment to a glass of red wine.

MAKES ABOUT 20

1 pound (450 g) boiling potatoes, peeled and quartered

Salt and freshly ground black pepper

1 egg

½ pound (225 g) Greek feta cheese, crumbled

⅓ cup finely chopped fresh flat-leaf parsley

⅓ cup finely chopped fresh mint

Pinch of freshly grated nutmeg

All-purpose flour, as needed

Olive or other oil, for frying

In a pot, cover the potatoes with cold salted water and bring to a boil. Reduce the heat and simmer the potatoes until fork-tender, 20 to 25 minutes. Drain into a colander and set aside to cool completely.

Transfer the potatoes to a bowl and mash with a fork or handheld potato masher. Mix in the egg, feta, herbs, nutmeg, and salt and pepper to taste. Mix well. Add flour if necessary to bind the mixture, kneading in 2 tablespoons at a time, until the mixture is solid enough to hold its shape.

Shape the croquettes into 1½-inch (4 cm) oblong or round patties. Place on a plate, cover with parchment then foil, and refrigerate for 1 hour to firm up.

Spread about 1 cup of flour into a plate.

In a heavy nonstick skillet, heat 1 inch (2.5 cm) of oil over medium to high heat. Test to see if the oil is hot enough by tossing in a piece of bread. It should crisp up in about 10 seconds. When the oil is ready, start dredging the croquettes lightly in flour, shaking off any excess. Fry in batches in the hot oil, turning once with a slotted spoon, until golden. Remove and drain on paper towels. Repeat until the entire mixture is used up.

Serve hot.

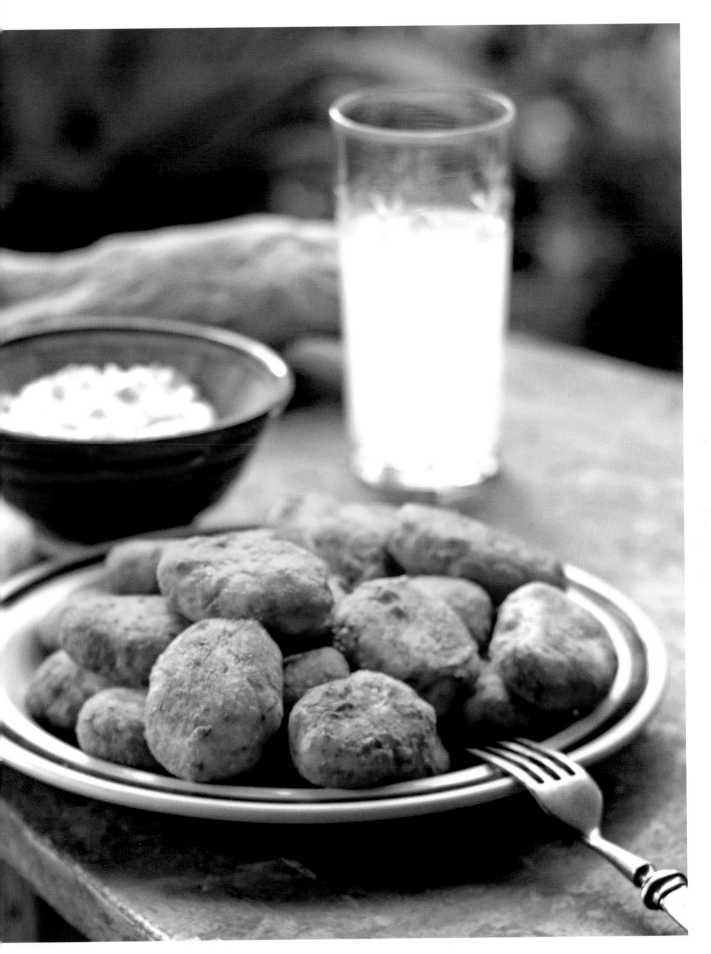

OMELET WITH WILD ONION STALKS

Omeleta me Karonoi

On Ikaria, onions that are not harvested but instead are left in the ground for the next year sprout delicious stalks (called *Karonoi*) in the spring, and these are collected and enjoyed in a variety of ways, from omelets to fritters to salads. They have a mild, discreetly onion-like flavor. You can also try blanching, patting them dry, then lightly frying them. When cooked this way and served with a little extra virgin olive oil and vinegar, they make for one of the spring season's best and most unique salads. Because nothing quite like *Karanoi* exists in American markets, I have adapted the recipe to use either ramps (wild leeks) or spring onion stalks.

MAKES 4 SERVINGS

1 cup chopped tender spring onion stalks or ramps

Sea salt and freshly ground black pepper

2 tablespoons extra virgin olive oil

4 eggs

Place the ramps in a nonstick skillet over low heat with a little sea salt. Cover and heat until they exude their own liquid, 3 to 4 minutes. Add the olive oil and swirl the pan back and forth.

Lightly beat the eggs with a little salt and pepper. Pour into the skillet and tilt it back and forth so that the eggs cover the surface. Cook, covered, until the eggs are set. Remove the omelet to a large plate and cut into strips or wedges. Serve hot.

VARIATION

You can add a little goat cheese or feta to the omelet, too, right after adding the egg, before they set.

MUSHROOMING IN THE MOUNTAINS

An old book on the folklore and agrarian life of Ikaria lists at least 25 varieties of edible wild mushrooms that grow on the island, categorized either by their shape or by the tree or bush they grow under. Add to that accounts of truffles that our friend Yiannis Koutoufaris, a shepherd who spends many hours a day in the woods, has recounted, with some finds, at least if his tales are to be believed, up to 10 and 12 inches in diameter. Ikaria is a mycological dream, and islanders take full advantage of the island's most delicious, if potentially dangerous, treats.

Mushrooms sprout after the first heavy, drenching rains of autumn. But the rain has to stop for the mushrooms to come up. Although they sprout all winter long, most are found in October, November, and December. My daughter, who spent her first New Year's on the island in 2014, noticed that nary a home she visited as part of the cavorting and caroling tradition was without mushrooms on the table.

The most preferred ones grow deep inside the forest, for example: on the steep slopes above Frandato, toward Arnopeza, an area in the middle interior of the island. There, the vegetation is a dense, sometimes impassable mix of pine trees and andraklo trees as well as bushes like arbutus, heather, and rock-rose. The mushrooms grow under the wet carpet of leaves, lichen, and pine needles that covers the forest floor. They are certainly not visible. Instead, as Yiannis Pedos, an experienced 'shroomer, described to me, "you go a-looking for bumps and humps on the forest floor."

My husband, Vassilis Stenos, describes his experience with Yiannis one November day: "Where we started, which was near the road, it was obvious that people had already been there. The 'shrooms had already been unearthed and you could see the indentations. In order to find mushrooms, we had to go deeper and deeper, where there are no footpaths, and actually crawl between the bushes and woods. In the beginning, I couldn't notice the bumps. My eye wasn't trained."

If the mushrooms manage to break through the thick forest carpet, they're probably already too big, past their prime, and maybe even rotten. They grow incredibly fast. They can double in size in a day. "We spent about an hour and a half there. Yianis collected 6 or 7 kilos [about 15 pounds]. Some were really large, maybe even half a pound each."

Mushroom Varieties on Ikaria

That day they collected chanterelles, called *pefkites*, after the Greek word for "pine," because they are found under pine trees; *kalamares*, *Coprinus comatus*, or shaggy ink caps; and *fouskes*, or puffballs, *Lycoperdum perlatum*.

Other delicious edible mushrooms on the island include many different varieties of boletus: *perdikopodares*, or partridge feet; *Ramaria aurea*; *kopromanites*, or common field mushrooms (*Agaricus campestris*); *voidoglossa*, which translates as "cow's tongue" and is not too different in

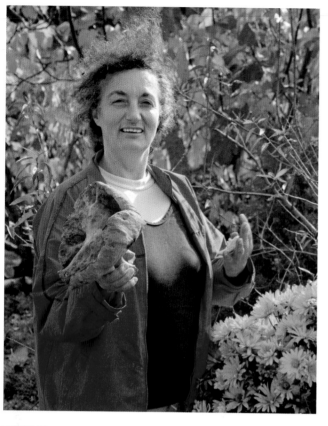
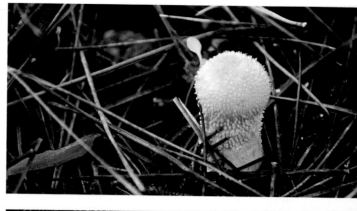
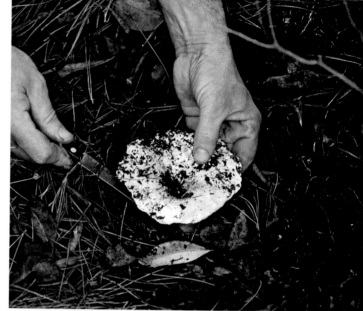
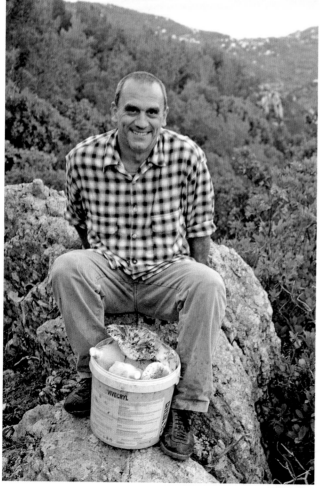
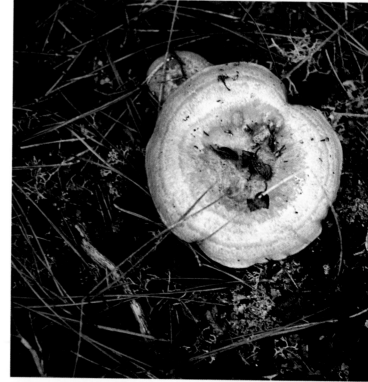

English—"beefsteak," or *Fistulina hepatica*; *hondritis*, a thick-stemmed, delicious white mushroom, whose scientific name is *Tricholoma columbetta*. There are also morels, which the Ikarians call *sfougarites*, or "sponge mushrooms," and several types of fungi in the Terfezia family, which are trufflelike, including the potato-shaped *laorkia*, or *Terfezia leonis* rhizopogon, and the *gaidourohondrines*, or "fat donkey."

At least two are deadly, but I could not find their scientific names. Ikarians simply call them *familites*, literally because their consumption has been known to kill off, well, entire families.

How to Cook Mushrooms Like an Ikarian

Ikarian cooks do not want to adulterate or camouflage the inherent flavor of the mushrooms, so they usually opt for one of several very basic preparations.

- ◈ **Grilled Mushrooms.** Typically, large mushrooms are grilled and served with olive oil and lemon juice.

- ◈ **Roasted Mushrooms.** Another treat, usually reserved for large mushrooms, which are tossed in olive oil and sea salt and roasted in the oven.

- ◈ **Fried Mushrooms.** Dredged or batter-fried chanterelles, ink caps, boletus and more make for some of the best on-the-spot *mezedes*. The mushrooms are dusted in flour and fried in olive oil, then salted; or dipped in a simple, thick batter of flour, water, and salt and then fried in olive oil.

- ◈ **Preserved Mushrooms.** Grilled mushrooms are preserved in olive oil.

- ◈ **Mushrooms "*Marinatoi*."** *Marinatoi* mushrooms are made by flouring then frying any variety of wild mushroom, removing them from the skillet, and then adding garlic, red wine vinegar, and rosemary to the oil and flour already in the skillet and cooking on low heat to get a thick sauce, which is poured over the mushrooms. It's a way to preserve them for a few days. A similar dish is made with small fried fish such as bogue (page 218).

Mushroom Nutrition

Mushrooms are chock-full of protein, vitamins B_1, B_2, B_3, B_5, B_6, folate, vitamin D, phosphorus, iron, zinc, potassium, copper, magnesium, and selenium. They also possess cancer-fighting and heart-healthy properties and hardly have any calories.

As if that's not enough, they also contain compounds that help us fend off the winter blues.

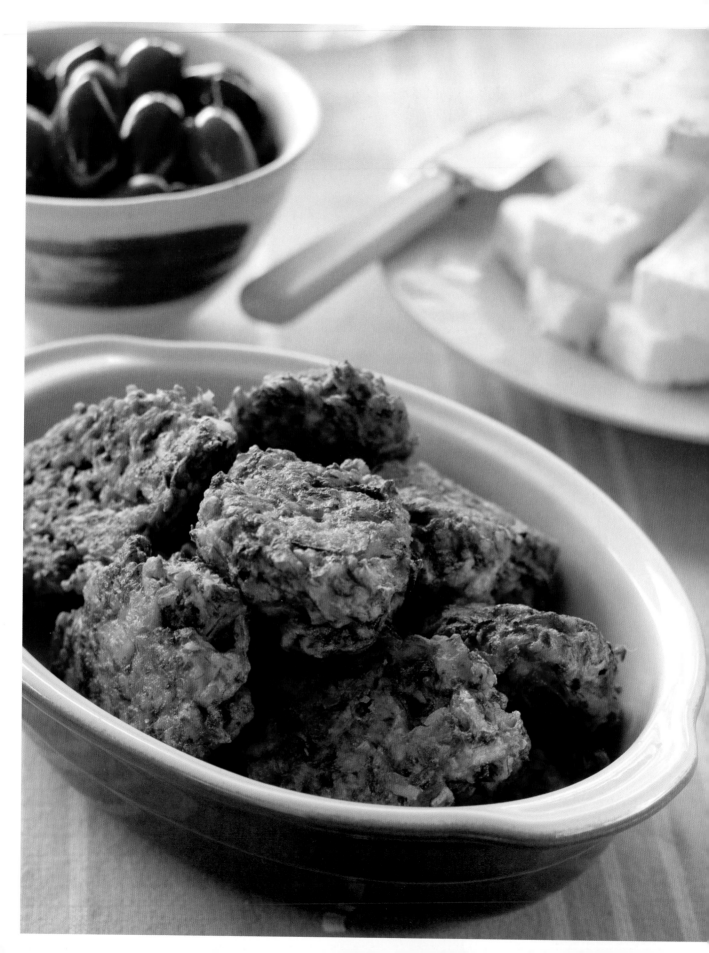

IKARIAN WILD GREENS PANCAKES WITH CAROB FLOUR

Tiganites me Horta

This old recipe harks back to another era, when even wheat flour was expensive, but carob flour, or powder as it is called now, was something even the poorest islander could access. Carob trees grow all over Ikaria and until World War II were an important source of food. Patties, fritters, and flat-cakes made with greens, herbs, and vegetables abound in Ikaria and on the Aegean islands in general. If you make these with the addition of carob flour, they will be dark brown. The carob flour imparts a subtle sweetness, too. You can also make these the way contemporary cooks do with plain, all-purpose flour. Either way, they are delicious with plain Greek yogurt or feta.

MAKES 24 TWO-INCH (5-CM) PANCAKES (6 TO 8 SERVINGS)

1½ cups chopped fresh mint leaves

1½ cups chopped fresh dill

1 cup chopped wild fennel*

3 cups chopped fresh spinach

3 red onions, minced or grated

Salt and freshly ground black pepper

1 cup spelt flour or whole wheat flour

1 scant teaspoon baking powder

½ teaspoon baking soda

½ cup carob powder

1 cup water

1 large egg, lightly beaten

Olive or other oil, for frying

In a bowl, combine the mint, dill, fennel, spinach, and onions. Season with salt and pepper to taste.

In a bowl, mix together the flour, baking powder and baking soda, carob powder,** and a little salt and pepper. Whisk in the water and egg to make a thick batter. Pour the batter into the greens mixture and stir to combine.

In a nonstick skillet, heat 2 to 3 tablespoons olive oil over medium-high heat. Working in batches of 4 to 6 pancakes at a time, drop heaping tablespoons of the batter into the hot oil. When the bottom sets, flip over to cook on the other side and remove when crisp and dark, 4 to 6 minutes total.

Drain on paper towels and serve.

*If you can't find wild fennel, use a fennel bulb instead. Chop it very finely and add it to the mixture together with the onions.

**You could use 1½ cups all-purpose flour for the spelt flour/carob blend.

SEA FENNEL IN BRINE

Samphire

One of the best things to do on Ikaria in spring and summer is to comb the rocks along the coast for rock samphire, one of the season's most nutritious plants. It is also known as sea fennel and in Greek is called *kritamo*, from the ancient Greek word for barley, *krithmon*, because apparently the seeds of both plants resemble one another. Its scientific name is *Crithmum maritimum*.

Rock samphire isn't unique to Greece. Indeed, it grows wild along the coasts of the entire Mediterranean as well as in Britain and Ireland. Its English name comes from the word "sampiere," which is from the French Saint Pierre (Saint Peter), the patron saint of fishermen. On Ikaria, *kritama* (plural of *kritamo*) are used in lieu of capers, very few of which grow wild on Ikaria. One local dish is *fava* (puree of yellow split pea) topped with *kritama*, and most people just mix *kritama* into summer tomato salads.

Samphire is one of the healthiest greens. Its therapeutic values have been known since antiquity. Both Dioscorides, the father of pharmacology, and Pliny, renowned botanist, wrote about its medicinal properties. Hippocrates recommended it for its diuretic and detoxifying abilities. It is chock-full of antioxidants and has use as such in cosmetics, too. It is said to brighten age spots and to lend a healthy glow to skin.

It is rich in iodine and packed with phytochemicals that protect the liver, heart, and cellular DNA. It is also rich in vitamins A, C, B_2, B_5, and D; amino acids; and minerals, such as iron, calcium, magnesium, phosphorus, silica, zinc, and manganese.

When you collect the sea fennel leaves, collect only the most tender leaves and buds. The time to do this is in May and early June in Greece.

Wash them very well.

MAKES ABOUT 2 QUARTS

---

1 pound (450 g) samphire (sea fennel) leaves	Vinegar
6 tablespoons plus 2 teaspoons salt	Olive oil

Add the 6 tablespoons salt to 1½ quarts (1.5 liters) water and bring to a boil. Blanch the samphire for 3 to 5 minutes, just to soften. The leaves will still be bright green and crunchy.

Rinse and cool.

Pack the leaves tightly in jars, then add the 2 teaspoons salt and fill the jars with vinegar. Close the lids, turn over a few times, then let stand for 24 hours. Drain, place back in the jars, and cover with olive oil. Let the pickled leaves stand for a month before consuming them.

PICKLED WILD HYACINTH BULBS

Volvoi

Volvoi are the small, bitter bulbs of the grape hyacinth, *Muscari comosum*, an ancient food that is still enjoyed in Ikaria, throughout Greece, and in Apulia, Italy.

When I started to read up on the nutritive value of these bulbs, it struck me, as it has many times when thinking about Ikarian food traditions in the context of local culture, religious practices, and seasons, that it makes perfect sense for people to seek them out during Lent. They are, in fact, a classic Lenten meze, and are often served side by side with a steaming plate of lentil soup, together with which they become a nutritional powerhouse. The bulbs are known empirically to be a natural way to detox; they are packed with minerals and soluble fiber, so leave you feeling full after eating them. The need to purify and the gift of feeling full on very little are both necessary if one is fasting, as many people still do, for the full 48 days of Lent. When served as an accompaniment to iron-rich lentils, they make for a perfect food.

MAKES 18 TO 24 SERVINGS

3 tablespoons coarse sea salt

3 pounds (1.5 kg) grape hyacinth bulbs (see page 299 for sources) or red or white cipollini onions, about 1 inch (2.5 cm) in diameter, peeled

2 cups white wine vinegar

6 garlic cloves, peeled and whole

1 small bunch fresh dill, chopped

1 scant teaspoon black peppercorns

Greek extra virgin olive oil

If using onions, peel but keep whole.

Bring a large pot of water to a boil and add 1 tablespoon of the salt. Blanch the hyacinth bulbs for 4 to 5 minutes. Strain and repeat process with fresh water and salt two more times. This process helps leech out the inherent bitterness in the bulbs. If you are using onions, you only need to blanch once and will need a total of 2 tablespoons of coarse sea salt.

In a large saucepan, bring the vinegar, garlic, dill, and peppercorns to a boil over medium heat. Remove and cool slightly.

Have a sterilized 1-quart canning jar ready. Place the bulbs or onions in the jar and pour in the vinegar mixture. Top with olive oil. Let cool completely and screw on the top. Refrigerate for at least 3 days but preferably a week before opening.

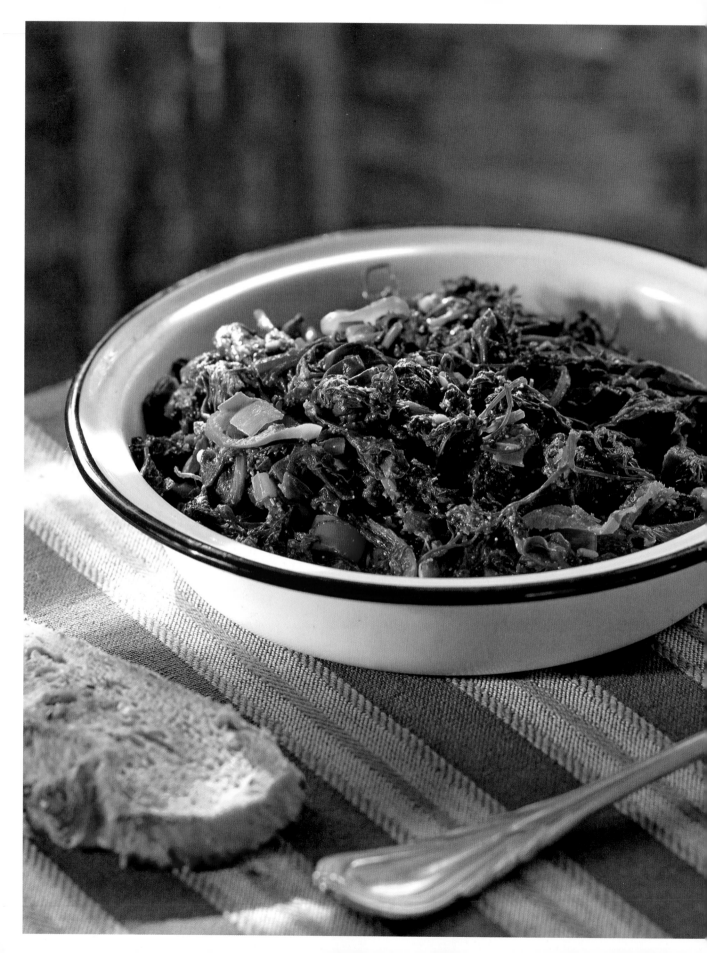

AROMATIC GREENS COOKED WITH ROE AND CHILE PEPPER

Sfouggato

Sfouggato is the name given to various egg-based dishes throughout the Greek islands; some are essentially omelets, while others are more like croquettes. But among older Ikarians, *sfouggato* was a dish that called for quite a different egg than that of the hen: fish eggs, or roe, called *tarama* in Greek. According to Myrsina Roussou, a sharp-witted woman well into her eighties who recalled her father making this for his male friends, it was (and is!) *"the* meze for *tsipouro* [grappa]."

MAKES 4 SERVINGS

- 2 tablespoons Greek extra virgin olive oil
- 1 bunch scallions, white and tender green parts, chopped
- 1 fresh green or red chile pepper (optional), seeded and chopped
- ½ pound (250 g) sorrel, spinach, or chard, chopped
- 2 cups chopped fresh wild fennel leaves*

- 1 bunch flat-leaf parsley, chopped
- 1 cup chopped fresh chervil or mint
- 2 tablespoons Greek *tarama*
- ¼ cup water
- 8 thick slices (1 inch [2.5 cm]) country bread, preferably sourdough, optional

---

In a large, wide pot or deep skillet, heat the olive oil over medium heat. Add the scallions and cook, stirring, until soft, about 8 minutes. Add the chile pepper, if using, and stir all together.

Add the sorrel (or spinach or chard), stirring until it wilts. Add the wild fennel, parsley, and chervil (or mint). Cook until all the greens are wilted.

Dilute the *tarama* with the water and stir it into the greens. Reduce the heat to low and simmer, partially covered, until the mixture is thick and creamy. Serve, if desired, with grilled bread.

*If you can't find wild fennel, substitute 1 large fennel bulb, trimmed and finely chopped. Add the chopped fennel when you cook the scallions. Or substitute 1 cup chopped dill and 3 tablespoons ouzo, adding the dill when you would have added the wild fennel. Pour the ouzo into the pan after the greens are wilted; increase the heat a little so that the alcohol can burn off.

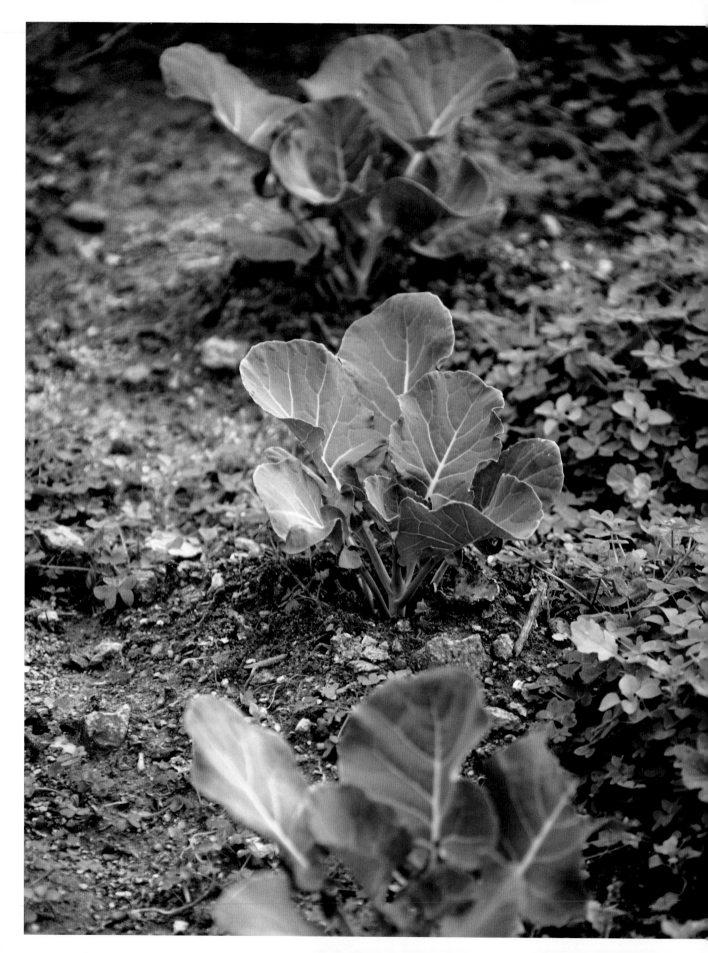

SALADS

RAW AND COOKED

SALAD ON THE TABLE IS JUST A GIVEN IN IKARIA and throughout Greece, regardless of the season. Dishes like *horiatiki* (what Americans call Greek salad, for example, brimming with tomatoes, peppers, onions, cucumbers, and olives) are actually what promoted the important health aspects of the Mediterranean diet, because traditional Mediterranean eating is based on a variety of bright, colorful, and flavorful foods that are high in nutrients and low in animal fats.

In Greece, a salad can be almost anything, so long as it is in season and fresh. It can be hot, as in boiled greens or boiled cruciferous vegetables like broccoli and cauliflower; room temperature, as in the myriad bean salads that are part of the Greek culinary repertoire; and, of course, refreshing—but typically also at room temperature, not chilled—as in the *horiatiki*, crunchy spring lettuce salads, and shredded winter cabbage and carrot salads, all three Greek classics.

Somewhere along the line in the long history of the Greek table, the suffix *salata* (which means salad) was appended to the gamut of well-known spreads, such as *taramosalata* (fish roe spread), *melitzanosalata* (roasted eggplant "salad"), and *tyrosalata* (cheese spread), all very typical Greek recipes. How this came to be is a mystery and to my mind these are not salads at all but *mezedes*, and as such I have included these diplike "salads" in the *mezedes* chapter.

On Ikaria, where so many people grow their own food, the salads are exceedingly fresh and delicious. There is nothing to compare the flavor of a just-picked Ikarian tomato, which is typically thick-skinned, fleshy, and very sweet; or homegrown lettuce, crisp but also soothing and somewhat lactic in flavor; or potatoes fresh out of the ground, boiled and served with little else besides olive oil pressed from the trees outside one's window.

In the following recipes I've tried to give as wide a variety as possible of salads both raw and cooked (but always seasonal) that grace the tables on Ikaria throughout the year.

SPRING LETTUCE SALAD WITH GREEN ALMONDS

Salata me Marouli kai Tsagala

This is not a traditional Ikarian dish. Instead it's my homage to the seasonal foods that are on island tables in spring, including tender, crisp romaine lettuce. This salad is refreshing, almost cleansing to the palate. You can substitute a handful of blanched, sliced almonds if you can't find the raw fresh nuts.

MAKES 4 SERVINGS

1 large head romaine lettuce, coarsely chopped or torn

⅓ cup finely chopped fennel fronds

⅓ cup chopped fresh dill

4 scallions, chopped

6 raw green almonds, rinsed and julienned

⅓ cup Greek extra virgin olive oil

2 tablespoons fresh lemon juice, strained

Sea salt

In a salad bowl, toss together the lettuce, fennel, dill, scallions, and almonds. In a small bowl, whisk together the olive oil, lemon juice, and salt to taste. Pour into the salad, toss, and serve.

LITTLE GREEN WONDERS: YOUNG ALMONDS

Green almonds are in season April, May, and June and are picked before the shell and the nut harden.

Ikarians enjoy them whole, fuzzy green soft shell and all, or cleaned, eating only the kernel within. The shelled fresh nut is dewy and mildly tart. "They were our candy when we were kids," my neighbor Stephanos explained.

The small green wonders are a nutritional powerhouse. They contain: flavonoids and vitamin E for the heart and to fight bad cholesterol and phosphorous, for bones and teeth. Green almonds help regulate blood sugar after a meal and are loaded with antioxidants that help flush the toxins out of our bodies. They help us maintain pH balance, protecting against a number of ailments, most impressively against osteoporosis. Finally, they contain brain and nerve food in the form of riboflavin and L-carnitine.

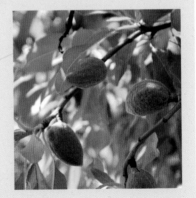

CLASSIC SPRING LETTUCE SALAD

Anoixiatiki Maroulosalata

Romaine lettuce is the salad green of choice on springtime tables on Ikaria and throughout Greece, too. At Easter time, people sometimes add quartered hard-boiled eggs to the salad. The result tastes like Greek spring: herbal, a little grassy, filled with sweet aromas and the crisp, faint bitterness of very fresh romaine lettuce.

MAKES 4 TO 6 SERVINGS

---

2 heads romaine lettuce, coarsely shredded

4 scallions, cut into thin rounds

1 bunch dill, chopped or snipped

5 tablespoons Greek extra virgin olive oil

3 tablespoons fresh lemon juice or red wine vinegar

Sea salt

Place the lettuce, scallions, and dill in a salad bowl. In a small bowl, whisk together the olive oil, vinegar (or lemon juice), and salt to taste. Pour into the salad, toss, and serve.

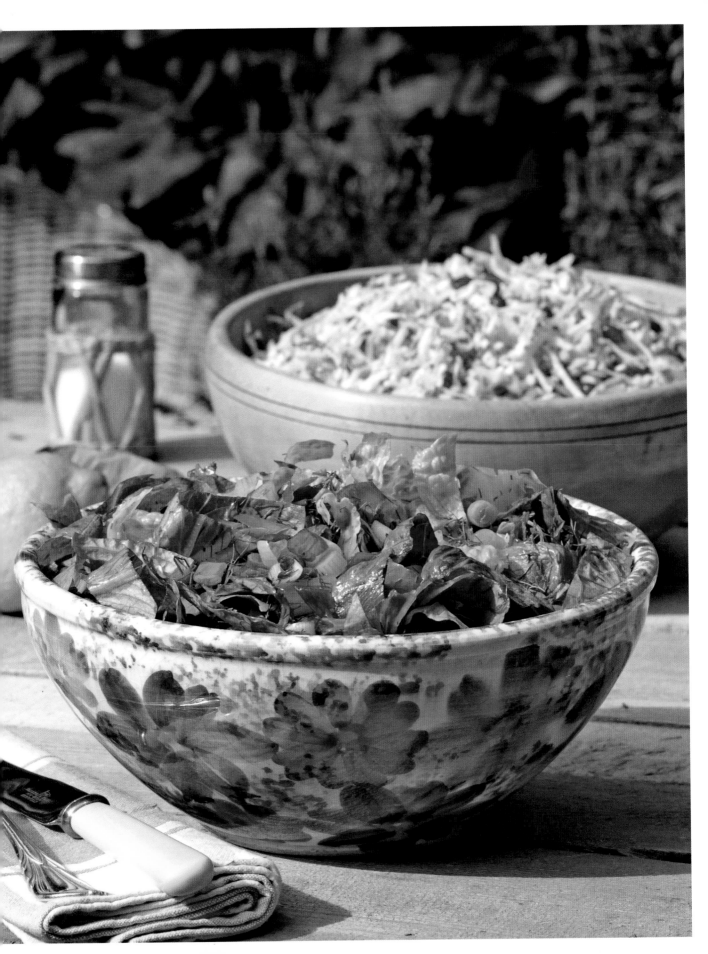

GARDENS OF LONGEVITY

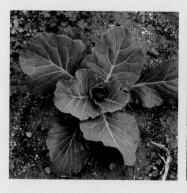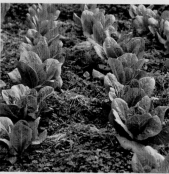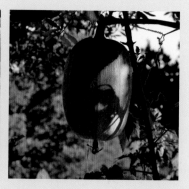

My friend David Kahn, obviously not Ikarian by ethnicity, nonetheless retired on the island with his wife, Robyn, both California transplants, one rainy March about 6 years ago as of this writing. They rent a very old stone house on the northwestern side of Ikaria, in a remote part of Raches, surrounded by plum and cherry trees, and over time have transformed their once fallow land into one of the most beautiful gardens in the area. It is so neat and organized and well-kept, that I once commented to him that he knows more than the locals about how to grow things. It was a conversation piece that stuck, unbeknownst to me until I saw him the summer I finished this book, at a local wedding. He pulled me aside to correct that assumption. "There is no way I know more than the people who have been doing this their whole lives. These people, they have roots here, like the plants do. They just know things about the land that I can never know."

Gardens to Ikarians were never a hobby, but always a necessity, and they still are for most of the 8,000 people who inhabit Ikaria year-round. Every home was surrounded by its olive, almond, and mulberry trees (for berries and excellent shade). Most families also had apricot, lemon, orange, quince, apple, and wild pear trees, if not on their land per se since not all of them flourish in one place, then somewhere accessible. Young and old tend the land, a point well made in the scientific research with regard to the natural exercise of the over-80 set, many of whom will bend, dig, plant, pluck, prune, and pick their way to ruddy-cheeked longevity.

But what they also do is scrutinize, slowly, constantly—the "just knowing things" that David was talking about.

"The old gardeners and farmers, they observed," says Thodoris Tsimbides, another friend and the founder of Archipelagos, an internationally recognized environmental preservation effort. Gardens were by necessity planted on small patches of land—remember, Ikaria is all mountains, valleys, and ravines, with very little arable land. The terraces carved into mountain slopes were largely used to plant barley, the predominant grain on the island until the 1970s. (Barley needs much less water than wheat, which was planted sparingly, milled and used mainly for holiday breads and pastries.)

One rarely, if ever, saw the neat, organized gardens like the Kahns' or our own or our elderly neighbors' a generation ago. "Everything was planted together," says Tsimbides. "Bean stalks between tomato plants, corn, peppers, eggplants, herbs, all in one garden patch, hodgepodge by design, which keeps the bugs away. The varieties were sturdier a generation ago, too, and naturally more resistant to pests. But even now, when I watch my mother, who is an excellent gardener, I am in awe of how she moves in the garden, how she observes things. She never sprays anything. When she picks beans, she'll just use her apron to wipe off the aphids or beetles or mites, whatever there is, from the tomato plants. She does this consistently, whenever she is in the garden. And that's a lot, all year round.

People rotate their garden plots and have a great source of fertilizer in goat manure and dead leaves. Composting is a natural, daily habit as nothing goes to waste in a village home.

But easy access to water changed Ikarian gardens. In the mid-1990s, a dam was built north of Raches, which has ended up being both a blessing and a curse. For one, the piping is not quite the same as in urban water systems. Only as recently as 2013 was town piping laid underground for more reliable distribution. Most people still have to drop and drag their own thick black hoses from the water source to their homes and gardens, which run in tangled messes along the roadsides for kilometers, not exactly doing justice to the natural beauty of the place. Wells and springs have also been left unattended; when I was a kid and until the dam came, Ikaria had amazing water, real mountain spring water that was delicious. Sure, it was untreated, so the lack of fluoride made for some awkward smiles, and one sometimes had to manually collect water from nearby springs and store it, usually in large clay jugs, where it was always cool. Now, the water supply is more convenient, but it's also fraught with technical problems and the water just doesn't taste the same.

Access to relatively unlimited water has also made people "less observant," as Tsimbides says. "Up until a generation ago, people planted their gardens close to streams and rivulets, so they'd have access to water. These were wooded, much shadier places. Plants stress out if they're exposed to the sun all day. The result is that gardens are just not as efficient. People have become less aware of the value of water, too."

But gardens are still an extremely important and integral part of life on the island. They take hard work, dam or no dam. The early fall was and still is a time of intense agricultural activity: Farms and fields are tilled; wheat and barley, for those who still grow it, as well as peas and favas were sowed so that they could germinate and sprout before the heavy rains. Overripe grapes and figs are picked and dried. Then, before you know it, it's olive season.

The fruits of all that labor are also a source of endless pleasure and pride. I can't count how many times I've relied on friends to share seeds and done the same, of course, or how often in the course of a summer I find bags and baskets full of fruits and vegetables or marmalades that friends and neighbors just leave outside our door, or the number of times I've heard Stefanos say to my lovely neighbor, Titika, his significant other, that he's brought her an amazing gift: the first cherries; the biggest, sweetest peaches, *apidia* (local pears that go by their ancient name); zucchini the size of footballs—all that and more are better than gold to someone who's chosen village life on Ikaria.

GRILLED ZUCCHINI SALAD WITH LOTS OF GARLIC

Kolokythakia stin Schara me Poly Skordo

Here's an old island way to cook zucchini that seems uncannily modern. The recipe is described in a small book on Ikarian food lore and recipes, mainly from the villages of Manganitis, Karkinagri, and Plagia on the south side. The original cooking method, which was on an iron hot plate over hot embers, intrigued me. Wood-fired cooking is still popular on Ikaria and adds a flavor dimension to a whole range of Ikarian dishes, including Spoon Sweets (see page 296), which were simmered in old pots in the hearth. All of this food is absolutely delicious. I have tried to recreate the effect so that a modern cook can also enjoy the outcome.

MAKES 6 TO 8 SERVINGS

6 large zucchini, ends trimmed

6 tablespoons Greek extra virgin olive oil

3 to 4 garlic cloves, cut into paper-thin slivers

3 tablespoons good-quality red wine vinegar

Sea salt

Preheat a grill to medium.

Rub the zucchini with 3 tablespoons of the olive oil and place in a shallow baking pan. Cover with foil. Place the baking pan on the grill over indirect heat. Close the lid and cook the zucchini until tender, about 20 minutes.

Remove and cut into 1-inch (2.5-cm) rings. Transfer the hot zucchini to a serving bowl.

Add the garlic, vinegar, salt to taste, and the remaining 3 tablespoons olive oil to the zucchini. Toss gently and serve.

NOTE: *You can also make a smoked chunky eggplant salad or turn grilled red or green peppers into a salad using the same seasonings.*

VASSILI'S CABBAGE SLAW

Lahanosalata tou Vassili

This is our standard winter salad, not quite an Ikarian tradition but one that many Ikarian friends have certainly enjoyed over the years. Cabbage, with its unique, slightly sweet taste, is perked up even more with the sour-sweet flavor of pomegranate seeds, the refreshingly grassy taste of snipped dill, and the earthy flavor of pine nuts and sunflower seeds. You can add even more color by mixing red and green cabbages. One key to making this as good as possible is to finely shred or grate the cabbage so that there is more surface area to absorb both the dressing and the flavors of everything else in the bowl.

MAKES 4 TO 6 SERVINGS

4 cups finely shredded green cabbage or a combination of finely shredded red and green cabbage

⅓ cup chopped fresh flat-leaf parsley

⅓ cup chopped fresh dill

⅔ cup pomegranate seeds

3 tablespoons pine nuts, toasted

2 tablespoons sunflower seeds, toasted

DRESSING

½ cup Greek extra virgin olive oil

2 tablespoons red wine vinegar

2 tablespoons fig balsamic vinegar, Greek honey, or grape molasses

Salt

In a serving bowl, toss together the cabbage, parsley, dill, pomegranate seeds, pine nuts, and sunflower seeds.

For the dressing: In a small bowl, whisk together all the ingredients for the dressing.

Pour the dressing over the salad and toss. Serve immediately.

HOW TO PREPARE HORTA (GREENS) FOR SALADS

Boiled greens, called *horta*, are considered salads in Greece and may be eaten either hot, warm, at room temperature, or cold.

Different types of greens are cleaned differently. For example, the wild chicories, with their knobby root and spiky leaves, need first to be trimmed with a sharp knife at the root end and kept whole before washing in cold water; other leafy greens, such as sorrel, need to be steeped in cold water, swished around, then removed by hand and drained, several times, until there is not a trace of dirt in the water.

Sweet greens (such as chard) and bitter greens (such as dandelion) are enjoyed as salads in Greece and on Ikaria, but never together in the same dish. To cook them, simply bring a pot of salted water to a rolling boil and drop the washed greens in. Boil for 5 to 20 minutes, depending on your own taste and on the toughness of the particular greens. Then, drain and let cool slightly.

Dress sweet or bitter greens with sea salt, good extra virgin olive oil, and either red wine vinegar or fresh lemon juice, again, to taste. A general rule is that bitter greens are dressed with vinegar, whereas sweet greens are seasoned with lemon juice.

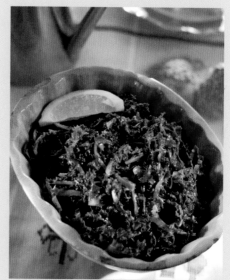

bitter greens are dressed with vinegar, whereas sweet greens are seasoned with lemon juice

PURSLANE AND OLIVE SALAD

Salata me Glistrida kai Elies

Purslane is a miracle weed that grows rampant in summer tomato and vegetable gardens in Greece, North America, and elsewhere. It has the highest amount of heart-healthy omega-3 fatty acids of any edible plant and more than even certain fish. It also contains 10 to 20 times more melatonin, an antioxidant that inhibits cancer growth. Its high content of pectin, a cholesterol-lowering soluble fiber, also makes it useful in thickening soups and stews. Purslane contains six times more vitamin E than spinach and seven times more beta-carotene than carrots. It's also rich in vitamin C, magnesium, riboflavin, potassium, and phosphorus. Its high content of B vitamins, which are important for carbohydrate metabolism, keeps the nervous system healthy. On top of all that, it tastes great, especially in salads like this, with flavors that are refreshingly acidic and textures that are a combination of succulent, crisp, and crunchy.

MAKES 6 SERVINGS

- ½ pound (225 g) purslane
- 2 large garlic cloves
- 1 cup small green olives, rinsed and drained
- 1 large English hothouse cucumber, peeled and coarsely chopped
- 1 bunch fresh flat-leaf parsley, finely chopped
- ⅓ cup Greek extra virgin olive oil
- 2 tablespoons red wine vinegar
- Sea salt

Wash and spin-dry the purslane. Trim away any tough stems. Coarsely chop and transfer to a salad bowl.

Crush the garlic with the side of a large chef's knife and scrape, along with its juices, into the salad bowl. Pit the olives, quarter lengthwise, and add to the bowl. Add the cucumber and parsley.

Pour in the olive oil, vinegar, and salt to taste. Toss and let sit at room temperature for at least 10 minutes before serving.

A WHOLE WORLD OF GREENS AND HERBS

Much has been said and written about the extensive variety of wild greens on Ikaria and the alacrity with which islanders consume them. They are, indeed, one of the roots of the longevity statistics, especially since wild foods—and by some accounts there are more than 300 edible wild plants on the island—were almost the only sustenance for the many nonagenarians who grew up in dire poverty.

A few years ago, as an exercise in "back to basics," I decided to try to survive and feed our family only on what I could pick wild, for at least a few days. It was late spring, right around Greek Easter, and we hadn't been to the island all winter. Our garden was knee-deep in weeds.

I was totally green back then, pun intended, a novice when it comes to what's edible and wild, so I called my friend Argyro, who agreed to give me a lesson in *horta* picking (*horta* being the Greek term for weeds, both edible and not). Within a 15-foot radius of our front door, Argyro helped me collect a mountain of wild greens that would become our family's meals for days: pies, purees, fritters, salads, and fare for the tossing with some steaming pasta, garlic, and olive oil. Wild carrot greens, poppy leaves, feathery fennel, and lemon balm were among the most memorable, the greens I could never before identify but that gave Argyro's own cooking its distinct flavor.

It was the beginning of a love affair that is still going strong, so much so that now, every time I am on the island, I relish the discovery of yet another wild thing to eat. Doing so makes me think of another friend, Yiannis Roussos, whose mother spoke almost endearingly of her childhood poverty, living six people strong on a diet almost exclusively based on the weeds and sprouts and snails and fish they could garner for nothing more than the family's own time and labor. "Weeds, weeds, weeds. That's what we ate," she told me emphatically one summer day in her garden, as I quenched thirsts both real and figurative while sipping her cool sour-cherry syrup mixed with ice water and scribbling down the recipes she recalled from another era.

Weeds are surely one secret to my fellow islanders' legendary life spans.

Lexicon of Edible Greens and Wild Herbs

In the following lexicon of greens and herbs, I have tried to document some of the hundreds of different edible and potable wild plants that carpet Ikaria. Many of these also grow wild in the United States.

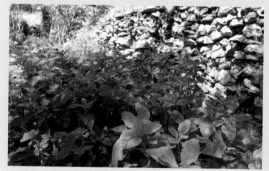
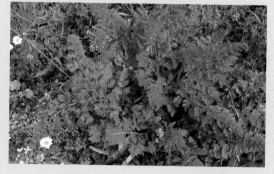

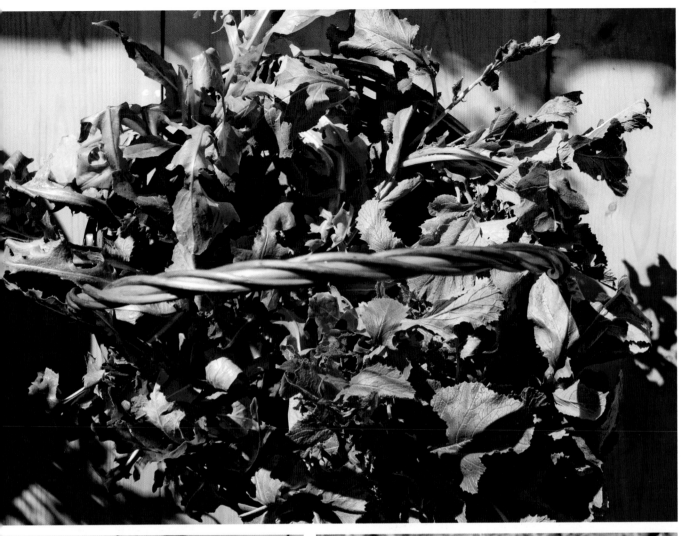

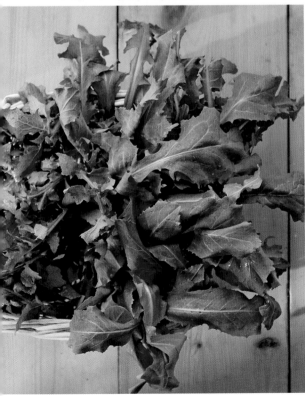

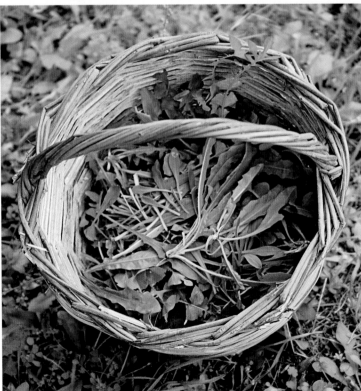

Sweet Greens

AMARANTH (*AMARANTHUS BLITUM*).
Vlita is the Greek name for this ubiquitous summer green, which is boiled for salads but also cooked into pies and vegetable stews, especially with zucchini. It is a different species of the same plant that produces the synonymous grain.

ASPARAGUS, WILD (*ASPARAGUS OFFICINALIS*). This is the kind of wild green that sends people to the hills with a sense of urgency, in search of it before the goats discover it. So was my experience trying to procure some awhile back only to learn that it had already been consumed. Nonetheless, wild asparagus, with its thin, flexible stalks, is one of the most delicious spring greens. They are blanched and enjoyed as a salad with a little olive oil and lemon juice or cooked in omelets.

BLUE MALLOW (*MALVA SYLVESTRIS*). Both savory pies and boiled greens salads are home to the *moloha* of the ancients. It has always been an important therapeutic herb and in Ikaria is still used dried as an infusion for chest colds and other maladies (see "Ancient Mallow," page 157).

BORAGE (*BORAGO OFFICINALIS*). Borage leaves go into salads and pies. In some parts of Greece its lavender flowers adorn salads, too.

BUR CHERVIL (*ANTHRISCUS CAUCALIS*). One of the most aromatic greens, with tiny tender leaves and a delicious, sweet flavor *kafkalithra* to the Greeks is used in salads and pies.

CARROT, WILD (*DAUCUS CAROTA*). It grows wild in many areas of Ikaria and two parts of the plant are used. The feathery greens at the top of the plant are snipped off to be mixed in savory phyllo pie fillings and the flowers, aka Queen Anne's Lace, are dipped in batter and fried.

COMMON REICHARDIA (*PICRIDIUM VULGARE*). The Greeks call this *pikralida* or *galatsida*, and love it, especially in boiled salads. It has a sweet taste and is one of the best winter greens.

FENNEL, WILD (*FOENICULUM VULGARE*). Perhaps no other green or herb is so closely associated with the cooking of Ikaria, for wild fennel, *maratho* locally, lends its perfume to countless local dishes. It is a favorite in fritters, savory pies large and small, and numerous stews.

FERNS. I am not sure if the variety of fern found on Ikaria is the esteemed ostrich fern (*Matteuccia struthiopteris*) from which the much-loved fiddleheads derive, but Ikarians do pick a wild, fiddlehead-shaped fern shoot in spring and they call it *vryha*. Blanched first, then either floured and fried, cooked up with eggs, or pickled, it is one of the most delicious, if ephemeral, springtime treats. During World War II, when wheat flour was scarce, the fiddleheads were coated in carob flour (ground from the many carob trees all over Ikaria).

GRASS LILY, OR STAR-OF-BETHLEHEM (*ORNITHOGALUM UMBELLATUM*). This thin-stalked green with its starlike flowers and long cluster of green buds is in season in the early spring.

LEMON BALM (*MELISSA OFFICINALIS*). This is *melissohorto* to the Ikarians, is one of the best greens for springtime savory pies. It could be the honey-leaf mentioned by the ancient Greek philosopher and botanist Theophrastus (circa 371 to circa 287 BC), in his *Enquiry into Plants*. Its slightly unctuous leaves are highly aromatic.

MEDITERRANEAN HARTWORT (*TORDYLIUM APULUM L.*). The Greeks call this *kafkalida* and consider its mild, sweet flavor ideal for savory pie fillings. It has soft, parsleylike leaves, thin stems, and a very faint fuzz.

NETTLES (*URTICA DIOICA*). *Tsouknida* is the term for stinging nettles, which are used in pie fillings and in some soups and cooked dishes.

PAPAVER RHOEAS. Known as *paparouna* or *koutsounata* to the Ikarians, this is a subtle, delicious spring green that is none other than the leaves of a species of wild poppy. It's one of the best greens for savory pies.

PURSLANE (*PORTULACA OLERACEA L.*). *Glistrida* is the Greek word, which means "slippery," because they say purslane loosens the tongue and makes people chatter. Greeks add it to salads and also cook it, especially with garlic and yogurt.

REDSTEM STORK'S-BILL (*ERODIUM CIRCUTARIUM L.*). This green, which in Greek is *kalogeros* and means "monk," is mainly cooked into pie fillings. It also goes by another name, roughly translated as "the partridge's nail," arguably after the long, needlelike shape of its shoots.

SHEPHERD'S-NEEDLES (*SCANDIX PECTIN-VENERIS*). This aromatic green, *myroni* in Greek, is eaten raw in salads as well as part of the filling mix in springtime savory pies.

SPINACH. You can find wild spinach around the island and plenty of people cultivate it, too. It is typically cooked with rice in a classic pilaf as well as being the basis for many savory pies.

TARO LEAVES. Although most people associate taro, *kolokasi* in Greek, with its corm or tuberlike root, a few of the older Ikarians I spoke to mentioned that they used to pick the leaves, too, and boil them as *horta*. The leaves actually contain more protein than the corms and are rich in vitamins A and C.

WHITE UPRIGHT MIGNONETTE (*RESEDA ALBA*). The Greek *rezeda* is a rare green found along rocky coasts. It is mainly used in boiled salads and in mixed-green savory pie fillings.

YELLOW SALSIFY (*TRAGOPOGON DUBIUS*). The name in Greek, *tragopogon*, means the ram's beard, for the long, wispy shape of this springtime shepherds' favorite. It is delicious both raw and cooked; its tender buds are one of the great country pickles of Greece.

Bitter Greens

BITTER DOCK (*RUMEX OBTUSIFOLIUS*). In Greece, *lapatho* is a green savored inside savory pies.

BLACK BRYONY (*TAMUS COMMUNIS*). *Avronies,* in Greek, are one of the most sought-after wild greens, a harbinger of spring that looks like thin-stalked asparagus but with a bitter taste. Greeks sauté them in olive oil and cook them in omelets.

BLACK NIGHTSHADE (*SOLANUM NIGRUM*). *Styfno*, which grows as a garden weed, is common in the early summer. It's boiled for salad.

CHICORY (*CICHORIUM INTYBUS*). *Radiki* in Greek, this is one of many wild chicories. It is mainly boiled in salads.

(continued)

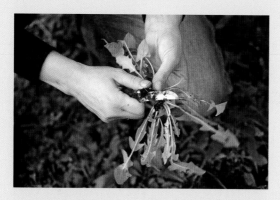

DANDELION (*TARAXACUM OFFICI-NALE*). *Radiki* in Greek, dandelion greens are eaten raw in salads and also boiled.

GARDEN CRESS (*LEPIDIUM SATIVUM L.*). *Kardamo* in Greek, this peppery green is one of the few enjoyed almost exclusively raw in salads.

GOLDEN THISTLE (*SCOLYMUS*). By far one of the most ancient wild prizes in the Greek flora, *askolymbrus*, as the golden thistle is called in Greek, is delicious as a boiled salad or as a green in stews, especially with avgolemono sauce.

LEONTODON TARAXACUM. This is *pikralida* to the locals. This spiky-leafed wild green is pleasantly bitter and great boiled in salads.

MEDITERRANEAN MUSTARD (*HIRSCHFELDIA INCANA L.*). The leaves and shoots of *vrouves* make excellent boiled salads.

PRICKLY GOLDENFLEECE (*UROSPER-MUM PICROIDES*). *Agriozohos* in Greek, this green is eaten mainly boiled in salads. Its shoots are also savored.

PRICKLY LETTUCE (*LACTUCA SERRI-OLA*). The tender shoots and thin, rounded leaves of *petromaroulo*, as it's called in Greek, are typically boiled into salads.

QUEEN ANNE'S LACE (*DAUCUS CAROTA*). On Ikaria, the plant known locally as *agrio karoto*, or wild carrot, has several uses in the kitchen: connoisseurs of savory phyllo pies use both the small, corrugated leaves and delicate flowers in fillings; an old Ikarian recipe calls for batter-frying the delicate, almost spongy flowers but only when they are young and still cup-shaped. Beware: Queen Anne's lace resembles deadly hemlock, so if picking wild, be sure it's the right plant. Otherwise, consider ordering the flower from a good, organic supplier.

ROCKET (*ERUCA SATIVA*). *Roka* is the Greek name for rocket, and it is exceedingly peppery, especially compared to the flavor of rocket in the United States. In Greece, *roka* is eaten raw in salads and sometimes cooked with black-eyed peas and other legumes.

SHEPHERD'S PURSE (*CAPSELLA BURSA-PASTORIS*). Called *kardamo* or *agrio-kardamo* in Greek, this peppery green is typically boiled up for salad.

SOW THISTLE (*SONCHUS OLERA-CEUS*). *Zohos*, to the Greeks, makes for one of the best salads, especially mixed with other greens.

WHITE MUSTARD (*SINAPIS ALBA*). A spicy green whose Greek name sounds like its Latin nomenclature, *sinapi* is boiled into salads.

Shoots

Shoots—called *tsimbita*, which means anything you can pinch or snap off—were and still are an important part of the wild food pantheon of Ikaria. Vine shoots, chickpea shoots, wild carrot tops, and more are among the young, energy-rich wild plants that are used in salads or savory pies.

Drinking Herbs

One of the habits common to all Ikarians, from the very young to the very old, is the consumption of herbal and other plant-based teas culled from the vast wild flora on the island. Many of these infusions, as Dan Buettner writes in *The Blue Zones*, "act as mild diuretics and so lower blood pressure."

In fact, the folk pharmacopoeia on Ikaria offers much more than a few herbal teas that act as diuretics. Ikaria's flora is surprisingly varied, given the size of the island, and herbal infusions were the medicines of yore. When I visited Dr. Ioanna Chinou of the University of Athens School of Pharmacy, she corroborated the medicinal value of the herbal and plant-based infusions so many Ikarians drink by noting that they are loaded with antioxidants and have many other salutary characteristics. Some, like pennyroyal and other mints, promote gum health and soothe stomachaches; others, like rosemary, combat gout. The diuretic effect of most of these natural beverages combats hypertension, perhaps one reason why the incidence of cardiovascular disease on Ikaria is so low.

Older people belong to a generation that remembers the time when there was no such thing as a pharmacy on the island and so grew up close to a source of folk knowledge—the therapeutic value of specific plants to help alleviate specific ailments—that has been all but lost. This was knowledge passed down from generation to generation. There was always a cupboard full of dried herbs and other plants stored away for use as medicines. That is still the case, to an extent; most people have little

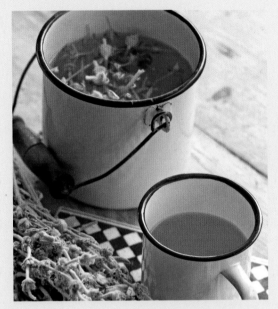

jars or muslin pouches filled with dried chamomile, oregano, thyme, rosemary, pennyroyal, sage, *Sideritis* (aka mountain tea), and more on hand at all times, ready for the steeping in a pot of boiling water, to be sipped for everything from stomachaches and colds to headaches and angina. Today, a handful of younger people on the island are resuscitating the knowledge and have started a cottage industry cultivating or, when permitted, collecting herbs and drying them for use as teas, infusions, and poultices.

In the following list, I have tried to give a sense of the variety, both among common and rarer potable plant-based remedies. Some, like mallow and purslane, I have already touched upon in the list of edible greens, for many of these plants are used both as infusions and in cooking, especially as fillings for savory pies.

To make an infusion, place a teaspoon or two of the dried herb in a tea strainer, and pour a cup of boiling water over it. Steep, covered, for 10 minutes. Strain and drink. You can sweeten the infusions with honey.

The most common herbal teas:

CHAMOMILE, OR *CHAMOMILI*. Chamomile is the infusion given to babies with colic and to help treat insomnia. In spring when it flowers, the whole island is perfumed with it, an aroma faintly reminiscent of green apples. Indeed, in Greek its name means "low apple," for the way it spreads, like clover, all over the surface of the ground. It is also made into a poultice for eye inflammations and rashes and is a natural expectorant.

THE MINT FAMILY. There are many different species of mint that have crossbred over thousands of years. On Ikaria, the most common species are *dyosmos* (spearmint), *menta* (peppermint), and *fliskouni* (pennyroyal).

◈ Spearmint is the best known and mainly used in cooking, although locals dry it and drink it as an antidote to upset stomachs.

◈ Peppermint is also dried and drunk as a calming tea for stomach cramps, menstrual pains, fevers, and colds. Older Ikarians say it's good for men with prostate issues.

◈ Pennyroyal, the smallest member of the mint family, grows wild and is also cultivated in gardens on the island. It can be used to treat the same kinds of tummy aches as the other mints, as well as something to soothe colds and flulike symptoms. It has been used since ancient times to help stimulate the menstrual process and locals say that pregnant women should not drink it.

OREGANO, OR *RIGANI*. Locals drink oregano tea to sooth indigestion and stomachaches.

ROSEMARY, OR *DENDROLIVANO*. Ikarians know that rosemary makes an excellent tonic and has antiseptic qualities. Older Ikarian women would infuse water with rosemary and use it as shampoo. I've done this—my hair was never shinier! It's a salve against colds, the flu, headaches, and stomachaches.

SAGE, OR *FASKOMILO*. Ikarians swear by sage and use it to treat a large range of ailments, especially colds and flu.

SAVORY, OR *THRIMVI* (in the local dialect). Found in the mountains all over Ikaria, savory is not only a favorite cooking herb but also a local medicinal herb. Locals consume it as an infusion and antidote to coughs, bronchial problems, and as a diuretic, helping the body to detox. It is supposed to be good for arthritis, and poultices of savory are sometimes used to heal skin rashes.

SIDERITIS. Called mountain tea, or *tsai tou vounou*. This is said to be an excellent antidote for upset stomachs, colds, and coughs, and a good diuretic. In addition, *sideritis* has many antiinflammatory properties. Consumed with lemon and honey, it makes a good salve for sore throats and coughs.

THYME, OR *THIMARI*. My friend Yiorgo told me that thyme is said to help make fatty foods less, well, fatty, and that is one reason why it is often used in meat cookery. As an infusion, Ikarians drink it for bronchitis, colds, sore throats, and to help digestion after a meal. Thyme infusions are said to be calming and cleansing and locals sometimes drink them to combat the occasional blues.

Lesser Known Plant Infusions

ABSINTHE WORMWOOD. Called *apsithia* in Greek, wormwood is the bitterest of all herbs, surpassing even rue. It is not used in the kitchen, but up through the 1950s the bitter absinthe leaves and flowers were dried, mashed, and mixed with honey to make the folk medicine called *mazoumi*, which was given to children and adults alike as a tonic.

BORAGE. The fresh leaves and flowers are a little reminiscent of cucumber, fresh and almost grassy. Leaves and seeds were made into an infusion that was said to help the onset of milk in nursing mothers. Borage is thought to help overtaxed adrenal glands and is drunk as a general detoxifying tonic and as a salve for colds, bronchitis, even pneumonia.

CHASTE TREE (*LIGARIA* in the local dialect, *Vitex agnus-castus* botanically). This plant grows literally everywhere on Ikaria and is a kind of miracle pest! On Ikaria, people use the leaves to relieve asthma. Its berries have medicinal properties that help relieve menstrual and menopausal hormonal issues. It grows near streams and by the roadside all over the island.

ELDER. Older Ikarians know this plant as *sambucos* and plant it outside their homes as a fly and mosquito repellent. The berries are a good source of vitamins A and C and are a natural laxative. An infusion made with the flowers helps treat colds and the flu.

HAWTHORN. Goats love what the Ikarians call *perikathe*, a tree that bears mealy, deep-red fruit and small, white flowers, which locals say are very good for the heart, as well as for diarrhea, dyspepsia, kidney stones, and sore throats.

PLANTAIN (NOT RELATED TO BANANAS!). I bought a bag of this most unusual herb, called *pentanevro*, or "five nerves" in Greek, at the annual show of local products that is held in the village of Christos, Raches, every summer. On Ikaria, it is one of a number of plant infusions used to cure kidney stones.

RUE OR HERB-OF-GRACE, called *apigano* in Greek. Rue has long been recognized for its cathartic qualities. Rue is extremely bitter and no longer used in the kitchens of Ikaria, although elsewhere in the Mediterranean it is sometimes used sparingly in salads. But older Ikarians drop a few sprigs into a bottle of *tsipouro* (the local firewater, like grappa) and sip it a few times a year to cleanse the blood. Like basil, rue is also known as an insect repellent.

ST. JOHN'S WORT. Its local, Ikarian name means "balsam weed," and almost no home is without a bottle of ruby-red olive oil that has been infused with the yellow-and-rust-colored feathery leaves and slim stalks of St. John's wort. We use it all the time to help heal cuts and other topical problems, and it works beautifully. I have used a few drops of the oil to help sooth earaches and have taken a teaspoon or two to help with various ailments that women in their fifties confront. Ikarians hold this herb in the highest esteem and use it, either steeped in olive oil or infused as tea, for a wide range of ailments, from burns and cuts to depression and even childhood incontinence. To make a cold infusion: Simply steep 2 teaspoons of the dried flowers in a cup of cold water for 8 hours. To make a warm infusion: Pour 1 cup of boiling water over 2 teaspoons of dried flowers, steep for 15 minutes, then strain.

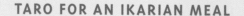

TARO FOR AN IKARIAN MEAL

On Ikaria, taro root is still one of the main sources of starch, especially in the winter months. It was the food of sustenance during the Occupation. Taro root is boiled for salads, stewed with goat or pork, cooked with beans, and even pureed for *skordalia*.

"It was our umbrella and our drinking cup," says my neighbor Titika Karimali, who recalls folding up taro leaves to form a bowl from which to catch spring water in the wild. Konstandina Koxyla, my friend Argyro's 90-plus-year-old mother, was one of the few people who confirmed that its leaves were also eaten as one of dozens of different wild greens on the island.

On Ikaria, taro grows wild near riverbanks and streams. It's easy to recognize by its big, floppy leaves.

It's no wonder the taro was such a life-giving plant for poverty-stricken Ikarians. It contains three times more dietary fiber than a potato. A 1-cup serving contains about 11% of our daily recommended requirements for vitamin C, 20% of our vitamin E requirements, and 22% of our vitamin B_6 needs. Taro is low on the glycemic index. It is also an excellent source of minerals, especially magnesium, potassium, phosphorous, copper, and manganese.

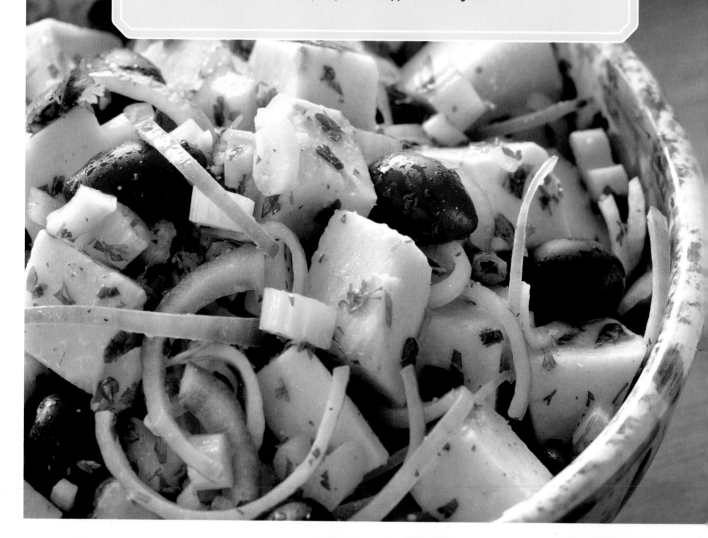

TARO ROOT SALAD

Salata me Kolokasi

This salad is the most common way to cook taro root on Ikaria. It is sometimes served with a side helping of bread-based *skordalia* (pages 9 and 10), defying most modern cooks' sense of starch overload.

MAKES 6 TO 8 SERVINGS

4 pounds (2 kg) taro root, peeled

Sea salt and freshly ground black pepper

1 red onion, halved and chopped (about 1 cup)

1 celery stalk, chopped

1 cup chopped fresh flat-leaf parsley or dill

10 kalamata olives

½ cup Greek extra virgin olive oil, or more, as needed

3 to 4 tablespoons fresh lemon juice or red wine vinegar (to taste)

Scrub the taro roots under cold running water. Peel the roots with a paring knife or vegetable peeler. Cut off the stem end. Cut the taro roots into 2-inch (5-cm) cubes.

Place in a pot with cold salted water. Bring to a boil. Reduce heat and simmer until fork tender, about 15 to 20 minutes. Drain and rinse the taro pieces in a colander.

Add the onion, celery, parsley (or dill), olives, olive oil, lemon juice (or vinegar), and salt and pepper to taste. Toss carefully. Serve either warm or at room temperature.

SWEET POTATO AND ARUGULA SALAD

Salata me Glykopatates kai Roka

Several farmers on Ikaria mentioned to me the sweet potatoes they remember as children, in the 1940s and '50s, and that most were grown on the terraced steps in the windswept southern town of Manganitis. My neighbor Titika, for example, recalled the simplest and most desired "dessert" of her youth: "We had sweet potatoes. That's it. With nothing on them. Just baked under the ashes in the fireplace. What a treat."

Sweet potatoes were also the tuber of choice for a salad, recounted to me by Myrsina Roussou, native of Manganitis. The addition of goat cheese or feta is mine, and totally optional. The original version is typical of the simple, pared-down dishes that nourished the generation that today is reaching triple-digit ages uniquely sound of mind and body. But the combination of dense, creamy sweet potatoes and sharp, peppery arugula seemed surprisingly sophisticated to me, even though this was the food of dire poverty.

MAKES 4 TO 6 SERVINGS

- 1½ pounds (750 g) sweet potatoes
- Salt, preferably sea salt
- 1 large red onion, halved and thinly sliced, or 1 bunch scallions, sliced
- 2 bunches fresh arugula, trimmed and coarsely chopped

- ½ cup Greek extra virgin olive oil
- 3 to 4 tablespoons red wine vinegar (to taste)
- 1 cup crumbled Greek feta cheese or goat cheese (optional)

In a large pot, cover the sweet potatoes with 2 inches (5 cm) cold salted water. Bring to a boil over medium heat. Reduce the heat to low and simmer until fork-tender but al dente, about 15 minutes. Remove, cool slightly, peel, and cut into 1½-inch (4 cm) chunks. (Alternatively, you can either roast or grill the sweet potatoes, peeled, sliced, salted, and tossed with ½ cup olive oil under the broiler.)

Transfer the sweet potatoes to a serving bowl. Add the onion (or scallions) and arugula to the bowl. Season to taste with salt and toss with the olive oil and vinegar. If desired, add the crumbled feta cheese (or goat cheese) and serve.

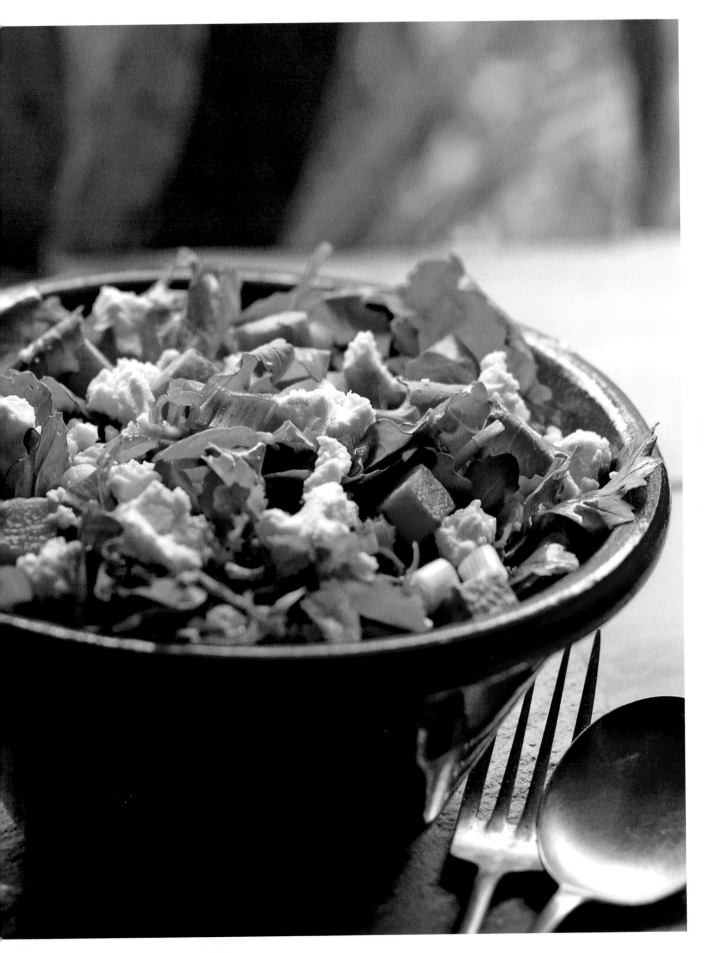

POTATOES ON THE IKARIAN TABLE

Potatoes and sweet potatoes were and still are basic foods on the island, something that flies in the face of current nutritional trends.

Potatoes are controversial, thanks to the way they are consumed in the United States: as fries, chips, and baked potatoes loaded with butter, sour cream, melted cheese, and bacon bits. A bit of ancient Greek wisdom could easily apply to the New World potato: *pan metron ariston*, or "nothing in excess."

Potatoes are a very good source of vitamin B_6 (important in athletic performance, cardiovascular protection, brain cell and nervous system activity, and building cells), vitamin C, various other B vitamins, potassium, copper, manganese, phosphorus, and dietary fiber. They also contain a variety of phytonutrients with antioxidant activity. As a matter of fact, potatoes' phytochemicals rival those in broccoli. New research has identified 60 different kinds of phytochemicals and vitamins in potatoes, making them a healthy food worth reconsidering, so long as you cook them right. The nutrients in potatoes help lower blood pressure and so protect against cardiovascular disease and may be beneficial for staving off respiratory problems and certain cancers.

Potatoes have an abundance of complex carbohydrates, important as a source of energy for the body, which are released slowly in the bloodstream, reducing overeating.

Sweet potatoes, the dessert of wartime inhabitants on Ikaria, flourish in the mineral-rich soil of Manganitis on the south side of the island. Like their savory cousins, sweet potatoes are nutrition bombs because they are:

- High in vitamin B_6 linked to the prevention of heart attacks

- A good source of vitamin C—producing collagen, which helps maintain youthful and elastic skin

- Rich in vitamin D, which plays an important role in energy levels and moods; helps to build healthy bones, heart, nerves, skin, and teeth; and fosters thyroid health

- High in iron, which is good for the production of red and white blood cells, improves resistance to stress, fosters proper immune functioning, and helps in metabolizing protein

- A good source of magnesium, which is the antistress mineral, very Ikarian!

- A source of potassium, which regulates heartbeat and nerve signals

- Are naturally sweet-tasting but with sugars that are slowly released into the bloodstream, ensuring a constant source of energy without the spikes in blood sugar levels that are linked to fatigue and weight gain

- Rich in carotenoids (such as beta-carotene), which help ward off cancer and protect against the effects of aging

IKARIAN POTATO SALAD

Kariotiki Patatosalata

One of the surprising findings of the Ikaria study was the frequency with which Ikarians ate—and still eat—potatoes. Surprising because the spud has been much maligned for its high carb content—and for the way it is consumed in the United States and Western Europe, in the form of fries and chips.

Ikaria has particularly good soil and climate for growing potatoes. There are two potato sowing seasons on the island, one in April and another in August. People in their eighties remember two varieties, the "Cretan" type, which was very hard with lots of eyes, and the "French" variety, which was well suited to boiling.

As for the salad below, it's simple enough. What distinguishes it is the fact that the potatoes are warm while every other vegetable is chilled or at room temperature.

MAKES 4 TO 6 SERVINGS

---

1 pound new potatoes

Sea salt

1 medium red onion, halved and sliced

2 medium firm-ripe tomatoes, cut into 1-inch (2.5 cm) chunks

2 Kirby cucumbers, halved lengthwise and cut crosswise into ⅛-inch-thick half-moons

1 large bunch purslane, trimmed

½ cup Greek extra virgin olive oil

3 tablespoons red wine vinegar

2 teaspoons dried Greek oregano or 2 tablespoons chopped fresh oregano

---

Scrub the potatoes clean but do not peel. Place in a large pot and cover with cold water by 2 inches (5 cm). Bring to a boil, add salt, and cook, skimming the foam off the surface of the water, until fork-tender, 25 to 35 minutes. Drain and transfer to a large bowl.

While the potatoes are cooking, prep all the vegetables.

Toss the warm potatoes with the onion, tomatoes, cucumbers, and purslane. Add the olive oil, vinegar, oregano, and salt to taste. Toss again and serve.

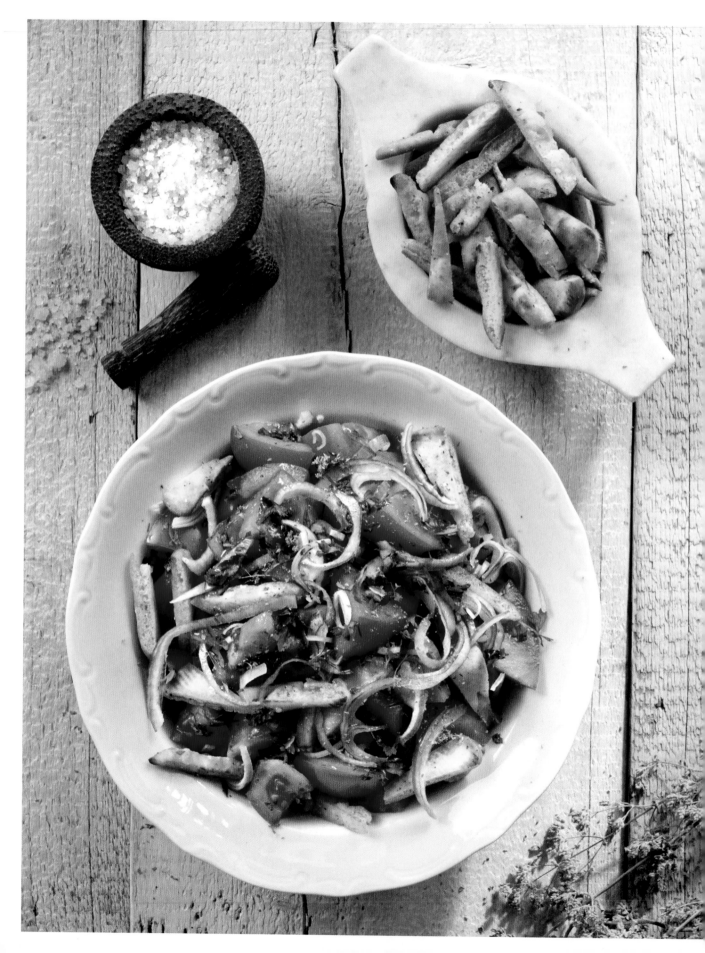

THEODOSI'S TOMATO AND PITA SALAD

Salata tou Theodosi

Theodosi runs the Filitsa taverna up in Carres, a mountain village about 3 kilometers from us in Raches. This salad is one of his signature dishes and we can't stop eating it whenever we order it. The grilled pita adds an irresistible smoky note to the succulent salad and makes for the perfect way to soak up all its delicious juices. Look for the best possible ripe tomatoes.

MAKES 4 TO 6 SERVINGS

2 (8- to 10-inch) pita, grilled or toasted well

3 large firm-ripe tomatoes, cut into 1½-inch (4 cm) chunks

2 red onions, halved and thinly sliced

1½ cups chopped fresh flat-leaf parsley

2 teaspoons dried Greek oregano

6 tablespoons Greek extra virgin olive oil

Sea salt and freshly ground black pepper

Cut the toasted pitas into strips about ⅛ inch (3 mm) wide and 2 inches (5 cm) long.

In a bowl, toss together the pita strips, tomatoes, onions, herbs, olive oil, and salt and pepper to taste. Serve immediately.

DO YOURSELF A LOT OF GOOD WITH A TOMATO

Tomatoes, so much a part of the Ikarian and greater Greek traditional diet, are loaded with vitamin C and are prime sources of beta-carotene lycopene, which helps strengthen the immune system. But beta-carotene must be consumed with fat for it to be well absorbed. In the context of the Mediterranean diet, that means olive oil, of course. With just ½ teaspoon of mono-unsaturated fat (the good fat in olive oil), the body is able to absorb five times more beta-carotene from vegetables such as tomatoes.

GREEK SALAD WITH AN IKARIAN TOUCH

Horiatiki opos tin Kanoun sto Nisi

Even a classic Greek salad—that intoxicating, irresistible combination of juicy tomatoes, kalamata olives, cucumbers, pungent onions, feta, oregano, and olive oil—has some regional variations. Greek salad on Ikaria often comes tossed with *kathoura*, the local goat's milk cheese, although feta (which is made with sheep's and some goat's milk) is a perfectly suited and more familiar addition for American cooks. A small handful of pickled sea fennel, obscure for most Americans, typically tops the salad. Capers will do the trick, too, adding just the right amount of salty, briny sharpness to this otherwise succulent seasonal salad. You can also add a hefty bunch of purslane to the tomato salad for an added touch.

MAKES 4 SERVINGS

3 large beefsteak or other meaty, fleshy tomatoes in season, cut into wedges

1 large, fat cucumber, peeled and sliced into 1/8-inch rounds

1 large red onion, halved and sliced

8 kalamata olives, rinsed

2 teaspoons dried savory or Greek oregano

Coarse sea salt

4 ounces Greek feta, preferably made from 100% goat's milk

1/2 cup pickled sea fennel (see Note) or pickled watercress, drained, or 1/3 cup capers, rinsed and drained

1/3 cup Greek extra virgin olive oil

In a serving bowl, combine the tomatoes, cucumber, and onion. Add the olives, savory (oregano), and salt to taste. Top with the feta and pickled sea fennel (or pickled watercress or capers). Add the olive oil. Toss the salad at the table, just before serving.

NOTE: *Sea fennel, or kritama, grows along the rocky coasts of Ikaria and is picked in spring and early summer, blanched, and pickled in brine. See Sea Fennel in Brine (page 32).*

A GREEN BEAN SALAD BORN IN MY GARDEN

Mia Salata me Fasolakia apo ton Kypo mou

A few summers ago, we had two interns who were siblings, Alana and Alex Eckhart, at our cooking classes on Ikaria. Alana saw my husband, Vassili, come into the kitchen with his arms wrapped around a bundle of fresh beans. She whipped up this salad and I've been making it ever since. Fresh beans are so sweet. When you mix them with tangy lemon juice and feta and temper all of that with sweet fresh basil, it's hard to want to eat anything else on a hot summer day.

MAKES 6 SERVINGS

1 pound yellow wax beans, trimmed

½ pound runner beans, trimmed

½ pound haricots verts or string beans, trimmed

2 lemons

2 cups crumbled Greek feta cheese

⅓ cup Greek extra virgin olive oil

2 garlic cloves, minced or slivered

⅓ cup slivered fresh basil leaves

Freshly ground black pepper

1 red onion, halved and sliced

⅓ cup chopped fresh flat-leaf parsley

1 teaspoon pink peppercorns

Set up a large bowl of ice and water. In a large pot of boiling salted water, blanch the beans for 3 to 4 minutes. Drain and transfer the beans to the ice water to cool down immediately. Drain.

Preheat a grill, the broiler, or a stovetop ridged grill pan. Grill the whole lemons until very lightly charred, a few minutes. Let cool slightly and grate the peel. Juice the lemons and set aside.

In a food processor, pulse together the feta, 2 tablespoons of the olive oil, 2 tablespoons of the lemon juice, the garlic, half the basil, and black pepper to taste.

Toss the green beans with the feta mixture, onion, parsley, pink peppercorns, remaining olive oil, remaining basil, lemon peel, and salt and pepper to taste. Adjust the seasoning with additional lemon juice, if desired. Serve.

BLACK-EYED PEA SALAD WITH SPRING HERBS

Mavromatika Salata me Myrodika

Black-eyed peas grow in the gardens of many Ikarians, a food of sustenance that comes chock-full of great nutritional components. Like others, we dry them, too, watching their bright green pods turn the color of hay as they dry. Black-eyed peas provide an excellent source of potassium, which is important for the proper function of cells, tissues, and organs. They contain zinc, which is important in cell metabolism, immune function, protein synthesis, and healing wounds. Like other legumes, they are also a great source of iron, as well as vitamin C, which helps our bodies absorb that iron. But beyond their health benefits, they taste great. Black-eyed peas are especially easy to pair in salads, their earthiness holding up well to pungent onions and intensely flavored spring herbs.

MAKES 4 TO 6 SERVINGS

2 cups dried black-eyed peas

1½ cups chopped wild fennel fronds*

1 large red onion, finely chopped (about 1 cup)

3 spring onions or scallions, sliced into thin rounds

2 garlic cloves, minced

½ cup Greek extra virgin olive oil

Juice of 1 to 2 lemons (to taste), strained

Salt

Place the beans in a pot with enough water to cover by 3 inches (7.5 cm). Bring to a boil, remove from the heat, drain, and repeat the process with fresh water. As soon as the black-eyed peas start to simmer again, reduce the heat and simmer until tender but al dente, 35 to 40 minutes.

Drain the black-eyed peas and toss with the fennel fronds, onions, and garlic. Add the olive oil, lemon juice, and salt to taste and serve.

*If you can't find wild fennel fronds, substitute 1 fennel bulb and fronds, finely chopped, plus ½ cup chopped dill.

A WORD ABOUT LUPINES

Lupines, one of the oldest edible legumes in the Eastern Mediterranean, are still part of the Ikarian diet. In my "neighborhood"—a short walk, in other words, from my front door on Ikaria, down a foot-path into the Platanidi valley below, lupines grow wild everywhere. The plant produces beautiful purplish blue flowers, and the beans are nestled in thick, almost fuzzy brown pods.

They have always been the Lenten snack on Ikaria and elsewhere in Greece, most likely because they are an incredible source of protein. My friend Lefteris, a local naturalist, believes that ancient lupines are poised to become the bean of the future, supplanting soybeans as a protein source, because they are not GMO. Indeed, on Limnos (an island farther to the north in the eastern Aegean) as well as in Holland, a few forward-thinking farmers are already starting to cultivate them.

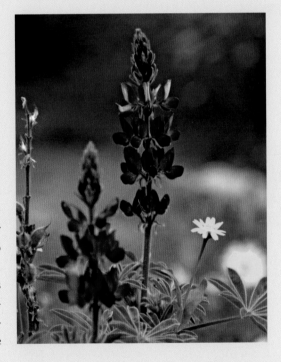

However, lupine beans contain an alkaloid that renders them poisonous (and bitter) unless "cured." To do this, the beans are first boiled until soft, then soaked in salt water. Ikarians use the salt water that is most available to them: the sea. Specifically, after they collect the beans in late February (just before Lent) and boil them, they traditionally tie them up in small muslin bags, which they then submerge in the hot springs on the south side of the island, where the combination of heat and salt expedites the whole process of transforming them from acrid to edible. Alternatively, farmers also submerge them inside their wells, where the constant rush of fresh water also does the job of curing.

Stefanos, my 75-year-old neighbor Titika's significant other, once told me they were the "popcorn" of his generation! People here know to harvest only the smallest lupines, for these are the most tender.

Once boiled they lose their bitterness and can be eaten as a salad. Here are two options for a late winter salad of lupine beans, Ikarian style. (You may find protein-rich lupine beans ready to eat, in brine, in both Greek and Italian grocery stores; in the latter, they are known as *lupini*.) Or you may substitute fava beans for the lupine beans.

LETTUCE AND LUPINE BEAN SALAD

Maroulosalata me Loupina

Greeks eat lupine beans during times of fasting, especially during Lent, when the beans are in season. And it's no accident why. Lupine beans are made up of 38% protein, 24% complex carbohydrates, and almost 8% minerals, especially iron (twice the amount in spinach), as well as calcium, zinc, magnesium, and copper.

The flavors in this salad are a nice mix of sharp and briny, thanks to the pickled cornichons, sweet from the fleshy red peppers, a little bitter, which is what really fresh romaine lettuce should taste like, and somewhat mineral-y, which is what the subtle lupine bean imparts. It is an unusual combination.

MAKES 4 SERVINGS

- 1 head romaine lettuce, torn
- 1 large red onion, coarsely chopped (about 1 cup)
- 1 cup canned or bottled *lupini* beans,* rinsed and drained
- 6 small cornichon pickles, cut into thin rounds
- 1 roasted red pepper in brine or olive oil, drained and chopped
- ½ cup chopped fresh dill
- ½ cup Greek extra virgin olive oil
- 2 to 3 tablespoons red wine vinegar (to taste)
- Salt

In a salad bowl, combine the lettuce, onion, *lupini* beans, cornichons, roasted pepper, and dill. In a small bowl, whisk together the olive oil, vinegar, and salt to taste. Pour this into the salad, toss well, and serve.

*You may substitute cooked fresh fava beans for *lupinis*. People with a peanut allergy should avoid lupines completely, however, as they tend to trigger an allergic reaction.

LEEK AND LUPINE BEAN SALAD WITH CAPERS

Prasosalata me Loupina kai Kapari

I love this between-the-seasons combination of ingredients. There are many dishes like this, which bridge the gap between winter and spring or summer and fall, combining late-harvest produce, leeks in this case, with the first of the next season's delicacies. Capers and sea fennel, both harvested in summer and pickled, are year-round treats.

MAKES 2 TO 4 SERVINGS

1 large leek

Salt

2 cups canned or bottled *lupini* beans,*
rinsed and drained

½ cup finely chopped fresh flat-leaf parsley

⅓ cup chopped fresh mint leaves

2 garlic cloves, minced

¼ cup capers or 1 cup Greek *kritama* (Sea Fennel in Brine, page 32), rinsed and drained

½ cup Greek extra virgin olive oil

2 to 3 tablespoons red wine vinegar (to taste)

Halve the leek lengthwise and rinse under cold running water to rid it of any sand or dirt. Cut the white part only crosswise into thin half-moons. Bring a small pot of salted water to a rolling boil and blanch the leeks for 2 minutes, just to soften. Remove and rinse immediately under cold tap water in a colander.

In a salad bowl, combine the leeks, *lupinis*, parsley, mint, garlic, and capers (for *kritama*). Add the olive oil and vinegar. Adjust the seasoning with extra salt if desired. Serve immediately.

*You may substitute cooked fresh fava beans for *lupinis*. People with a peanut allergy should avoid lupines completely, however, as they tend to trigger an allergic reaction.

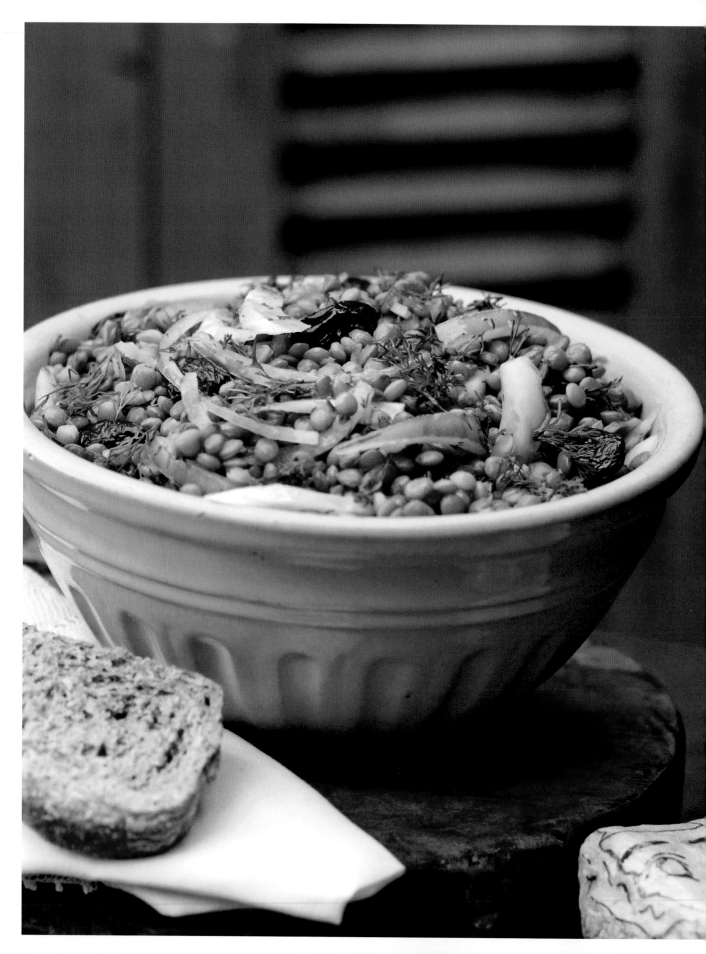

LENTIL SALAD WITH FENNEL, ONIONS, AND LOTS OF HERBS

Fakes Salata me Maratho, Myrodika kai Kremmydia

Lentils are one of the oldest pulses in the Eastern Mediterranean and one of the most important on Ikaria. Mostly people cook them up in simple soups. This salad is a bit of a hybrid, something we eat in our home in the spring and early summer, when there is still plenty of feathery wild fennel around. You can substitute dill instead, and the salad may be served warm or at room temperature.

MAKES 4 TO 6 SERVINGS

2 cups small lentils, rinsed

1 fennel bulb, trimmed and chopped or thinly sliced

1 large red onion, halved and thinly sliced

½ cup chopped fennel fronds or snipped fresh dill

½ cup chopped fresh Chinese celery or regular celery leaves

⅓ cup chopped fresh mint leaves

2 teaspoons dried Greek oregano

10 olives: kalamata or wrinkled (salt-cured) black olives such as Greek *throumbes* or Moroccan

½ cup Greek extra virgin olive oil

¼ cup red wine vinegar

Salt

Place the lentils in a pot with enough cold water to cover by 3 inches (7.5 cm). Bring to a boil over medium heat. Reduce to low and simmer, uncovered, until the lentils are tender but al dente, 25 to 35 minutes. Drain and rinse.

Transfer the lentils to a serving bowl and add the fennel, onion, fennel fronds (or dill), celery, mint, oregano, and olives.

In a small bowl, whisk together the olive oil, vinegar, and salt to taste. Pour into the salad, toss well, and serve.

FAVA BEAN SALAD WITH FENNEL AND SCALLIONS

Koukia Salata me Maratho kai Kremmydaki

Fava beans, one of the oldest and most intriguing legumes in the Eastern Mediterranean, were forbidden by Pythagoras because their embryonic shape was thought to contain the souls of the dead. They are also the source of much controversy in Greece, where many suffer from favism, a hereditary disease in which ingesting favas can be dangerous. Nonetheless, those of us whose bodies do contain the enzyme that can metabolize fava beans wait for them with alacrity each spring. This salad is not an Ikarian dish per se, but rather a composite of dishes found all over the Greek islands. If anything, the profuse use of fennel gives it an Ikarian flair.

Fava beans have a unique flavor, almost musky and sweet and sour at the same time. They come alive with all the herbs, robust scallions, and fresh lemon juice in this salad.

MAKES 4 SERVINGS

2 pounds (1 kg) fresh young fava beans in the pod

½ cup chopped fennel fronds or dill

5 scallions, cut into thin rounds

½ cup Greek extra virgin olive oil

Juice of 1 lemon (or more to taste), strained

Salt and freshly ground black pepper

Shell the beans: Using a small, sharp paring knife, snip off the ends of the pod and pull back along both seams, taking the fibrous thread with the knife. Discard the thread and pod.

Bring a large pot of salted water to a rolling boil and blanch the beans for a few minutes, until tender but al dente. (Greeks like their vegetables very well cooked.) Drain the beans into a colander and rinse under cold water.

Transfer the beans to a bowl. Toss in the fennel or dill and scallions. In a small bowl, whisk together the olive oil, lemon juice, and salt and pepper to taste. Add to the salad. Toss and serve.

ARUGULA, MINT, AND FRESH FAVA BEAN SALAD

Roka Salata me Koukia kai Dyosmo

The arugula that grows in Ikarian gardens is almost as spicy as chile peppers. I love the combination of ingredients in this dish. The mint cools and balances the spiky heat of local arugula, while the fava beans, with their earthy flavor, are a grounding force.

MAKES 4 SERVINGS

2 cups fresh or frozen shelled fava beans*

2 bunches arugula, torn

4 scallions, cut into thin rounds

1 whole green garlic (optional), chopped

½ cup chopped fresh mint leaves

3 tablespoons capers, drained

5 tablespoons Greek extra virgin olive oil

3 tablespoons fresh lemon juice

Salt

Blanch the fava beans in salted, boiling water for 5 minutes, or until tender but al dente. Drain in a colander and rinse immediately with cold water. If using fresh beans, take a paring knife and remove the little black "eye" from the beans.

In a salad bowl, toss together the beans, arugula, scallions, garlic (if using), mint, and capers. In a small bowl, whisk together the olive oil, lemon juice, and salt to taste. Toss into the salad and serve.

* If using fresh fava beans, shell them but do not peel them.

DRIED FAVA BEAN SALAD
WITH SAGE AND LOTS OF ONIONS

Xera Koukia Salata me Faskomilo kai Kremmydia

Dried fava beans are totally different in taste, texture, and color from their fresh counterparts. They have always been an important part of the Greek larder, despite the fact that a large number of people in this part of the world cannot eat them because they lack the enzyme that enables their bodies to metabolize the beans. This is called favism and people in Greece are tested for it at birth. However, the dried beans are a terrific source of protein and minerals like calcium and phosphorus for those who can enjoy them.

MAKES 4 TO 6 SERVINGS

1 pound (450 g) dried fava beans

4 fresh or dried sage leaves

3 red onions, halved and thinly sliced

3 garlic cloves, minced

Salt and freshly ground black pepper

⅔ cup Greek extra virgin olive oil

1 tablespoon dried Greek oregano

Juice of 2 lemons

Soak the beans for 8 hours or overnight in ample cold water.

Drain the beans and transfer to a pot with fresh water to cover by 3 inches (7.5 cm). Add 2 sage leaves. Simmer until soft, about 1 hour 30 minutes. Remove, cool slightly, and, using a sharp paring knife, remove the leathery membrane and the dark "eye" on one side of each bean.

Heat the onions and garlic in a dry skillet over low heat. Season with a little salt and cook, covered, until the onions exude their own juices and are tender, about 8 minutes. Check and stir frequently; add a little water if necessary to keep them from burning. Add half the olive oil, half the oregano, and the remaining sage leaves and keep cooking over low heat until the onions are lightly golden. Remove and discard the sage leaves.

Transfer the beans to a serving bowl. Add the onion mixture, lemon juice, the remaining olive oil and oregano, and salt and pepper to taste. Toss well and serve.

VARIATION

Fava bean salads were also—actually, more typically—served with pickled bulbs. You can substitute whole Pickled Wild Hyacinth Bulbs (page 33) for the onions in this recipe. Toss them in at the end.

COOKED SALAD OF AMARANTH AND ZUCCHINI

Vlita kai Kolokithakia Vrasti Salata

This simple dish is a summer meal that simmers in the pots of every Ikarian home. The zucchini is typically large enough to hold up during boiling; keep in mind that Ikarian zucchini, which is only cultivated in the summer and watered very sparingly, doesn't exude nearly as much liquid as its American counterpart. You may have to adjust the cooking time as a result.

Simple as this dish is, when you serve it with feta or another goat's milk cheese and good sourdough whole-grain bread, it is much more than just a salad. It really becomes a proper meal.

MAKES 4 SERVINGS

⅓ cup Greek extra virgin olive oil, plus more for dressing

1 garlic clove, sliced

1 pound (450 g) amaranth or other sweet greens, such as chard

2 medium zucchini, about 2 inches (5 cm) in diameter, cut into 3 pieces each

Sea salt

Juice of 1 to 2 lemons (to taste), strained

In a large pot or Dutch oven, heat the olive oil over medium heat. Add the garlic and swirl in the oil for a minute or so, being careful not to let it burn.

Add the amaranth (or other greens) and stir. Add the zucchini. Cover and steam the greens and zucchini over low heat in their own juices. If they don't exude enough, add a touch of water, just enough to keep the mixture moist. Cook until the greens and zucchini are tender, about 15 minutes.

Remove, transfer to a plate, and season with salt, extra virgin olive oil, and lemon juice to taste. Serve hot or at room temperature.

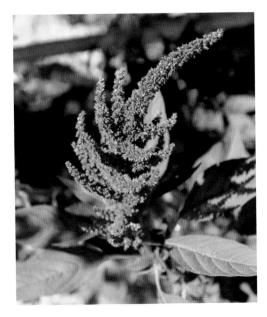

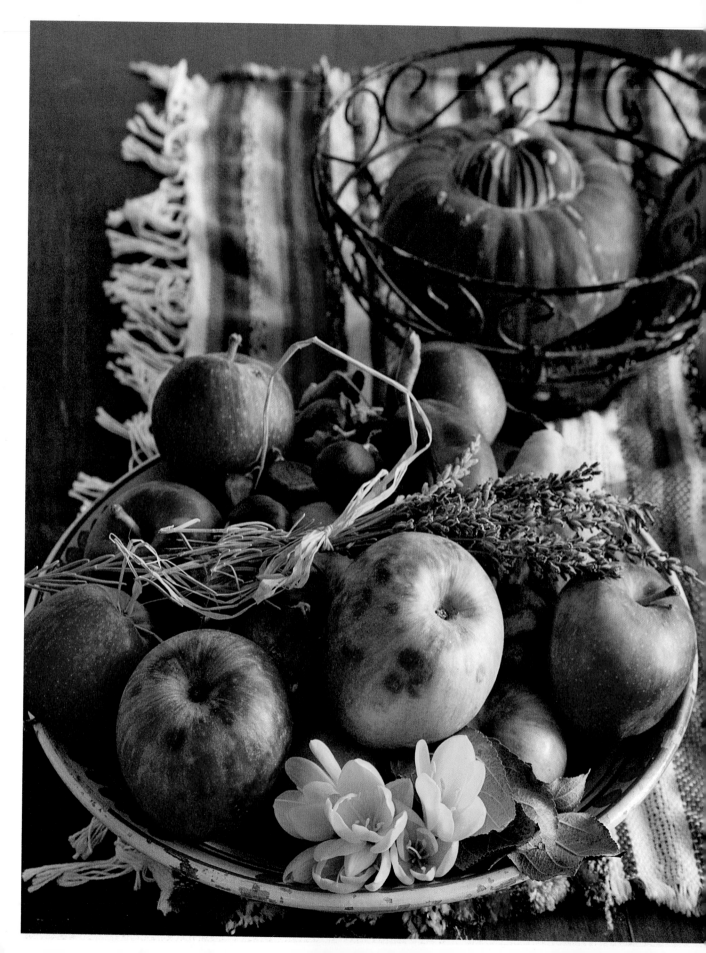

COMFORTING
SOUPS

HOW MANY TIMES HAVE I SAT AROUND THE TABLE with friends on Ikaria, wineglasses spread out all about the table, bread torn into chunks, a platter of fish poached and white as alabaster in the middle, and the soup made with it steaming in bowls? Fish soups probably top the list of favorite Ikarian dishes, and together with the poached fish themselves and boiled vegetables from the pot, make a main meal. But then again most soups are a main course in this traditional "poor man's" kitchen.

The variety of soups in Greece is not vast, generally speaking. There are no veloutés, no creamed soups, not too many hearty meat soups. But on the island, especially in winter—when it can rain for a month on end, and the fog is thick and chilling, and where the wind can blow up to many miles an hour—hot soup is a welcome meal.

Ikarian cooks make most of the same traditional soups that are found all over Greece: lentil, bean, bulgur-tomato, and more. They season them with the herbs they love and have on hand, like wild sage and oregano for lentil soups, oregano or savory for white bean soups, maybe with the addition of a heat-inducing chile pepper. Simple bulgur-tomato soup is an old recipe, and the goat meat soup, whether boiled in cauldrons for a thousand people at one of the island's *panygyria* (feasts) or made at home, is the meat soup specialty of the island. Goat meat is preserved in salt and shredded to add to bean soups for flavor, too.

IKARIAN FISH SOUP WITH AVGOLEMONO

Psarosoupa Avgolemono

It is rare to see fish soup avgolemono, a Greek classic, made with potatoes, as it is traditionally on Ikaria, instead of with rice or orzo, attesting to the importance of the humble tuber in the local diet. Avgolemono soup is a rich source of protein, derived both from the egg and from the fish (or chicken, another classic), and is also a good source of carbohydrates, making it the ultimate comfort food!

"Boil fish soups without any water! Or with very little and never rinse the fish lest you wash away its flavor," says Yiorgos Stenos, a fount of knowledge about life on his native island.

MAKES 6 TO 8 SERVINGS

2 to 2½ pounds (1 to 1.25 kg) fresh whole soup fish (includes rock fish like scorpion fish and stargazers, plus combers and grouper), scaled and gutted

Salt and freshly ground black pepper

2 large potatoes, peeled and cut into 1-inch (2.5 cm) cubes

2 large red onions, coarsely chopped (about 2 cups)

3 large carrots, cut into pieces to match the potatoes

1½ cups chopped Chinese or regular celery

6 cups water

2 large eggs

Juice of 2 lemons, strained

1 cup Greek extra virgin olive oil

⅓ cup fresh lemon juice

Season the fish with salt inside and out.

Place the vegetables in a soup pot large enough to hold all the fish. Place the fish over the vegetables, placing the large fish in first and the smaller ones on top. You can also place the fish in a clean cheesecloth, tied loosely, to prevent bones from breaking into the soup.

Pour in just enough of the water to barely cover the fish. Season with salt and pepper and bring to a boil. Reduce heat, cover, and simmer until the fish is cooked, 20 to 25 minutes. Carefully remove the fish with a slotted spoon and set aside, covered, to keep warm. Add the remaining water to the broth and bring to a boil.

In a large, preferably stainless steel, bowl, whisk the eggs until very frothy, about 5 minutes. Slowly drizzle in the lemon juice, whisking constantly. Take a ladleful of the hot fish broth and drizzle it in a slow, steady stream, whisking vigorously all the while, into the egg-lemon mixture. Repeat with two more ladlefuls of the broth. Pour this mixture back into the soup pot and tilt the pot back and forth so that the egg-lemon mixture is evenly distributed. Serve immediately.

Serve the fish separately on a platter. Whisk together the oil and juice; serve on the side.

SALT COD AND CELERY SOUP AVGOLEMONO

Kakavia me Bakaliaro, Selino kai Avgolemono

Ikarian fishermen salted the catch from local waters to eat in winter, when the sea is often too rough to go fishing. They'd cook salted mullet, bream, and more in a simple tomato sauce, or on the grill, or serve them as part of a salad. But salt cod, smoked herring, and other preserved fish from far-off waters have long been a part of the local cuisine. Salt cod was known as the fish of the mountains, because it travels well and was sold inland by itinerant fishmongers. Like smoked herring, a traditional poor man's *meze*, cod was sold in local *pantopoleia*, or small general markets, like the one Yiorgos Stenos ran for decades in the heart of Christos, Raches, the main village on the north side of the island. Indeed, this recipe came from him; it's a dish he remembered his mother making.

MAKES 6 SERVINGS

1 pound (450 g) salt cod, soaked to desalt (see Note on next page)

½ cup Greek extra virgin olive oil

1 large onion or 5 scallions, chopped (about 1 cup)

1 small bunch Chinese celery or 3 stalks regular celery, trimmed and chopped (about 1½ cups)

1 cup long-grain rice

6 cups water

Freshly ground black pepper

3 egg yolks

Juice of 2 lemons

Drain and shred the cod.

In a large soup pot, heat the olive oil over low heat. Add the onion (or scallions) and cook, stirring occasionally, until wilted and soft, about 10 minutes.

Add the celery and stir to coat in the olive oil. Continue cooking over low heat for a few minutes, to soften.

Add the shredded cod and the rice and stir to coat. Add the water and bring to a boil. Season with pepper to taste, and simmer until the rice is cooked, about 20 minutes.

In a medium glass or stainless steel bowl, whisk the egg yolks until frothy. Slowly drizzle in the lemon juice, whisking constantly until the mixture is very thick. Take a ladle at a time of the soup liquid, trying not to get any solids, and drizzle into the egg-lemon mixture drop by drop to temper the mixture. Repeat with a second ladleful.

Pour the tempered egg-lemon into the soup pot and tilt back and forth to distribute evenly. Serve immediately.

NOTE: *To desalt the cod, start 2 days ahead. Cut the cod into large serving pieces. Place in a large pot of cold water, keep refrigerated, and change the water every 4 to 5 hours.*

SEAWATER AS A CONDIMENT

"The sea was so clean, kids would dampen their *paximadia* [rusks] in it. We'd wash our fruit in the sea when I was little," writes John Chrysochoos in his book *Ikaria: Paradise in Peril.*

Seawater has long been a source of great flavor to local cooks. They scooped it up in ladlefuls to make their classic fisherman's soup, *kakavia.* They added it to dishes like Periwinkle Pilaf (page 195). They used it as a natural brine, sometimes even storing cheese in it (a practice that at least until 10 years ago I had also seen alive and well on nearby Limnos island).

But things have changed. Ikaria's coasts are still very clean, comparatively speaking. But in the summer it's not unusual to see the occasional stretch of tar marring the sand, or debris, having been washed ashore by errant boats.

Ikarians still cling to their love of the sea and all its edible life, which they search out, if a little more assiduously than once, when things were purer, in isolated parts of the coast. Seawater isn't used for much of anything in July and August, when the beaches are packed with people, but if you are lucky enough to find yourself on Ikaria in the off months, you might just happen across a fish soup seasoned with the sea or enjoy the tangy sweetness of an early June apricot washed in the waves.

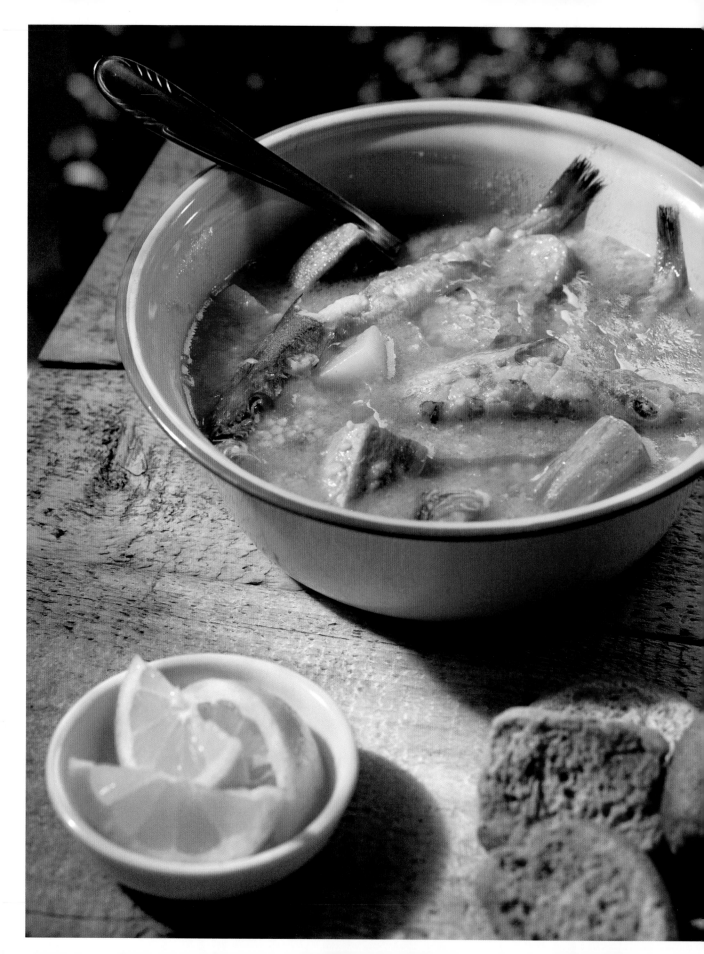

IKARIAN FISHERMAN'S SOUP WITH TRAHANA

Psarosoupa me Trahana

Before rice became a common grain in Greece, village cooks on Ikaria relied on wheat in all its manifestations to make soup more filling: bulgur or cracked wheat; *trahana* (see page 96), an ancient, granular fermented grain product made from either bulgur, cracked wheat, or flour and whole goat's milk, buttermilk, or yogurt; and sometimes the local ribbon-shaped pasta called *matsi*. Today, all over Greece, fish soup is almost universally enriched with rice.

MAKES 6 TO 8 SERVINGS

1½ cups Greek extra virgin olive oil

2 medium red onions, finely chopped (about 2 cups)

2 large boiling potatoes, peeled and cut into ½-inch (2 cm) cubes

2 small zucchini, cut into 2-inch (5 cm) rounds

1 large firm-ripe tomato, peeled, seeded, and chopped

Salt and freshly ground black pepper

Juice of 3 large lemons, strained

5 cups water

3 pounds fresh whole soup fish (a combination of sea bass, red snapper, scorpion fish, rockfish, grouper, bream, and/or red mullet), dressed

⅔ cup sweet or sour *trahana*, store-bought or homemade (page 98)

In a large heavy pot, heat ½ cup olive oil over medium heat. Add the onions, cover, and reduce the heat to very low. Steam the onions in the oil until wilted and soft, about 15 minutes. Add the potatoes, zucchini, and tomato. Season with salt. Add one-third of the lemon juice and 1 cup of the water. Cover, bring to a boil, reduce the heat to low, and continue cooking for about 10 minutes.

Place the fish in the pot in order of size, with the larger ones on the bottom and building upward so that a mullet or any other small fish are on top. Season each layer with salt and pepper as you go. (You can also place the fish in a clean cheesecloth, tied loosely, to prevent bones from breaking into the soup.) Add enough water to the pot to cover the fish by about 1 inch (2.5 cm). Cover the pot and cook the soup until the fish is fork-tender and the potatoes done, 20 to 25 minutes. Remove the fish and vegetables from the pot with a slotted spoon and place on a serving platter.

Bring the broth back to a boil, replenishing with the remaining 4 cups water. Add the *trahana* and simmer until tender, about 12 minutes. Season the soup with ½ cup olive oil and half of the lemon juice.

Whisk the remaining ½ cup olive oil together with the remaining lemon juice until the mixture emulsifies. Serve this as a sauce for the fish.

Serve the broth and fish and vegetables separately.

MIGHTY OAKS FROM LITTLE ACORNS GROW—AN UNUSUAL SOUP

"My uncle had grapevines in Cambos, and I used to walk there to work [about 25 miles from his home in Raches]" says Yiorgos Stenos, our dear friend who is a very young 83. "My job was to help him graft the vines. I was 9. I remember it all very well. I learned to cook there, too! We ate acorns then. In fact, we ate them a lot during the Occupation," he says. "We'd boil them, then soak them for about 10 days, which made them sweeter because they can be quite bitter, then peel the hulls away by hand, bake them to dry and, finally, grind them to flour in a stone mill. Acorns were our source of starch during those years, because we saved the barley and what little wheat there was for bread. We made soup with acorn flour and tomatoes and I always heeded my uncle's advice: 'Save a little of the soup to eat before you leave, so you can climb back up over that steep mountain easily like a partridge.'"

Mighty oaks from little acorns grow! There is nothing diminutive about this old Ikarian survival food, as our friend Yiorgos pointed out. On lush Ikaria, oaks grow mighty indeed, and their humble fruit has helped the islanders through times of severe dearth.

Acorns are very rich in complex carbohydrates and fiber, but very low in sugar and are arguably one of the best foods for controlling blood sugar levels. They are a great source of minerals (especially manganese, calcium, potassium, phosphorus, and iron) and vitamins, mostly from the B complex, and they are lower in fat than most other nuts.

One thing to remember, though, about acorns, or *velanidia*, is that they are very tannic. Most of the tannins are contained in the cap. Acorns were always soaked, then roasted, as part of the process to make them less bitter. The tannic water is itself a salve, both antiviral and antiseptic, and can be sipped as a tea for diarrhea or used as a gargle for sore throats.

Acorns are seeing a revival in Greece. At least one enterprising farmer, on the island of Kea, has built a thriving cottage industry out of farming and processing them for food. And, because they are gluten-free, the flour from acorns could be appealing even to Americans, as wheat allergies and celiac disease seem to be running rampant.

Acorn flour was not the only base for old-fashioned Ikarian soups and porridges. Cornmeal, local noodles (*matsi*) cooked with milk, and *trahana* (page 96) were, too. These are recipes that hark back to another era for sure, but I've included them in these pages, knowing that these were among the few foods that nourished the generation of 100-year-olds that today has captured the news.

OLD IKARIAN TOMATO-ACORN SOUP

Hilos me Tomata kai Velanidia

The idea of cooking with acorns is about as far from the mainstream American kitchen mind-set as it gets! But this simple soup provides quick, easy nutrition. Acorn flour tastes nuttier than wheat flour and does not get as pasty. This soup tastes like the forest with tomatoes! It is hearty, with a subtle, enigmatic flavor. It is also great chilled. You can source acorn flour online (see page 299).

MAKES 6 TO 8 SERVINGS

½ cup Greek extra virgin olive oil, plus more for serving

2 large onions, finely chopped (about 2 cups)

1 cup acorn flour*

6 large tomatoes, grated or pureed in a food processor, or 4 cups of canned tomato purée

6 cups water

2 to 3 sprigs fresh savory, oregano, basil or thyme

Sea salt and freshly ground black pepper

In a large, wide pot, heat the olive oil over medium heat. Add the onion and cook until soft. Add the acorn flour and stir to coat in the oil. Add the grated or puréed fresh tomatoes or the canned tomato purée, water, herb sprigs, and salt and pepper to taste. Bring to a boil, reduce the heat to low, and simmer until thick, 15 to 20 minutes.

Remove the herb sprigs. If desired, serve with a drizzle of olive oil on top. This soup is also lovely with a dollop of Greek yogurt or crumbled feta.

*You may substitute the acorn flour with chestnut flour.

CORNMEAL AND GREENS SOUP

Tsorvas

I have been hearing about *tsorvas* and the use of corn kernels and cornmeal in the Ikarian diet ever since my Aunt Mary, who passed away several years ago at the age of 97, mentioned the corn-stuffed cabbage leaves she remembered as a child. Other nonagenarians have talked to me about *tsorvas*, which was either some kind of cream (akin to polenta) or soup, or pilaf made with either the dried, milled corn kernels of a sweet white corn that is still grown on the island, or with a meal or flour made with the same corn. I have never been able to find either an exact definition or an exact recipe, so I tried my best to approximate what *tsorvas* was in the recipe below. Whatever it was exactly, corn was an important part of the diet before the advent of rice and it was one of the major foods of sustenance. It's also quite delicious!

MAKES 6 SERVINGS

6 tablespoons Greek extra virgin olive oil

2 red onions, finely chopped (about 2 cups)

2 garlic cloves, smashed with the side of a knife

1 pound (450 g) Swiss chard

1 cup coarsely chopped fresh mint leaves

1 cup coarsely chopped fresh chervil

6 cups (or more) water or low-sodium chicken broth or vegetable broth

1 cup polenta (coarse cornmeal)

Sea salt and freshly ground black pepper

Crumbled goat's milk cheese or Greek feta cheese, for garnish (optional)

In a large, wide soup pot, heat 3 tablespoons of the olive oil over medium-low heat. Add the onions and garlic and cook until wilted, about 5 minutes.

Add the chard and half the herbs to the mixture and stir until wilted. Add 4 cups of the water or broth, bring to a boil, and in a slow, steady stream add the cornmeal, stirring vigorously with a wooden spoon all the while. Season to taste with salt and pepper.

Add the remaining 2 cups water (or broth) and simmer the soup until thick and creamy, about 30 minutes total. About 5 minutes before removing from the heat, add the remaining herbs and, if necessary, additional water or broth to maintain the soup's liquid, creamy consistency.

Drizzle in the remaining 3 tablespoons olive oil just before serving. If desired, garnish the soup with a little crumbled cheese.

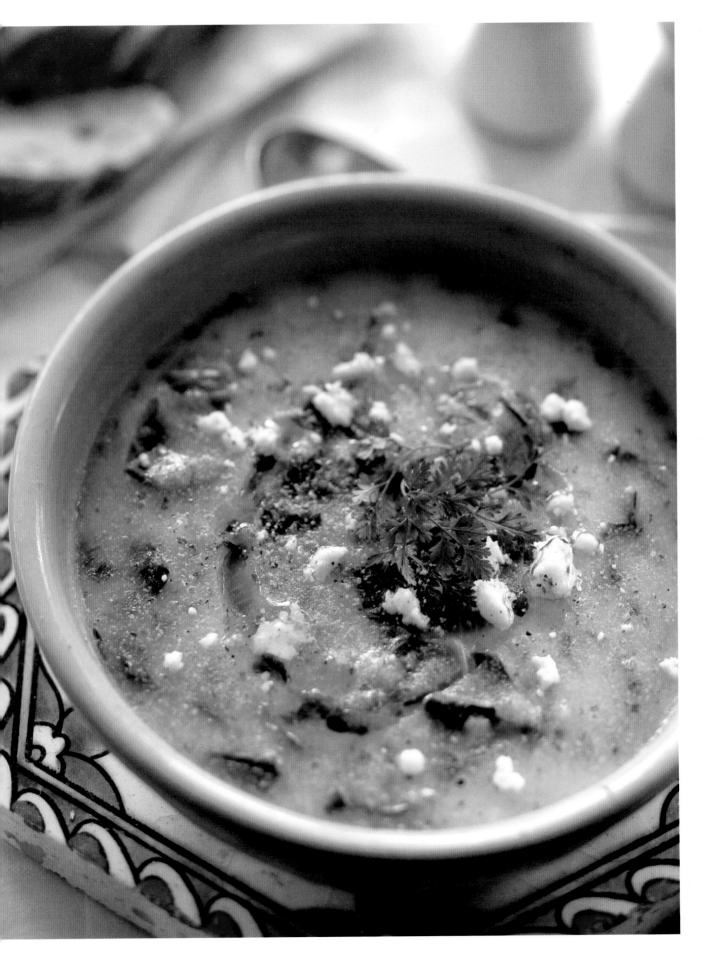

IKARIAN MILK SOUP

Matsi me Gala

This is a very old Ikarian recipe and was both a breakfast dish and an easy evening meal. It was traditionally prepared with *matsi*, the fresh or dried noodles that are the local pasta. It is rare to see this recipe in the island cooking today, but it played a role in the diets of the very old.

MAKES 4 TO 6 SERVINGS

4 cups water

Salt and freshly ground black pepper

½ pound Greek *hilopites*, tagliatelle, or fettuccine noodles (preferably fresh)

4 cups goat's milk

2 to 3 tablespoons olive oil or sheep's milk butter

Freshly grated nutmeg

In a large pot, bring the water to a boil over medium heat and add salt. Add the pasta.

Meanwhile, in a separate pot, heat the milk. When the pasta is about two-thirds of the way cooked, pour in the hot milk.

Continue to simmer until the pasta is soft. Stir in the olive oil (or butter). Adjust the seasoning with salt, pepper, and nutmeg. Serve hot.

COMFORTING PORRIDGE

Porridge made either from corn or *trahana* was eaten for breakfast, and was ideal for keeping bellies filled and blood glucose low.

There are a lot of old wives' tales surrounding porridge—in some places in Greece it was believed that you had to stir it clockwise to ward off the devil, or that you had to eat it standing up. Nowadays, as nutritionist Maria Byron Panayidou mentioned to me, "It has the power to vacuum up cholesterol, boost testosterone, fend off heart disease, and suppress appetite."

IKARIAN FAVA BEAN SOUP WITH FRESH OR DRIED BEANS

Soupa me Koukia

Local cooks like to mash a portion of this soup, right inside the pot using a fork, to achieve a thick, hearty consistency. The flavors are subtle, delicate, and herbaceous. If using dried favas, the soup will taste much earthier and denser than when using the fresh beans.

MAKES 6 TO 8 SERVINGS

- 2 cups frozen or fresh fava beans (if using fresh, shell but do not peel) or 1 pound dried favas (see Note)
- 1 cup Greek extra virgin olive oil
- 2 leeks, white and light green parts only, cleaned and sliced
- 1 large onion, chopped (about 1 cup)
- 2 medium or large carrots, diced
- 1½ cups chopped Chinese or regular celery, including the leaves
- 2 small potatoes, peeled and diced
- 1½ cups chopped canned plum tomatoes
- 1 large fresh or dried chile pepper (optional)
- 2 quarts water
- 3 bay leaves
- ⅓ cup chopped fresh flat-leaf parsley
- ½ cup chopped fennel fronds
- Salt and freshly ground black pepper
- Juice of 1 lemon, strained

Blanch the fresh or frozen fava beans.

In a large, heavy soup pot or Dutch oven, heat ⅓ cup of the olive oil over medium heat. Add the leeks, onion, carrots, and celery. Cook, stirring, until vegetables are just tender, about 8 minutes. Add the potatoes, favas, tomatoes, chile pepper, water, bay leaves, parsley, fennel, and salt to taste. Bring to a boil, add ½ cup of the olive oil, reduce the heat, cover and simmer until the vegetables are tender, about 45 minutes. (If using peeled dried favas, the cooking time will be closer to 1 hour; if using unpeeled, it will be closer to an 1½ hours.)

Remove the soup from the heat and discard the spice bag (if it was used).* Pour in the remaining olive oil and the lemon juice, adjust the seasoning with additional salt and black pepper, and serve.

*At this point you can puree about 2 cups of the hot soup and add it back into the pot, stirring to blend, for a creamier, denser texture.

NOTE FOR DRIED FAVAS: *There are two varieties, peeled and unpeeled. You can find both in Greek and Middle Eastern food shops. Peeled dried favas will cook up in less time and look better, and have an attractive cream color. Unpeeled dried favas have a dull green, leathery skin and need to be soaked overnight or for 8 hours in ample water before cooking.*

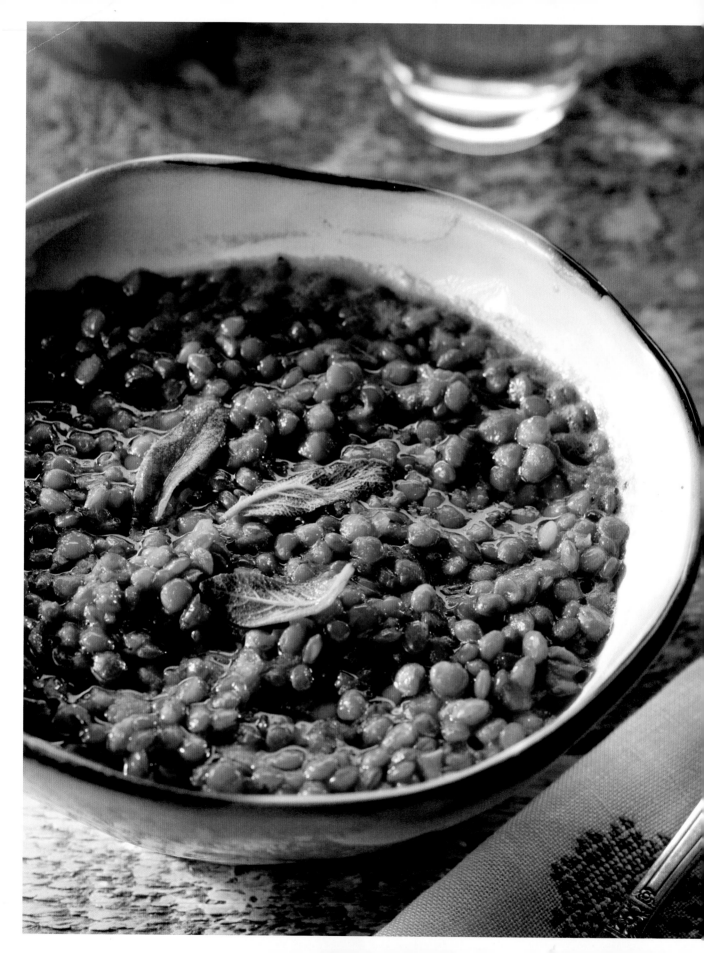

LENTIL SOUP WITH SAGE AND CHILE PEPPER

Fakes me Faskomilo kai Kafteri Piperia

As unexpected (and seemingly Southwest American) as the use of sage and chile peppers might seem in this Ikarian soup, cooks from a generation or two ago on the island used both to flavor lentils. "We put chile peppers in bean soups in general, because black pepper was too expensive," my neighbor Titika explained one day. The chile peppers generally grown in Ikarian gardens resemble the long, thin cayenne variety. Another addition to any kind of bean dish were the *tsifia* (page 16), or salted, dried summer vegetables, such as zucchini and eggplants. This lentil soup is thick and comforting.

MAKES 6 TO 8 SERVINGS

2 large red onions

Salt

2 medium garlic cloves, minced

1 pound small brown lentils

½ cup chopped or pureed tomatoes

4 fresh sage leaves

2 sprigs dried oregano

2 bay leaves

1 fresh or dried chile pepper,* such as bird's eye, Medusa, Fresno, de árbol, or cayenne

½ cup Greek extra virgin olive oil, plus more for serving

¼ cup red wine vinegar, plus more for serving

Coarsely chop 1 onion. Place in a large, heavy pot, sprinkle with a little salt, and cook, covered, over very low heat until tender, 6 to 8 minutes. Add the minced garlic and stir.

Rinse the lentils in a colander. Add the lentils, tomatoes, sage, oregano, bay leaves, and chile pepper to the pot, and toss all together for a few minutes over low heat. Pour in enough water to cover the contents of the pot by 3 inches (7.5 cm). Increase the heat to medium, bring to a boil, reduce the heat to low and simmer, partially covered, until very tender, about 1 hour.

Season to taste with salt. Pour in the olive oil and vinegar just before serving.

To serve: Discard the bay, oregano, and sage leaves. Slice the remaining onion. Sprinkle a few onion slices over the top of each soup portion. Drizzle in additional olive oil and vinegar if desired.

*Almost any chile will do. Sizes and heat levels vary, of course, so choose according to personal taste.

GOAT AND VEGETABLE SOUP

Aiga Vrasti me Lahanika

This comforting soup is something home cooks make fairly often. Goat meat is the most prevalent animal protein on Ikaria. You may substitute lamb for goat.

—————————— **MAKES 6 TO 8 SERVINGS** ——————————

2 pounds (1 kg) bone-in goat shoulder and leg, cut into serving pieces

Salt and freshly ground black pepper

4 large onions, peeled and left whole

3 large carrots, cut into 1/4-inch (1-cm) rounds

3 large potatoes, peeled and cubed

1 1/2 cups chopped Chinese celery

1/3 cup short-grain rice or bulgur

Juice of 2 lemons

1/2 cup Greek extra virgin olive oil

Whole-grain rusks or thickly sliced and toasted sourdough bread, for serving

Rinse the goat meat. Season well with salt and let stand for 30 minutes.

Place the goat in a large soup pot with enough water to cover by 3 inches (7.5 cm). Bring to a boil. Reduce the heat and simmer for 30 minutes, skimming any foam off the surface of the broth.

Add the onions, carrots, potatoes, and celery. Season with salt and pepper to taste. Simmer, partially covered, until the meat is falling off the bone, about 2 hours. About 20 minutes before the meat is done, add the rice and cook until tender.

Season with lemon juice, olive oil, and additional salt and pepper if necessary.

To serve the soup, place the rusks or toasted sourdough bread on the bottom of individual soup bowls and ladle the soup in, meat and all.

VARIATION

Chicken and Vegetable Soup: The same exact soup is also made with chicken on the island, specifically hens of a certain age! Look for large hens, preferably free-range. Trim excess fat, remove the neck and giblets, and add to the pot whole.

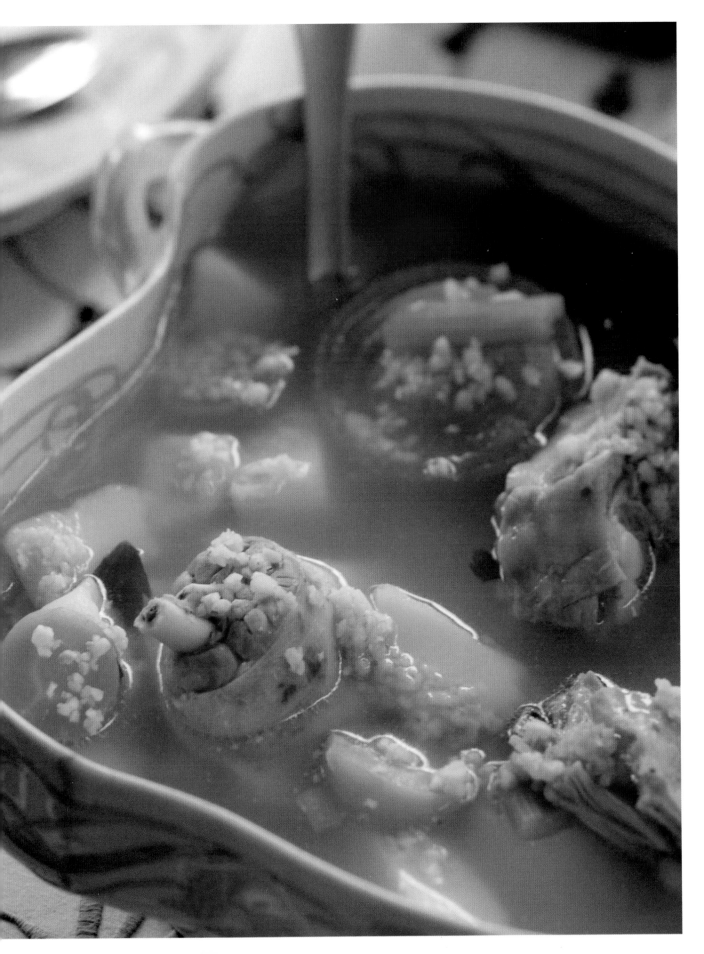

NAVY BEAN SOUP WITH SPECKS OF GOAT

Ikariotiki Fasolada me Katsikisio Pastourma

It's almost impossible to replicate this soup in its truly local rendition because it calls for Ikarian *pasturma*, which is salted, air-cured goat, an island specialty to this day, but made in ever more dwindling numbers. One could conceivably cure goat at home, if not the whole animal then certainly a leg; Italians sometimes do this, and call it *violino di capra*. There is also a goat meat prosciutto, called *moceto*, but it is about as hard to find commercially as the Ikarian version of *pasturma*. You can substitute a bit of cooked goat or lamb or Jamaican goat jerky, which tastes quite different. Leaving it out is also perfectly okay. This is delicious served with grilled sourdough bread or rusks, olives, or feta.

MAKES 6 TO 8 SERVINGS

- 2 cups dried navy beans, soaked for 8 hours or overnight
- 2 quarts water
- 1 cup Greek extra virgin olive oil
- 2 large onions, chopped (about 2 cups)
- 3 medium or large carrots, finely chopped
- 1½ cups chopped Chinese or regular celery, including the leaves
- 2 medium potatoes, peeled and finely chopped
- 1½ cups chopped canned plum tomatoes

- 1 large fresh or dried chile pepper, such as serrano or cayenne (optional)
- 3 bay leaves
- Salt and freshly ground black pepper
- ⅓ cup chopped fresh flat-leaf parsley
- 1 cup shredded goat pasturma, shredded cooked goat or lamb meat, or Jamaican goat jerky (optional)
- Juice of 1 lemon, strained

Place the beans in a large pot with the water and bring to a boil over medium heat. Simmer uncovered, until the beans are about halfway cooked, about 1 hour, skimming the foam off the top during the first 30 minutes or so.

Add ½ cup of the olive oil, the onions, carrots, celery, potatoes, tomatoes, chile pepper (if using), bay leaves, and salt and black pepper to taste. Cover and simmer for 25 minutes. Stir in the parsley and goat (if using) and continue simmering until the soup is thick and all the vegetables are tender, about 20 minutes longer.

Remove from the heat and stir in the lemon juice and remaining ½ cup olive oil.

Serve hot.

CURED GOAT FOR SUSTENANCE AND FLAVOR

Pasturma, or *bastirma* as it is also spelled, is a well-known spicy cured beef product traditionally made all over the Eastern Mediterranean. On Ikaria, *pasturma* is something else entirely: It is seasoned, air-dried goat meat.

I saw Ikarian goat *pasturma* prepared many years ago, when I visited the home of a local goat-herd and farmer named Yiannis Koutoufaris.

It was a late August day when I visited him. The clothesline in his yard was heavy with half carcasses of his own goats, which he had slaughtered several days earlier. They hung in rough-weave plastic construction sacks, which he had punctured from place to place to let air in. The day was windy, as so many are in August, when the *meltemia* whip up. On each breeze I could easily discern his spice paste of choice—a totally local blend of sea salt, dried oregano, and savory.

The yard was an obstacle course of hoses, crates, tools, baskets of blackberries, potatoes, and peppers. Long, twisted summer squashes rested here and there. But the drying goats were definitely the center of attention, a farm preparation that harks back to another era, really, before refrigeration.

Preserving the island's main source of animal protein was an end-of-summer job in most families, the cured goat (which is salty, tough, and chewy) providing necessary protein for winter. It was always consumed a little at a time, usually to enhance an otherwise all-plant-based meal of bean soups and other vegetable casseroles. It was also served with a few olives and bread as a meze.

Today, at least on the north side of the island, only one shepherd I know still makes it, Yiorgos Parikos, who runs the butcher shop in our village, Aghios Dimitrios.

The *pasturma* is always made with a large animal, either an old female goat or a ram. The legs are deboned and splayed while the spine is kept intact, which enables the animal to be suspended easily. It is heavily scented with salt, and the herb mixture mentioned above, then left for about 2 hours under the August sun (covered) so that the meat absorbs the salt thus kick-starting the drying process. *Pasturma* makers use reeds, an all-purpose material that grows rampant on some parts of the island, to keep the splayed meat butterflied, the better for drying. It takes 10 to 12 days to complete the drying process.

As for consuming this unusual charcuterie, it is either rehydrated and cooked as one would fresh goat, with potatoes, say, or with a tangy tomato sauce; or it is used in very small amounts to enhance bean and vegetable soups and casseroles.

Goat preserves don't end with this unusual *pasturma*, however. There is also the local *confit de chèvre,* aka *kaourma,* which is essentially goat simmered in salted water then put up in its own fat.

TRAHANA

Trahana is an ancient, granular wheat product made with milk or yogurt that is used as the main ingredient in porridgelike soups or as a way to thicken other soups. It is not unique to Ikaria. Indeed, home cooks all over the Eastern Mediterranean prepare trahana at the end of every summer, when it is hot and breezy enough for the pebbly grains to dry easily.

On Ikaria, we buy our *trahana* from Maria Kalimboukou, who is the caretaker of the Theoktisti Monastery in Pygi. She makes *trahana* as a way to support the monastery, which dates to the 14th century and is the oldest on the island.

There are many different versions of *trahana* all over Greece, some made with cracked wheat, others with flour; some with whole milk—almost always ewe's or goat's milk (called "sweet *trahana*")—others with yogurt or buttermilk (called sour *trahana*), or even vegetable pulp (a Lenten version); some are shaped into tiny granules, resembling bulgur, or in chunks about the size of a woman's pinky, or as shallow cups, the specialty on Lesvos, another eastern Aegean island.

On Ikaria, most people like and make the sweet version, with whole goat's milk and flour, although there are buttermilk- or yogurt-based sour *trahanas*, too.

Maria makes *trahana* during the whole month of August and we often bring friends and our cooking-school guests here to watch the process.

Her kitchen is primitive—two gas burners and a sink. To make *trahana*, she mixes flour, goat's milk, and a pinch of salt in an oversized pot and stirs this over low heat until the mixture forms a dense batter, a little like oatmeal. She lets it cool for several hours or overnight until it is solid enough to break into pieces, and then she sets it out on netting that she's draped over a small laundry stand. It takes a day or so for these chunks to dry out until they become hard enough to press through a metal sieve, the final process that renders them pebble-shaped.

Ikarian cooks use *trahana* in fish soup (page 77), in an old dish with pork, and as a simple porridge, boiled with plain water or tomatoes (see page 99), sometimes served with a little feta or *kathoura*, the local goat's milk cheese.

Maria Byron Panayidou, the nutritionist whom I consulted for the book, taught me that the nutrient content of *trahana* depends upon the yogurt or milk and flour ratios as well as other ingredients in the recipe. It is a useful high-protein dietary supplement with an average 15% to 16% protein content. Flour, which is high in complex carbodydrates, is known to be a poor source of essential amino acids, particularly lysine and threonine. However, the combination of flour and yogurt or milk proteins makes *trahana* a complete amino acid source, she explained.

Trahana is also a good source of calcium (although content is affected by the flour and yogurt ratio in each recipe, as well as by the type of yogurt used), iron, and zinc as well as other minerals. It is also a good source of B vitamins.

You can find *trahana* in Greek and Middle Eastern food shops. See page 299 for sources.

INSTANT ANCIENT TRAHANA SOUP

Trahanosoupa Paradosiaki

Here is the simplest and, to my palate, most delicious way to cook *trahana*. As I have mentioned earlier, sweet *trahana* on Ikaria refers to *trahana* that is made with whole goat's milk, which is strong and tart. Elsewhere, sweet *trahana* is made with cow's milk and has a much more subtle, almost bland flavor. Sour *trahana*, made with buttermilk or yogurt, is decidedly more acidic and very delicious, at least to my palate.

MAKES 6 SERVINGS

½ cup Greek extra virgin olive oil

1½ cups sweet or sour trahana, store-bought or homemade (page 98)

8 cups water or vegetable stock

Salt and freshly ground black pepper

Juice of 1 lemon, strained

6 tablespoons Greek yogurt or crumbled feta cheese

In a medium soup pot, heat 2 tablespoons of the oil over medium heat. Add the *trahana* and stir to coat in the oil for about a minute. Pour in the water (or stock). Reduce the heat to low, season to taste with salt and pepper, and simmer until the soup is dense, thick, and porridgelike, 8 to 12 minutes, depending on the variety of *trahana* you find.

Remove from the heat and stir in the lemon juice. Serve in individual bowls, topped with yogurt or crumbled feta and drizzled with the remaining 6 tablespoons olive oil.

HOMEMADE TRAHANA IN AN AMERICAN KITCHEN

Spitikos Trahanas

The traditional way to make *trahana* is to combine and cook bulgur with buttermilk, goat's milk, and/or yogurt, to take this dense mass, break it up into chunks, dry them in the sun, and then press them through a fine-mesh sieve until they become pebbly granules, larger than couscous and about the size of bulgur.

Making *trahana* the traditional way is all but impossible unless you happen to live in a hot, dry place, since the *trahana* has to be dried outdoors over several days. Instead, thanks mainly to my colleague Carlos Carreto (not Ikarian, not even Greek, but the executive chef at Molyvos Restaurant in New York City, which prepares trahana in-house), I co-opted this recipe.

MAKES 3½ POUNDS (1.6 KG)

12 cups coarse bulgur

4 cups plain Greek whole-milk yogurt

1 quart whole cow's milk

1 quart whole goat's milk

¼ cup fresh lemon juice

Salt and freshly ground black pepper, to taste

Place all the ingredients in a large, wide pot and cook over medium heat, stirring, until the mixture becomes a dense, solid mass, about 30 minutes.

Preheat the oven to 250°F (160°C). Line 4 baking sheet with parchment paper.

Spread the trahana mass evenly over the baking sheets to a thickness of about ¼ inch (6 mm). Bake it uncovered until it is cracker hard and brittle, 3 to 4 hours.

Let cool slightly, then break up into 1- to 2-inch (2.5 to 4-cm) chunks. Cool completely and store in jars or muslin bags in a cool, dry place.

WINTER PORK AND TRAHANA SOUP

Trahanosoupa me Hoirino

The original recipe for this soup calls for boiling big chunks of bone-in pork for several hours to get a flavorful broth, then adding *trahana* and onions. I have simplified it a little, by using bone-in pork chops.

MAKES 6 SERVINGS

2 quarts water

1 to 1½ pounds bone-in pork chops, trimmed of fat

2 large onions

1 carrot, whole

3 bay leaves

6 to 8 allspice berries

½ teaspoon black peppercorns

Salt and freshly ground black pepper

⅔ cup Greek extra virgin olive oil

1½ cups sour *trahana*, store-bought or homemade (page 98)

Juice of 1 to 2 lemons (to taste)

In a large pot, combine the water, pork chops, 1 whole onion, the carrot, 2 of the bay leaves, the allspice berries, and peppercorns and bring to a boil. Season with salt. Simmer until the meat is falling off the bone, about 1 hour.

Remove the chops and set aside to cool. Strain the broth and set aside. Discard the solids.

Finely chop the remaining onion. Wipe the pot clean and heat ½ cup of the olive oil over medium heat. Add the onion and cook until wilted and lightly colored. Add the *trahana* and toss to coat in the oil. Pour in the strained broth, remaining 1 bay leaf, and a little salt and pepper to taste. Bring to a simmer.

Meanwhile, shred the pork chop meat. Add this to the soup. Simmer the soup until the *trahana* has disintegrated and the soup is thick and hearty, like porridge.

Stir in the remaining olive oil and season to taste with salt, pepper, and lemon juice. Serve.

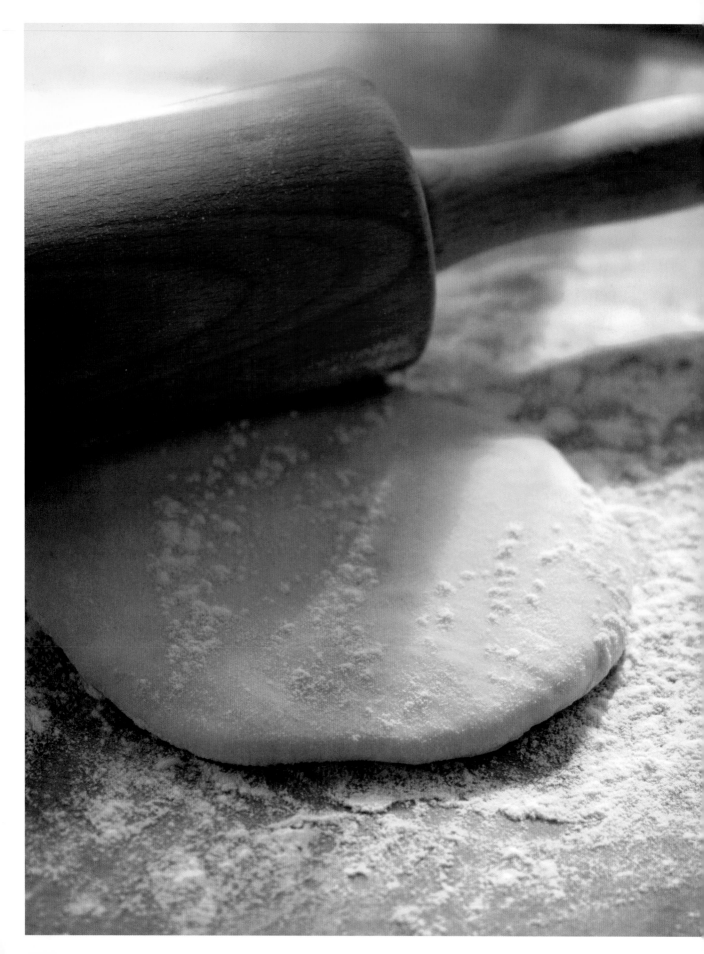

SAVORY
PIES AND BREADS

DOUGH IS COMFORT. EVERY DAY AROUND 11 A.M., I walk up the overgrown stone footpath that meanders past my home and make my way to Socrates' bakery. Like the village *cafeneio*, it's the gathering place, where picking up the daily loaf is also an excuse for picking up the daily news and gossip. I usually buy a *carvelli,* a one- or two-pound round loaf, since we're a family of bread eaters and in the summer the house is always filled with kids at that age when they're always hungry.

Socrates makes a few other things besides bread, so inevitably I also come back with rings of crisp *tyrokoulouro*—a twisted, round, sesame-covered cheese bread—or with flaky phyllo pies stuffed with greens and cheese under my arm.

Bread and savory phyllo pies are the soul of the Ikarian table. The island's traditional pies aren't as varied as the gamut of savory pies from central and northern Greece.

Ikarian phyllo pies tend to be individual pieces (called *pitarakia*) that look a little like empanadas. They are traditionally fried (wood was too precious to waste on lighting the outdoor oven, which many homes had, more than a few times a month). Preparing them turns into something like a small party and a reason for an invitation, to the tune of "My mom is making *pitarakia*. Come on over."

Wild greens, wild fennel, pumpkin, and zucchini are the vegetables Ikarian cooks like most to pack within envelopes of phyllo. There are other pies, too, of course, and I've offered a smattering of them in this chapter.

Note: Anyone can make phyllo the traditional Greek home cook's way. However, you can substitute the commercial variety for the homemade kind if you wish to. In a whole-pan pie, use 6 layers of phyllo on the bottom and 4 on top, brushing each layer with olive oil. For individual pies, cut the phyllo stack in half lengthwise and use 2 sheets at a time per individual pie. Brush each sheet with olive oil.

BASIC HOMEMADE PHYLLO DOUGH

Spitiko Filo

There are about as many recipes for homemade phyllo as there are regional cooks in Greece. The recipe below for homemade phyllo is my basic, all-purpose recipe. It makes for a malleable dough that is easy to work with and easy to roll. It may be used to prepare any of the pies in this book, and will be enough for either a 15-inch or 18-inch savory pie, which you can easily bake in a large paella pan. You can halve the recipe (and, by extension, individual pie and filling proportions) to make smaller pies in 8-inch or 10-inch round baking pans.

MAKES ENOUGH FOR A 15- TO 18-INCH PIE

3½ to 4½ cups bread flour or finely ground semolina flour from durum wheat*

1 scant teaspoon salt

1¼ cups water

½ cup Greek extra virgin olive oil

1 tablespoon red wine vinegar, balsamic vinegar, ouzo, *tsipouro*, or lemon juice

In a stand mixer fitted with a dough hook, beat together 3¼ cups of the flour and the salt for about 5 seconds. Add the water, olive oil, and vinegar (or other liquid). Mix on low speed for 3 minutes to combine, then increase speed to medium. Knead with the hook, stopping the mixer to add additional flour as needed, in ½-cup increments, until the dough is very smooth and pliant and balls up easily. The whole mixing process should take 10 to 12 minutes.

Transfer the dough to an oiled bowl. Cover tightly with plastic wrap and let stand for 1 hour at room temperature before using. You can prepare the dough and store it, either in the refrigerator, very well wrapped, for several days, or in the freezer, for up to 2 weeks. Always bring it back to room temperature before using. If it's frozen, thaw first overnight in the refrigerator.

Follow the directions in the individual pie recipes for rolling out the dough.

*Available online and in Greek food shops around the country

VARIATION

Whole Wheat Homemade Phyllo Dough. Replace 1½ cups of the bread flour with finely ground whole wheat flour.

GREEK PIE NUTRITION

The greens and vegetable pies on Ikaria are a great source of nutrition. Many of these Greek pies are actually vegan, but lacking in nothing in so far as flavor, texture, mouthfeel, and satisfaction go.

Healthy Pumpkins

One of the most beloved vegetables used in local phyllo pies is pumpkin, which is a nutrient-dense, very low-calorie vegetable—3½ ounces (100 g) of pumpkin has 26 calories and no saturated fats or cholesterol. Pumpkin is rich in dietary fiber, antioxidants, minerals, and vitamins. It is one of the food items recommended in cholesterol-controlling and weight-reduction programs.

Pumpkin brims with many antioxidants, such as beta-carotene and vitamins C and E. It is an excellent source of polyphenols, which protect against age-related macular degeneration. Copper, calcium, potassium, and phosphorous are among the many minerals found in pumpkin. And save the seeds! They're a terrific source of dietary fiber, heart-healthy monounsaturated fatty acids, protein, minerals, and vitamins.

Miracle Onions and Leeks

Cut or chop an onion or leek and you release their cancer- and diabetes-fighting compounds. A major phytochemical compound in onions, leeks, and their relatives is allicin, which helps fight cholesterol and has known antibacterial, antiviral, and antifungal properties. Onions are also a great source of chromium, which helps our tissue cells respond appropriately to insulin levels. Vitamin D and manganese, both antioxidants, are found in abundance in the humble onion.

Goodness in Swiss Chard and Spinach

Chard and spinach are excellent sources of vitamin C, which we need to absorb iron, explains Maria Byron Panayidou, the nutritionist who helped me on this book. A hundred grams, about 3 ounces, of chard provide 700% of the daily requirement for vitamin K, which helps strengthen bones and possibly fight Alzheimer's because vitamin K can help limit neuronal damage in the brain. (Ikarians do eat a lot of leafy greens like chard and spinach, and the level of dementia in the nonagenarian set on the island is impressively low.)

The list of good things in Swiss chard goes on: It is rich in B vitamins, which are essential for good metabolism. Finally, Swiss chard is a rich source of minerals like copper, calcium, sodium, potassium, iron, manganese, and phosphorus. Potassium is an important component of cell and body fluids that helps control heart rate and blood pressure, by countering the effects of sodium. Iron is required for cellular oxidation and red blood cell formation.

Regular inclusion of chard in the diet has been found to prevent osteoporosis, iron-deficiency anemia, and vitamin A deficiency; and it is also believed to protect from cardiovascular diseases and colon and prostate cancers.

LONGEVITY GREENS AND PUMPKIN PIE

Hortopita tis Makrozoias

There is no one recipe for this pie. Instead, there are seasonal variations depending on what one picks in the wild or, for a less peripatetic US cook, on what one can find either at the greengrocer, in Asian markets, or via professional foragers and/or specialty produce Web sites (page 299).

The greens in this recipe represent what is available from the fall to early spring on the island. There is only one rule when it comes to selecting which edible wild or cultivated greens to use in pies: They have to be sweet.

The amount of olive oil I use in my greens pie, having learned the recipe by watching many Ikarian women make it, is undoubtedly more than most American or non-Greek cooks are used to. But the copious amount of olive oil is really what makes this dish. Inside the filling, the olive oil lends both flavor and just the right silky texture that makes so many Greek vegetable dishes delicious and easily palatable. I douse the phyllo with olive oil, approximately 2 tablespoons (when I make this I really just eyeball it, as we say in restaurant-kitchen lingo) per layer. The result is that the pie is almost oven-fried. The layers of phyllo are crisp but the filling is soft and comforting.

You could very well use commercial phyllo for this, and I explain how to substitute at the beginning of the chapter, but it really does pale in comparison to a greens or other savory pie made with homemade pastry. You'll be surprised at how easy the pastry recipe actually is to work with.

MAKES 6 TO 8 SERVINGS

2 pounds pumpkin or butternut squash, peeled, seeded, and coarsely grated

Coarse sea salt

1¼ cups Greek extra virgin olive oil

1 leek, tough greens trimmed and discarded, whites and pale green parts rinsed well and chopped

2 large red onions, finely chopped (about 2 cups)

1 pound (500 g) spinach, coarsely chopped, washed, and well drained

1 pound (500 g) Swiss chard, preferably green-stemmed, coarsely chopped, washed, and well drained

1 bunch sweet sorrel, washed and coarsely chopped

1 small bunch chervil or bur chervil, chopped (about 1½ cups)

1½ cups snipped fresh dill

3 small bunches wild fennel, leaves only, chopped (about 2½ cups)*

1 small bunch flat-leaf parsley, chopped

1 small bunch fresh oregano, chopped

1 small bunch mint, leaves only, chopped

Freshly ground black pepper

Basic Homemade Phyllo Dough (page 103), at room temperature

Flour or cornstarch, for rolling out the phyllo dough

---

* If you cannot source wild fennel, one of the most characteristic herbs on Ikaria and throughout the Greek islands, chop 2 fennel bulbs and their leaves and add them to the pie when you sauté the onions and leek.

(continued on page 107)

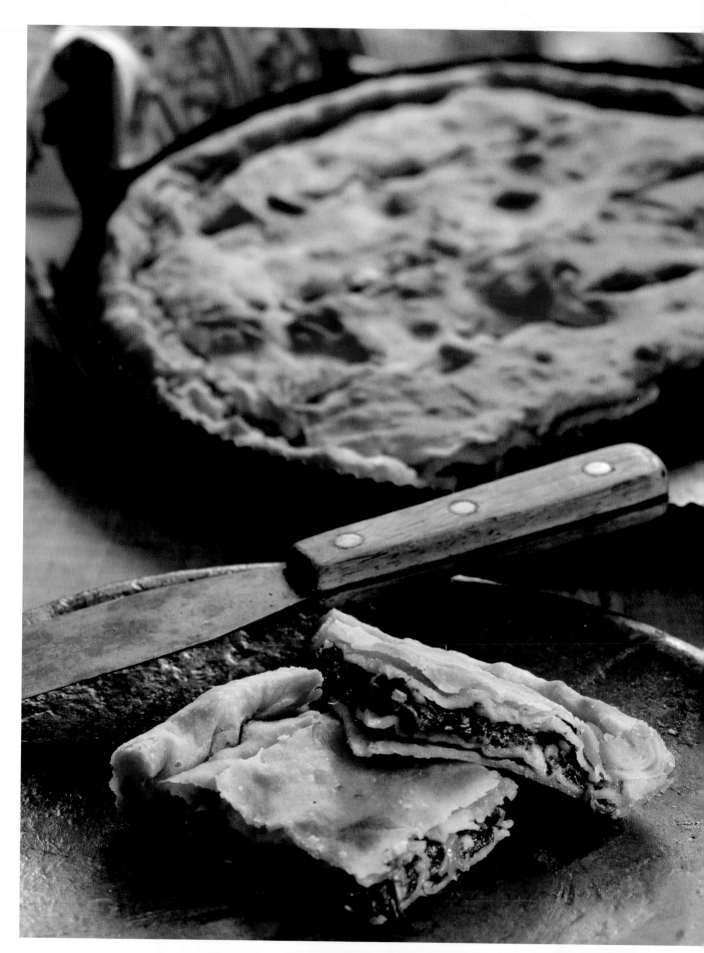

Place the coarsely grated pumpkin (or squash) in a colander. Salt lightly and toss. Place a plate on the pumpkin and weights, such as cans, on the plate, and leave to drain for about 1 to 3 hours.

Position a rack in the center of the oven and preheat to 350°F (160°C). Lightly oil a 15-inch (39.5 cm) round baking or paella pan or a shallow, rectangular roasting pan or rimmed baking sheet (16 x 12 inches [40 x 30 cm]).

Squeeze the pumpkin with your hands to get rid of as much liquid as possible.

In a large skillet or wide pot, heat 2 tablespoons of the olive oil over medium heat. Add the pumpkin and cook until it wilts and most or all of its liquid has evaporated, anywhere between 10 and 30 minutes, depending on the water content of the pumpkin. Transfer to a large bowl.

Wipe the same pan clean (or use a separate pan) and heat 2 tablespoons of the olive oil over medium heat. Add the leek and onions and cook until wilted. Transfer to the bowl with the pumpkin.

In the same pan, heat another tablespoon or two of olive oil and wilt the spinach and chard. Add to the bowl.

Add the sorrel and all the other chopped fresh herbs to the bowl. Season to taste with a generous amount of salt and a little pepper.

Set aside ½ cup of the olive oil for brushing the layers of phyllo and pour the remaining oil into the filling. Stir to blend.

Divide the phyllo dough into 4 equal-size balls. On a lightly floured surface, roll out the first dough ball, using the shape of your pan as the guide. For round pans, roll out to a round about 18 inches in diameter; for rectangular pans, roll out to a rectangle about 3 inches larger than the perimeter of the pan. Place the dough inside, leaving about 2 inches (5 cm) hanging over the edge. Brush with 2 tablespoons of olive oil. Repeat with the second piece of dough. Brush that, too, with olive oil.

Spread the filling evenly inside the pan, over the second layer of phyllo.

Repeat the rolling process for the third sheet, placing it over the filling, and pressing down gently. Brush generously with olive oil.

Finally, roll out the last piece of dough to a slightly smaller piece and place it over the surface of the pie. Join and fold in the bottom and top overhanging dough, rolling it decoratively around the perimeter of the pan to form a pretty rim. Brush the top of the pie generously with olive oil. Score the top of the pie into serving pieces, taking care to not draw the knife all the way through to the bottom of the pan.

Bake until the pastry is golden and crisp and the pie pulls away from the edges of the pan, 40 to 50 minutes. Remove, cool in the pan, and serve.

(continued)

Variations on a greens pie depend on the seasonal availability of greens and the personal taste of the cook. Pumpkin and greens such as the ones in this recipe, with the exception of wild fennel, which is wild only in the spring but cultivated in the fall, too, not on Ikaria per se but in Greece at large, are typical of cold-weather pies. Other greens you could include (and it's a more-the-merrier, or, rather, "more-the-healthier" approach that every home cook on Ikaria takes) are:

- Sweet dandelion
- All sorts of sorrels and docks (they're related)
- Mediterranean hartwort
- Fresh marjoram
- Grated carrot
- Mallow leaves

- Stinging nettles (they need to be cut and handled with gloves and blanched before use in the filling)
- A little bit of lavender
- A few fresh sage leaves, finely chopped
- Scallions and all manner of onions may be used, too

In the spring, other great greens grow wild on Ikaria, including poppy leaves, wild fennel, wild carrot, and lemon balm, all highly prized and aromatic additions to *hortopita*.

In summer, when the land dries up, Ikarians make greens pies with amaranth, parsley, dill, mint, and grated zucchini (see Summer Greens Pie with Zucchini and Herbs, opposite page).

SUMMER GREENS PIE
WITH ZUCCHINI AND HERBS

Hortopita Kalokairini

Zucchini, which grows in copious amounts in so many Ikarian gardens, is put to good use in many dishes, but by far this savory pie, an icon of summer on the island, is one of my personal favorites. A similar pie, but with pumpkin instead of zucchini, is made in the fall. This pie is delicious: It's herbaceous, sweet from the onions, and earthy from the flavor of the greens.

───── **MAKES 8 TO 10 SERVINGS** ─────

- 3 pounds (1.5 kg) zucchini, preferably large, coarsely grated
- Salt and freshly ground black pepper
- ½ cup plus 5 tablespoons Greek extra virgin olive oil, plus more for oiling the pan
- 3 large red onions, finely chopped
- ½ pound (250 g) amaranth leaves (if available) or Swiss chard, chopped
- 5 to 10 squash blossoms (if available), cleaned of pistils and finely chopped

- 2 cups finely chopped wild fennel*
- 1 cup chopped fresh mint leaves
- 1 cup chopped fresh flat-leaf parsley
- Leaves from 1 bunch fresh oregano, finely chopped
- 1½ cups crumbled Greek feta cheese
- Basic Homemade Phyllo Dough (page 103), at room temperature
- Flour or cornstarch, for rolling out the phyllo dough

Place the zucchini in a colander and toss with salt. Place a plate over the zucchini and a weight, such as cans, over the plate. Let the zucchini drain for 1 to 3 hours, or overnight. Squeeze bunches at a time in your hands to get as much liquid as possible out. It is important for the zucchini to be as dry as possible. Place in a large bowl.

Position a rack in the center of the oven and preheat to 375°F (180°C). Lightly oil a 15-inch (39.5 cm) round baking or paella pan or a shallow, rectangular roasting pan or rimmed baking sheet (16 x 12-inch [40 x 30 cm]).

In a large skillet, heat 2 tablespoons of the olive oil over medium heat. Add the onions and cook until soft, about 10 minutes. Add the zucchini and cook over low heat until it releases any remaining liquid. Add the amaranth (or Swiss chard) and cook down so that the greens also release their liquid and it evaporates. If there is still residual liquid in the pot, drain the vegetables in a colander for a few minutes.

*If you can't get wild fennel, substitute 1 large fennel bulb, finely chopped, and 1 cup snipped dill. Add the fennel bulb when you cook the onions. Add the dill when you add the mint and parsley.

(continued)

Transfer the onion-zucchini-greens mixture to a large bowl and combine with the squash blossoms (if using), herbs, and feta. Season to taste with salt and pepper and mix in 3 tablespoons of olive oil.

Divide the phyllo dough into 4 equal-size balls. On a lightly floured surface, roll out the first dough ball, using the shape of your pan as the guide. For round pans, roll out to a round about 18 inches in diameter; for rectangular pans, roll out to a rectangle about 3 inches larger than the perimeter of the pan. Place the dough inside, leaving about 2 inches (5 cm) hanging over the edge. Brush with 2 tablespoons of olive oil. Repeat with the second piece of dough. Brush that, too, with olive oil.

Spread the filling evenly inside the pan, over the second layer of phyllo.

Repeat the rolling process for the third sheet, placing it over the filling, and pressing down gently. Brush generously with olive oil.

Finally, roll out the last piece of dough to a slightly smaller piece and place it over the surface of the pie. Join and fold in the bottom and top overhanging dough, rolling it decoratively around the perimeter of the pan to form a pretty rim. Brush the top of the pie generously with olive oil. Score the top of the pie into serving pieces, taking care to not draw the knife all the way through to the bottom of the pan.

Bake until the pastry is golden and crisp and the pie pulls away from the edges of the pan, 40 to 50 minutes. Remove, cool in the pan, and serve.

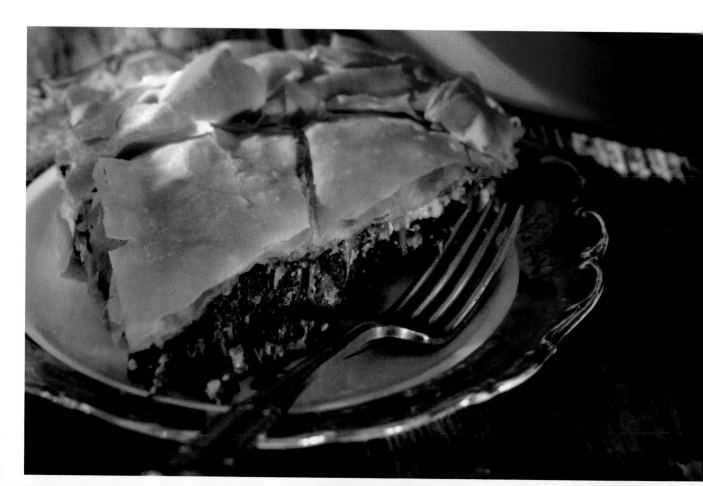

FENNEL: THE QUINTESSENTIAL FLAVOR OF IKARIA

Wild fennel is the herb that best defines local cooking and the aroma of Ikaria itself. It blankets the island from April through June and its licorice-like aroma is everywhere discernible. Ikarian cooks use fennel in pies, meat and fish dishes, as the base for fritters, as a seasoning in pasta and rice dishes, and more. I couldn't imagine Ikaria's table without the scent of fennel.

Fennel, like all herbs, has a host of therapeutic qualities. In folk medicine, fennel has been known to help treat amenorrhea, angina, asthma, anxiety, depression, heartburn, and water retention. It is said to help lower blood pressure and boost sexual desire.

Fennel is an excellent source of vitamin C, dietary fiber, potassium, molybdenum, manganese, copper, phosphorus, and folate. In addition, fennel is a good source of calcium, pantothenic acid, magnesium, iron, and niacin. Maria Byron Panayidou, the nutritionist who worked with me on the science data, notes that fennel is often used for colic; wind; irritable bowel; for healthy kidneys, spleen, liver, and lungs; suppressing appetite; breast enlargement; improving the digestive system; and increasing milk flow and urine flow.

Fennel's esteemed reputation dates back to the earliest times and is reflected in its mythological traditions. In the Greek myths, fennel was closely associated with Dionysus, the Greek god of food, wine, and revelry. It grew in the field in which one of the great ancient battles was fought and that was subsequently named the Battle of Marathon, after this revered plant, *marathos* in Greek. Fennel was also awarded to Pheidippides, the runner who delivered the news of the Persian invasion to Sparta.

Wild fennel has an abundance of feathery leaves that look a little like dill fronds but softer. The bulb of cultivated fennel, from which sprout far fewer leaves, is crunchy and slightly sweet. In either form, fennel adds a refreshing note to almost any food it touches. Although it is related to parsley, carrots, and dill, it tastes more like anise or licorice.

All the Ikarian home cooks I know pick mountains of wild fennel in April, May, and June, when it is in season, and blanch then freeze it so they can have it in their pies all year long.

In the United States, fennel grows wild in northern California. If you can't find the wild variety, in most recipes you can substitute fennel bulb and fronds (look for bulbs that have a lot of them), or even add a piece of star anise to a simmering pot to approximate the intoxicating aroma of this characteristic Ikarian herb.

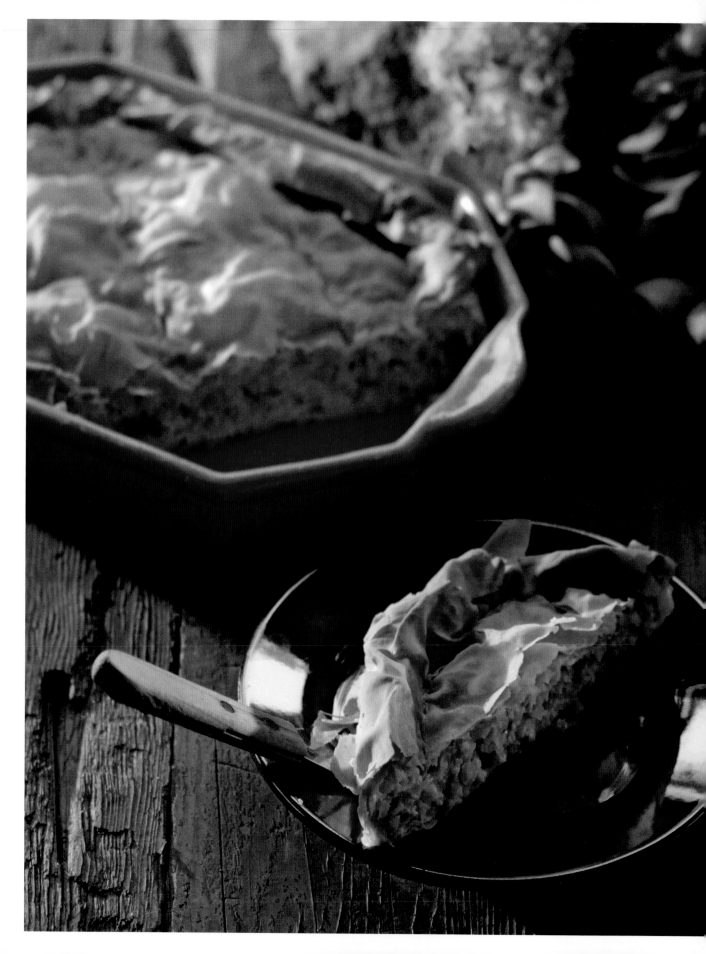

SIMPLE ONION PIE

Kremmydopita

I can't count the times I've enjoyed a bite of the simplest onion pie in the garden of my friend Eleni Karimali. This isn't exactly her recipe, but it's based on what she's told me she does, which is pretty much almost nothing save for sautéing a whole lot of coarsely chopped onions until they are sweet, and then spreading them between layers of phyllo. If you have a wood-burning oven, use it to bake this!

MAKES 8 TO 10 SERVINGS

12 tablespoons Greek extra virgin olive oil

8 large red onions, coarsely chopped (about 8 cups)

1 cup crumbled goat cheese or goat's milk feta cheese (optional)

Pinch of freshly grated nutmeg

Sea salt and freshly ground black pepper

Basic Homemade Phyllo Dough (page 103), at room temperature

Flour or cornstarch, for rolling out the phyllo dough

In a wide pot, heat 4 tablespoons of the olive oil over medium heat. Add the onions and cook, stirring occasionally, until they wilt and start to turn golden, about 30 minutes. Remove and set aside to cool slightly. Transfer to a bowl. Mix in the cheese (if using), nutmeg, and salt and pepper.

Position a rack in the center of the oven and preheat to 375°F (190°C). Lightly oil a 15-inch (39.5 cm) round pan or a rectangular roasting pan or rimmed baking sheet (16 x 12 inches [40 x 30 cm]).

Divide the phyllo dough into 4 equal-size balls. On a lightly floured surface, roll out the first dough ball, using the shape of your pan as the guide. For round pans, roll out to a circle about 18 inches in diameter; for rectangular pans roll out to a rectangle about 3 inches larger than the perimeter of the pan. Place the dough inside, leaving about 2 inches (5 cm) hanging over the edge. Brush with 2 tablespoons of olive oil. Repeat with the second piece of dough. Brush that, too, with olive oil.

Spread the filling evenly in the pan, over the second layer of phyllo. Repeat the rolling process for the third sheet, placing it over the filling, and pressing down gently. Brush generously with olive oil.

Finally, roll out the last piece of dough to a slightly smaller piece and place it over the surface of the pie. Join and fold in the bottom and top overhanging dough, rolling it decoratively around the perimeter of the pan to form a pretty rim. Brush the top of the pie generously with olive oil and score into serving pieces, taking care to not draw the knife all the way through to the bottom of the pan.

Bake until the pastry is golden and crisp and the pie pulls away from the edges of the pan, 40 to 50 minutes. Remove, cool in the pan, and serve.

SMALL SUMMER PIES WITH AMARANTH AND SCALLIONS

Hortopitakia me Vlita

Summer is the poorest time for greens all over Greece; there is virtually no rain, hence few wild greens besides the common amaranth (*vlita* in Greek), *styfnos*, or nightshade, which Greeks pick before the plant flowers and boil for salad, and purslane, one of the world's healthiest foods. Only amaranth is used in pies. It has a very subtle, almost smoky flavor when cooked and its leaves have a delicious, slightly rough texture. This pie is mild in flavor thanks to the amaranth, but it gets a flavor kick from copious amounts of robust herbs.

MAKES 40 PIECES

2¼ pounds (1 kg) amaranth greens, spinach, or chard, stemmed

⅔ cup Greek extra virgin olive oil, plus ample olive oil for frying

15 scallions or 3 large onions, finely chopped (about 3 cups)

2 garlic cloves, crushed in a garlic press

1½ cups finely chopped fresh flat-leaf parsley

2 cups chopped fresh mint leaves

1 cup chopped fresh oregano leaves

Salt and freshly ground black pepper

Basic Homemade Phyllo Dough (page 103), at room temperature

Flour or cornstarch, for rolling out the phyllo dough

Finely chop the amaranth greens (or spinach or chard), then wash and drain thoroughly.

In a large skillet, heat the olive oil over medium heat. Add the scallions (or onions) and cook until wilted. Add the garlic and greens and cook, stirring frequently until wilted and all the liquid has evaporated. Remove and cool for 10 minutes.

Combine the amaranth mixture with the parsley, mint, and oregano. Season generously with salt and pepper. Set aside.

Roll out, shape, and bake or fry the pies as directed in "Rolling Out Ikaria's Little Phyllo Pastries" on the next page.

ROLLING OUT IKARIA'S LITTLE PHYLLO PASTRIES

The shape of Ikaria's handheld small pies is typically a cylinder or flattened tube with crimped edges. The pies call for homemade phyllo pastry, which is quite different, sturdier, hardier, more pliant but not as flaky as commercial phyllo.

Once you prepare the dough and let it rest, you can roll out the phyllo in one of two ways: the traditional way with a rolling pin or dowel, or the more convenient way, using a pasta maker, which many home cooks on the island own and use.

If using a pasta maker, sprinkle cornstarch on a work surface and between the cylinders on the pasta maker. Divide the dough into 6 balls and keep covered with a kitchen towel. Working with one ball of dough at a time, roll out the dough, following the directions on the pasta maker, until you get a strip about 3 inches (7.5 cm) wide and 18 inches (40 cm) long and about as thin as a dime. Cut into 3-inch (7.5 cm) squares.

If rolling by hand, using a dowel or rolling pin, divide the dough into 6 balls and keep covered with a kitchen towel. On a work surface dusted either with flour or cornstarch, working with one ball at a time, roll out the dough to approximately a 12-inch (30 cm) square. Cut three 4-inch (10-cm) square pieces out of each sheet.

Place a heaping tablespoon of the filling in the center of each small square and roll up like a cylinder, flattening as you go. Press the edges together with the tines of a fork dampened in a little water.

Set the pies aside on a piece of parchment or wax paper. Continue with the remaining phyllo and filling. You can either bake or fry them right away, or freeze the pies and bake or fry them later, directly from the freezer.

To bake: Preheat the oven to 350°F (180°C). (Alternatively, if you have access to a wood-burning oven or an outdoor grill with a lid, you can preheat it. You may also place a pizza stone inside a conventional kitchen oven.)

Oil several baking sheets or line them with parchment paper or silicone baking mats. Place the pastries on the prepared pans, spacing them about 1½ inches (4 cm) apart. Brush the pastries with olive oil and bake, for 12 to 15 minutes in total, turning once, or until golden and crisp.

To fry: In a large nonstick skillet, heat about 1½ inches (2.5 cm) of olive oil. Fry the pastries, 4 or 5 at a time, without crowding the pan, until golden. Remove with a slotted spoon and drain on paper towels.

SMALL HERB AND GREENS PIES

Pitarakia and Marathopitarakia

Most home cooks on Ikaria uphold the island tradition of making small, handheld pies with all the same ingredients as mentioned in the recipes for *hortopita* (pages 105 and 109). Indeed, it is the handheld version—either fried in plenty of olive oil (best when the skillet is over a wood-burning flame as in a hearth) or baked—that is the real tradition on the island. There is a reason for that: In most of the Aegean Islands, wood, the main fuel from time immemorial until the 1960s, was in short supply. Even on Ikaria, which is blessed with pine forests, people did not—and still don't—cut down trees cavalierly. So, the fireplace or potbelly stove, both with the dual role of heating the home and providing a place to cook, was where most food was prepared. This stovetop tradition is still very much alive, even if the stovetop is now a gas or electric burner.

This recipe is for the most favored and characteristic filling, with wild fennel and onions, called *pitarakia me maratho* (small pies with fennel). But you can substitute the filling for any of the pies on pages 105, 109, and 113.

MAKES 30 TO 40 SMALL PIES

½ cup Greek extra virgin olive oil

3 large red onions, finely chopped

3 large bunches wild fennel, stems trimmed and discarded, feathery leaves chopped, or 2 large fennel bulbs, finely chopped, and 1 cup of fennel fronds, chopped

Sea salt and freshly ground black pepper

Basic Homemade Phyllo Dough (page 103), at room temperature

Flour or cornstarch, for rolling out the phyllo dough

In a deep skillet or wide, shallow pan, heat ¼ cup of the olive oil over medium heat. Add the onions and chopped fennel bulb, if using, and cook until wilted, about 8 minutes. Add the fennel leaves. (Alternatively, you can blanch them for a few seconds in salted boiling water. Remove and drain thoroughly. Then, add them to the sautéed onions.) Season with salt and pepper to taste. Mix in the remaining ¼ cup olive oil.

Roll out, shape, and bake or fry the pies as directed in "Rolling Out Ikaria's Little Phyllo Pastries" (page 115).

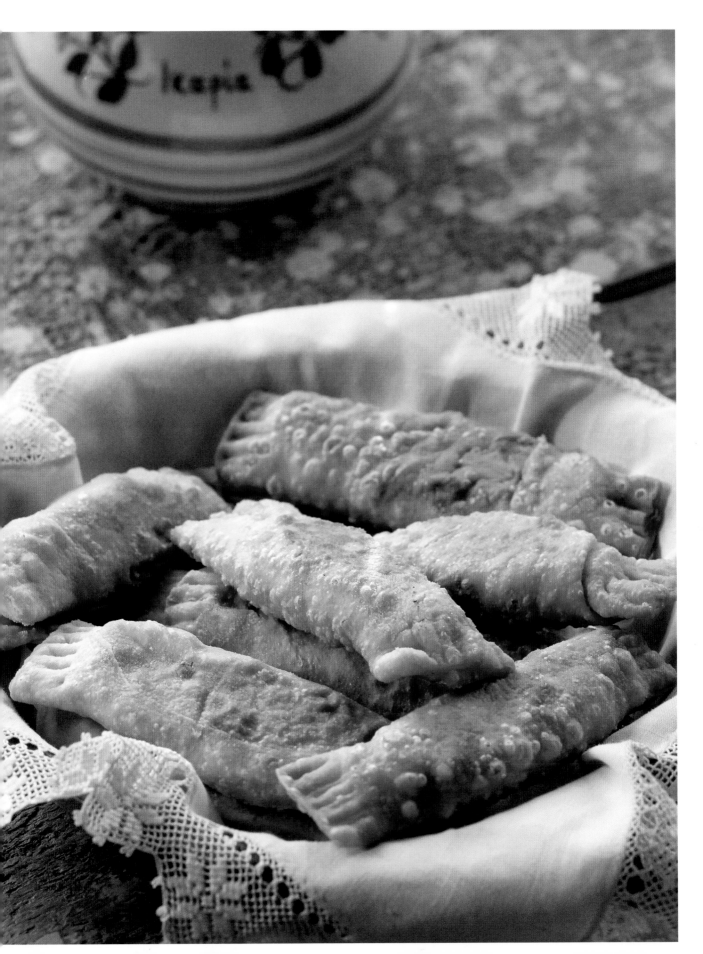

FINGER-SIZE CHEESE PIES

Kariotika Tyroboureka

The cheese pies on Ikaria are nothing like the rich whole-pan pies made in northern Greece, pies that sometimes have 12 to 15 layers of homemade phyllo. Ikarian cheese pies tend to be smaller, and meant for one. Local cooks prefer their own *kopanisti*, a spicy soft goat's milk cheese, to feta in this dish. You can use one of the *kopanisti* recipes in this book, goat's milk feta (such as *kalathaki Limnou* from the island of Limnos), or a combination of goat's milk feta and chèvre.

MAKES 36 TO 40 PIECES

3 cups Mary Safos's Ikarian-Style New York Kopanisti (page 6) or Whipped Feta Kopanisti (page 7), or traditional Ikarian *kopanisti* (page 7)

4 large eggs

Basic Homemade Phyllo Dough (page 103), at room temperature

Flour or cornstarch, for rolling out the phyllo dough

Place the *kopanisti* in a large bowl and stir in the eggs. Mix by hand with a wooden spoon. Set aside.

Roll out, shape, and bake or fry the pies as directed in "Rolling Out Ikaria's Little Phyllo Pastries" (page 115).

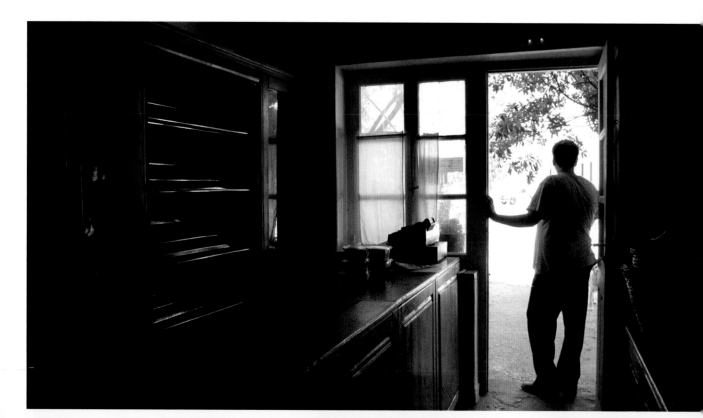

POPI'S SKILLET PUFF

"Fouskopita" tis Popis

Outside of the port of Evdilos, en route to our part of the island, is a small taverna right on the road in the village of Fytema, called Popi's. The food is simple. I've borrowed a recipe for Purslane and Olive Salad from Popi (page 47), as well as this one, for a puffy, crisp, cheese-stuffed skillet pie. You can also bake the pies. To do so, brush them with olive oil and bake them for 15 to 20 minutes in a preheated oven at 375°F (190°C).

MAKES 6

DOUGH

3 cups bread flour or fine semolina from durum wheat

2 teaspoons active dry yeast

1 teaspoon salt

⅓ cup Greek extra virgin olive oil

1 cup warm water

FILLING

4 cups crumbled feta, soft goat cheese, Ikarian *kathoura*, or Whipped Feta Kopanisti (page 7)

Olive oil and/or vegetable oil, for frying

For the dough: In a stand mixer fitted with the dough hook, combine the flour, yeast, and salt. Add the olive oil and warm water and mix with the dough hook until a ball forms. Increase the speed to medium and knead until smooth and silky, stopping the mixer now and then to push the dough down with a rubber spatula. Remove the dough, shape into 6 equal balls, and place in an oiled bowl. Cover tightly with plastic wrap and set aside for about 1 hour, to rise and almost double in bulk. Gently punch the dough balls down a little, cover, and set aside again for about 30 minutes to rest.

On a work surface dusted with either flour or cornstarch, roll out the first ball to a 12-inch round. Place ⅔ cup of the cheese filling on the center of the dough round and fold closed in the shape of a half moon. Press down gently with the rolling pin so that the cheese spreads as evenly as possible inside the pie. Press closed with dampened fingers or the dampened tines of a fork. Repeat with the remaining dough and cheese.

At this point you can fry them immediately or wrap well in plastic and freeze for later; fry directly from freezer.

In a 12-inch skillet, heat about 1½ inches (4 cm) of oil until almost at the smoking point. Add the first pie. Turn once. Remove with a slotted spoon as soon as it turns golden. Repeat with the remaining pies. Serve hot.

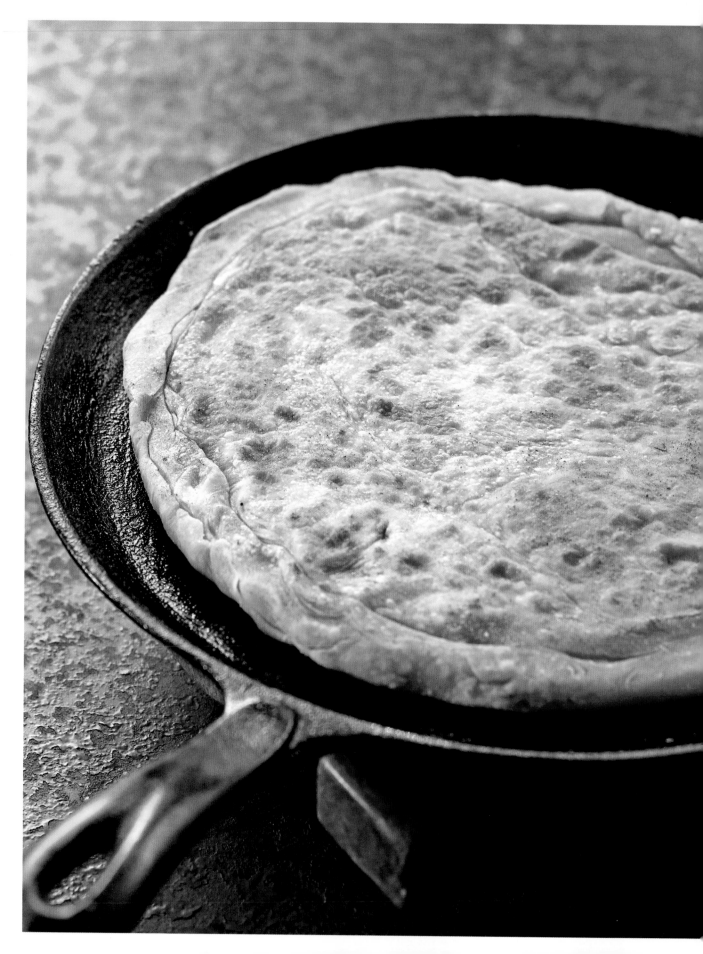

COLLARD, HERB, AND PORK GRIDDLE PIE

Pita me Lahanides kai Hoirini sto Satzi

This pie is the perfect example of a recipe from a particular place and time, produced and savored in a context that is very different from that of today. For one, it calls for the use of pork fat, or *ksingi*, in the local dialect, which, until the late 1960s, played a fairly important role in the local kitchen, despite the status of olive oil in the larger Mediterranean diet. Pork was a necessity and every family who could afford a pig kept one. In today's terms, we're talking about totally organic meat, raised on the refuse of families who ate mainly a plant-based diet. To toss a few cracklings in a frying pan full of wild greens was to make a treat, and I can only imagine that this pie, like most recipes with meat, was savored as such.

You'll need a large round cast-iron griddle (flat not ridged) for this.

MAKES 8 SERVINGS

DOUGH

3 cups bread flour or fine semolina from durum wheat

2 teaspoons active dry yeast

1 teaspoon salt

⅓ cup Greek extra virgin olive oil

1 cup warm water

FILLING

2 tablespoons lard* or 2 slices organic bacon, finely chopped

2 red onions, finely chopped

¾ pound collard greens (*lahanides* in Greek), trimmed and chopped

2 cups chopped fennel fronds

Leaves from 1 large bunch mint, chopped (about 1½ cups)

2 cups mixed wild greens and herbs such as Swiss chard, sweet sorrel, sweet dandelion, chervil, and parsley, or any combination of delicate, sweet herbs and edible weeds

Salt

Olive oil, for brushing the griddle and the dough

For the dough: In a stand mixer fitted with the dough hook, combine the flour, yeast, and salt. Add the olive oil and warm water and mix with the dough hook until a ball forms. Increase the speed to medium and knead until smooth and silky, stopping the mixer now and then to push the dough down with a rubber spatula. Remove the dough, shape into 4 equal balls, and place in an oiled bowl. Cover tightly with plastic wrap and set aside for about 1 hour, to rise and almost double in bulk. Gently punch the dough balls down a little, cover, and set aside again for about 30 minutes to rest.

*If cracklings are also available, chop about 2 tablespoons and mix them into the filling, but omit the bacon.

(continued)

For the filling: While the dough is resting a second time, in a large, deep skillet or wide pot, heat the lard or bacon and add the onions and fennel bulb, if using, cooking over medium heat until soft. Add the collards, fennel, mint and other greens or edible weeds, in batches if necessary, until wilted. Set aside to cool.

Take the first ball of dough and roll it into a round about 12 inches in diameter (or to a circumference slightly smaller than a large round griddle. Brush the surface of the dough round with a little olive oil. Fill it with half the greens mixture. Roll out a second ball of dough and place it over the greens. Press the top and bottom rims together and roll inwards to form a decorative edge. Set aside on a large plate or work surface sprinkled with cornstarch. Repeat the whole process to make a second 12-inch pie. Cover with a kitchen towel for 20 minutes.

Warm a round cast-iron griddle over medium heat, and brush with 1 teaspoon olive oil. Carefully slide the first pie onto the griddle. Grill over medium or medium-low heat until the bottom side is set and golden. Using a plate, flip it over and slide it back in on the uncooked side. When the bottom is golden and set, remove and repeat with the second pie.

VILLAGE BREAD AND/OR YIANNI'S CHEESE BREAD

Horiatiko Psomi y/kai Ta Tyrokoloura tou Yianni

Our bakery in the village of Aghios Dimitrios, just up the old stone path from our home, makes the most delicious feta-filled bread rings, not unlike the *kouloura Thessalonikis*, or sesame bread ring, that is sometimes called a Greek bagel and is otherwise known as *simit* in other parts of the Eastern Mediterranean. The *kouloura* dough has a subtle sweetness to it; Yianni's cheese-filled bread rings by contrast are crunchy and savory. On summer mornings, around 10 a.m., when they just come out of the oven, I send my son up the path, a few euro in hand, to go and fetch some. He returns a few minutes later, inevitably having eaten one on his way back home!

MAKES 2 LOAVES OR 12 CHEESE-FILLED BREAD RINGS

2 cups warm water

7 to 8 cups bread flour

1 envelope active dry yeast, or sourdough starter

2 teaspoons sugar

¼ cup Greek extra virgin olive oil

1 tablespoon salt

2 egg whites, lightly whisked with 2 tablespoons water

1 cup sesame seeds

1½ cups crumbled Greek feta cheese (optional)

In a stand mixer, combine 1 cup of the warm water with 1 cup of the bread flour, the yeast (or starter), and sugar. Tightly cover the top of the bowl with plastic wrap and then with a large kitchen towel, or better yet, with an old blanket, and let it stand in a warm, draft-free place for about 1 hour, until the mixture is thick and pasty and has begun to swell.

Attach the dough hook to the mixer.

Add the remaining 1 cup warm water, the olive oil, 5 cups of the flour, and salt to the bowl and mix on low speed until everything is combined. Slowly add enough of the remaining flour, stirring slowly and then on medium speed with the dough hook, until a smooth, silky dough takes shape. Using a rubber spatula, push the dough down on occasion as you mix it.

Remove the dough, knead it for a few minutes by hand on a floured surface, and place in an oiled bowl, preferably glass or ceramic. Cover tightly with plastic wrap and swaddle in a large kitchen towel or blanket. Let the dough rest until doubled in bulk, about 2 hours.

(continued)

Punch it down by hand in the bowl, or, alternatively, place it back in the clean mixer bowl and knead with the dough hook for a few minutes.

At this point, you can either shape the dough into 2 loaves and set them either free-form on an oiled baking sheet or in 2 oiled 10-inch loaf pans; or, you can divide it into 12 balls and let them rest, covered, on a floured surface or in an oiled pan, to make the bread rings.

If making loaves, preheat the oven to 450°F (230°C). If making cheese-filled rings, preheat the oven to 400°F (220°C).

For the loaves: When the loaves are almost doubled again in bulk, make 3 slits diagonally on the surface with a sharp paring knife. Brush with the egg white mixture and sprinkle generously with sesame seeds. Bake until golden brown and the bottom sounds hollow when tapped, 35 to 40 minutes. Remove to a rack and let cool.

For the cheese-filled rings: Take each of the 12 dough balls and shape each into a rope about 1 inch (2.5 cm) wide and 12 inches (30 cm) long. Flatten each rope using a rolling pin to a width of about 2 inches (5 cm). Sprinkle with 1 heaping tablespoon of crumbled feta. Roll lengthwise into a tight cylinder to a width of about 2 inches (5 cm), twist gently while holding both ends, then bring the ends together to form a 5- or 6-inch (12.5- or 15-cm) ring. Press to close. Place the rings on a floured surface, i.e., a table covered with kitchen towels. Let rise for about 15 minutes.

Place several rings on 1 or 2 large, oiled or nonstick baking pans (however many your oven will hold). Brush with the egg white wash and sprinkle with sesame seeds. Bake until puffed, golden, and crisp, about 20 minutes. Remove and serve hot or warm.

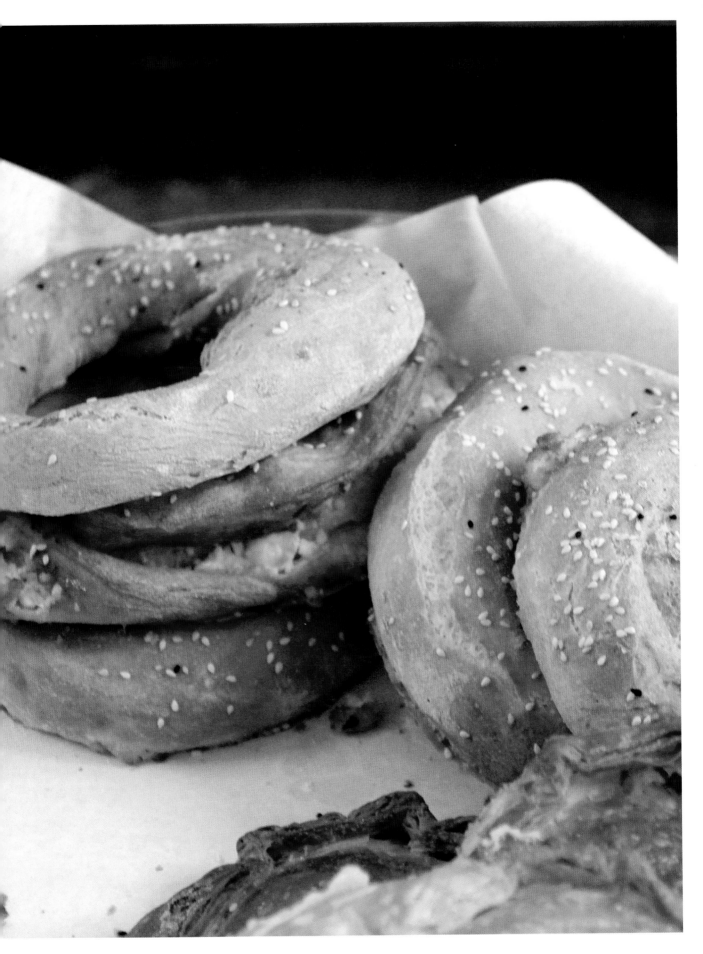

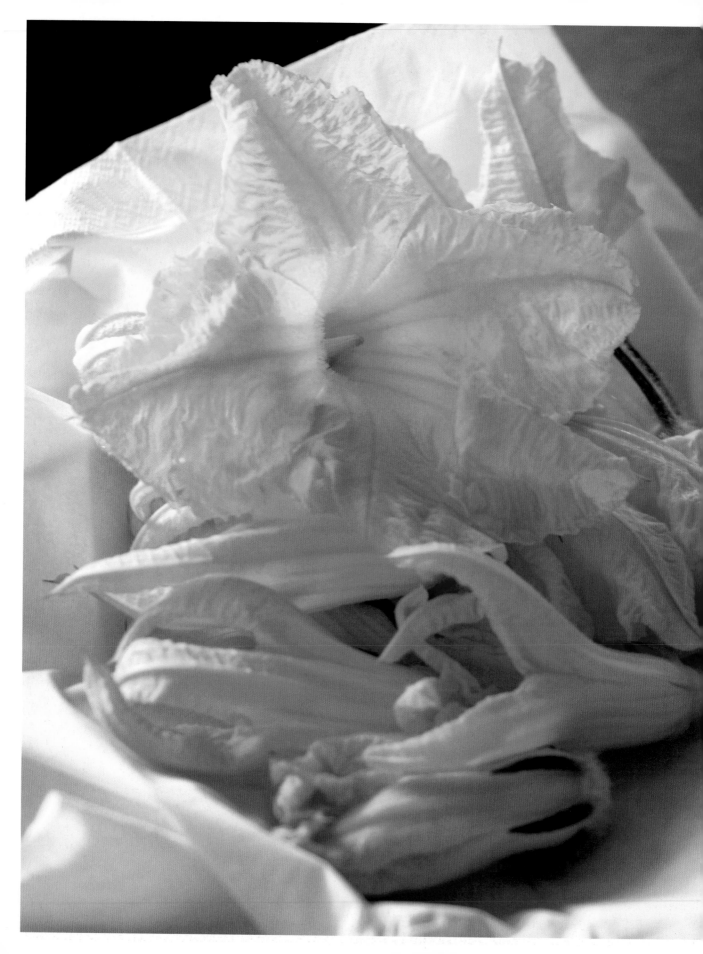

VEGETABLES

AS A MAIN COURSE

ABOUT A DOZEN YEARS AGO, WE OPENED A restaurant, Villa Thanassi, in the Ikarian village of Christos. Our good friend Yioula cooked for us, and her specialty was the island's national dish, *soufico*, the ultimate slow food: silky and unctuous, it's a soft, layered dish of all the summer vegetables, a little like ratatouille. For all its simplicity, a proper one might take hours to make, at least the way Yioula did it, salting and draining each vegetable separately, then pan-frying them in olive oil, again, separately; then, finally, layering everything in a Dutch oven and letting the flavors meld by slow-cooking the whole thing for about 45 minutes. The generous amount of olive oil that Yioula used and her unhurried approach to making *soufico* resulted in a dish where the vegetables were all very soft, almost caramelized in the sense that all the sweetness inherent in them had had time to develop. The soft, comforting texture bestowed by the olive oil made the vegetables more palatable. It was our bestseller. Then, one night, Yioula called in sick and the sous-chef made the *soufico*, shrugging off the slow cooking for expedience by cooking everything in a deep fryer. Oddly, it was as though our customers sensed that something was wrong; we didn't sell a single order that night!

This story always stayed with me because it is a paradigm for the care inherent in cooking even the simplest vegetable dishes. It's also a paradigm for the feel-good quality these dishes, when made well, inspire.

Vegetable cooking on Ikaria is totally dependent on the seasons. There is, for example, a summer and a winter version of *soufico*. Most islanders live by what their garden grows, and by what they can preserve from it, such as the *tsifia*, or sun-dried fruits and vegetables (page 16), which still see them through the long, wet winters.

But Ikaria's vegetable cookery, aside from a few local brushstrokes—i.e., the use of unusual herbs like pennyroyal here and there, the presence of long-forgotten ingredients like green almonds, the preference for slow stews, and the love of collards—really follows the same tenets as the vegetable cookery throughout Greece. That is, people take for granted the inordinate number of dishes that are main courses, plant-based and wanting in nothing so far as flavor, variety, and substance, because these dishes have always been and still are their daily sustenance. Olive oil in copious amounts is part of the vegetable cookery traditions; indeed, a whole category of plant-based dishes is called *ladera*, after the Greek word for olive oil, a nod to its use not only as a cooking fat but as a flavoring agent once the food is cooked. Almost all the recipes in both the vegetable and bean chapters fall into the category of *ladera*.

That said, eating more vegetarian meals can be a challenge when it comes to getting complete proteins, proteins that include essential and nonessential amino acids, which our bodies need for complete nutrition. It is no accident, then, that so many of Ikaria's, and indeed Greece's, plant-based dishes include the kinds of combinations that make for nutritionally complete meals. It's not by chance, for example, that so many of the greens and vegetable stews also include potatoes, which round out the nutritional profile; or that there are so many vegetable or legume and rice dishes.

With a piece of good whole-grain bread and perhaps some cheese or preserved meat or fish, most of the island's main-course vegetable dishes provide us with our daily nutritional requirements in one plate.

The best part is that they taste great.

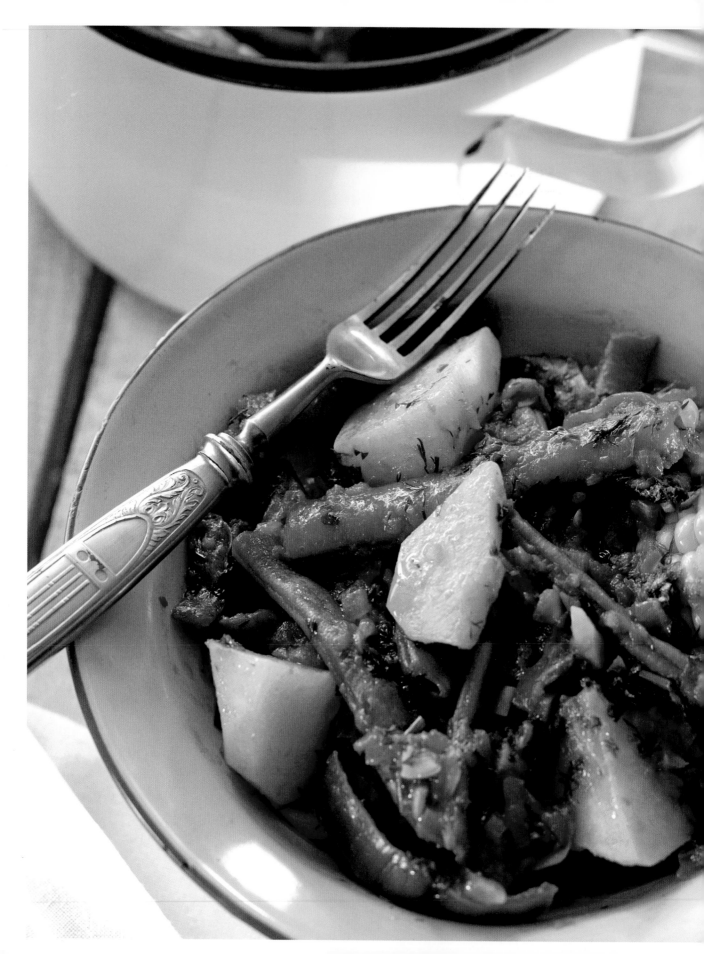

EVERYTHING SUMMER VEGETABLE STEW
Mageirio

Mageirio, after the verb, "to cook," *mageirevo*, is essentially an all-purpose summer stew, a kind of "throw-everything-in-one-pot," dish that almost every home cook makes at least once a week, making use of everything that grows in her garden. This and the next recipe offer slight variations on the theme. If amaranth greens are unavailable, you can use any sweet green, such as chard or dandelion.

In days gone by, Ikarian cooks used to add a bit of salted, cured goat, called *pasturma* (page 95), or bits of preserved pork to this.

MAKES 4 TO 6 SERVINGS

⅓ cup Greek extra virgin olive oil, plus more for serving

3 cups water

2 medium red onions, coarsely chopped (about 2 cups)

4 garlic cloves, chopped

2 pounds (1 kg) green beans, trimmed and halved crosswise

3 green bell peppers, cut into ½-inch (1.25 cm) rings or strips

1 fresh chile pepper (optional), whole

3 ears of corn, husked and halved

4 medium boiling potatoes, peeled and cubed

3 large firm-ripe tomatoes, chopped or grated

½ pound amaranth or sweet dandelion greens, trimmed and coarsely chopped

1 cup chopped fresh mint leaves

½ cup chopped fresh flat-leaf parsley

Salt

In a large pot, heat the olive oil and water over medium-high heat. As soon as the water simmers, add the onions, garlic, beans, bell pepper, chile pepper (if using), corn, and potatoes. Simmer until the potatoes and corn are firm-tender, about 25 minutes.

Add the tomatoes, greens, and herbs. Season with salt to taste. Stir gently to combine, cover, and simmer over low heat until all the vegetables are very tender, 20 to 25 more minutes. Serve warm or at room temperature, drizzled with as much additional olive oil as desired.

THE KNOT, THE PHARAOH, AND INFLATION:
AN ISLAND OF NICKNAMES

Our closest friends on the island are typically named after Greek saints, Biblical prophets, and, once in a while, ancient philosophers: John, Constantine, Nikolas, Elijah, Socrates, and others. But many have a whole other identity nowhere apparent on any official document: their nicknames. Quirky, impetuous, and yet spanning generations, nicknames are one of those local customs that evince both pragmatism and a certain humor.

For example, one of the best-loved villagers in all of Raches, and a real character, is Kostas Kohylas, 87, who is most commonly known as Combos, "the Knot," which in times gone by was also a unit of measure, roughly equivalent to an inch. Kostas, whose bright blue eyes seem to smile all the time, inherited the nickname from his grandfather, also named Kostas Kohilas. As Combo the younger explained, his *pappou*, or granddad, had a controlled hankering for wine. Whenever the elder would be served a glass, he'd inevitably qualify his portion by requesting "just a knot's length," and gesture the amount with his fingers. It stuck and it made its way past wars and famines and emigrations to land on the doorstep of his namesake two generations later. But there was a practical reason beyond sheer quirkiness. In the village there are at least a dozen other men all named Kostas Kohilas. So being able to make a distinction makes sense. What doesn't, though, is the case of Kostas the younger's brother, Yiorgos, born to the family with little competition on the given-name front. Yet, throughout his life pappou's moniker stuck and morphed so that he was known as Combo-Yiorgi, "George the Knot." On Ikaria, nicknames wend their way down the family tree in part out of reverence for those who have passed.

Another good friend, Ilias Moraiti, is known all over Ikaria and beyond, wherever Ikarians exist, as Pharaoh, a label he acquired as a young boy on a visit in the 1950s to Ikaria, his parents' birthplace, from Alexandria, Egypt, where his father was an affluent copper merchant. Everyone calls him Pharaoh, in the same way that everyone knows the local greengrocer as Arafat, because he once had to wear an eye patch for months, an occurrence that somehow made locals think of the face of the late Palestinian leader.

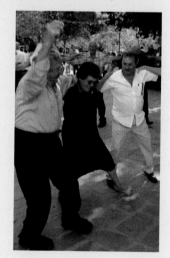

Another good friend is referred to as "Inflation," or Timarithmos in Greek, probably a lot more often than by his real name, Kostas Plakidas. He got stuck with Timarithmos in the summer of '83, when, at the age of 12, he seemed to grow by a couple of centimeters a day. Some old man noticed his speedy upward progress and commented that he grows as fast as the inflation rate. It stuck. To this day, to his face, people call him either the full, Timarithmos, or just . . . Tim!

COLLARDS COOKED WITH POTATOES

Lahanides me Patates

This simple dish is very much indicative of the lean, healthy traditional diet of islanders whose food supply was limited, families large, and waking hours filled with the survival chores inherent in village life. That this could be a main course, perhaps with a bowl of olives, a few specks of home-cured meat or cheese, and bread or rusks, speaks tomes.

MAKES 4 TO 6 SERVINGS

¾ cup Greek extra virgin olive oil

2 large red onions, coarsely chopped (about 2 cups)

2 pounds (1 kg) collard greens, stems removed and leaves cut into 1- to 1½-inch (2.5- to 3.5-cm) ribbons

4 large potatoes, peeled and quartered or cut into 6 chunks each

Salt and freshly ground black pepper

In a large wide pot, combine ¼ cup of the olive oil, the onions, and collards. Cover and cook over very low heat until both are wilted, about 10 minutes. Check every few minutes to be sure the vegetables aren't burning. Add a little water if necessary to keep that from happening.

Add the potatoes and another ¼ cup olive oil. Season with salt to taste and stir gently. Pour in enough water to come about one-third of the way up the contents of the pot. Continue cooking the vegetables until there is no liquid left in the pot and the mixture is soft, at least another 30 minutes. Season with additional salt and pepper to taste. Pour in the remaining ¼ cup olive oil and serve.

VARIATION

You can use other sweet greens in lieu of collards in this dish. Swiss chard, sweet sorrel, and spinach are all good candidates. You can also add 1 cup canned chopped tomatoes to the pot, right after adding the potatoes. Adjust the water content accordingly.

POTATOES BRAISED WITH WILD FENNEL

Patatato

Patatato on other Greek islands such as Amorgos is a meat and potato stew. When researching recipes for this book, I came across this dish, which is meatless, and cooked it one spring day as we were enjoying our annual Easter break on the island. I thought I had unearthed something old and unique, until my husband walked in the door, looked in the pot, and said, "Oh, *patatato*. I haven't seen that in a long time!" It is very common. *Patatato* is about as simple as simple gets, but the freshness of ingredients and the intense flavor of wild fennel make it uncannily sophisticated.

MAKES 4 SERVINGS

8 scallions, chopped

6 tablespoons Greek extra virgin olive oil

6 medium Yukon Gold potatoes, peeled and cut into 1½-inch (4-cm) cubes

½ cup white wine

Sea salt and freshly ground black pepper

1 cup chopped wild fennel or fennel fronds

Juice of 1 lemon

In a large, wide pot, combine the scallions and 3 tablespoons of the olive oil. Cover and cook over low heat until the scallions are soft and translucent, about 7 minutes.

Add the potatoes, wine, and enough water just to come about halfway up the contents of the pot. Season with sea salt to taste. Cover and simmer until the potatoes are almost cooked, about 25 minutes.

Add the wild fennel and a bit more water if necessary to keep the mixture moist. Cover and continue simmering until the potatoes are fork-tender, another 10 to 15 minutes. Just before serving, stir in the lemon juice, remaining 3 tablespoons olive oil, and pepper to taste. Serve hot or at room temperature.

OLD-STYLE IKARIAN TOURLOU: PAN-ROASTED POTATOES, ZUCCHINI, AND OREGANO

Tourlou tis Palias Epohis

Tourlou is typically a mixed summer vegetable casserole found all over the Eastern Aegean. The word is Turkish (*turlu*) and means a hodgepodge. There are many similar casseroles around Greece that go by different names. Even the *mageirio* recipe on page 131 is sometimes called *tourlou*.

What I like about this old Ikarian recipe is its utter simplicity. It also reminds me of a similar recipe with pumpkin, not zucchini, also made in a skillet, which is from neighboring Samos.

MAKES 4 TO 6 SERVINGS

1 pound (500 g) potatoes, peeled and cut into ¼-inch (60-mm) rounds

1 pound zucchini, cut into rounds to match potatoes

Sea salt and freshly ground black pepper

⅓ cup Greek extra virgin olive oil, plus more for serving

2 teaspoons dried Greek oregano, plus more for serving

Alternating between them, layer the potatoes and zucchini in overlapping circles in a large, wide pot or deep skillet. Season with sea salt and pepper. Add the olive oil and oregano. Cover the pot or skillet and cook the vegetables until tender and until the bottoms of the potatoes and zucchini are slightly charred. Flip over onto a plate, sprinkle with a little more oregano, drizzle (if desired) with olive oil and serve.

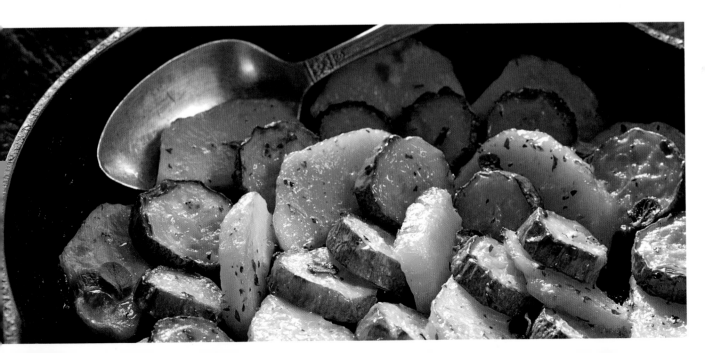

STEWED PEPPERS

Piperies Yiahni

This is a dish I make almost every summer when we have our cooking classes on the island because I like to show American guests that the simplest ingredients and techniques can often make for the most astonishing flavors, so long as everything is fresh and in season. You can serve this as a meze, too, and you can add a few fresh chile peppers to the lot for some kick.

MAKES 6 SERVINGS

1½ pounds (700 g) long green sweet peppers, such as cubanelles or Marconi peppers

1 large red onion, finely chopped (about 1 cup)

½ cup Greek extra virgin olive oil

2 garlic cloves, minced

Salt

1½ cups chopped plum tomatoes (fresh or canned)

1 tablespoon tomato paste

2 bay leaves

3 or 4 sprigs fresh oregano or 1 scant tablespoon dried Greek oregano

Whole-grain bread and feta cheese or goat's milk cheese, for serving

---

Remove and discard the pepper stems and seeds, but keep the peppers whole or halve lengthwise.

In a large, wide pot or deep skillet, combine the onion and 1 tablespoon of the olive oil. Cover and cook over low heat until wilted, 8 to 10 minutes.

Stir in the garlic. Add the peppers, season with a little salt, and cover. Cook over the same low heat until the peppers wilt, 10 to 12 minutes. Add the tomatoes, tomato paste, bay leaves, and oregano. Cook over low heat, covered, until the peppers are very soft and the sauce thick. Remove from the heat and discard the oregano sprigs and bay leaves. Stir in the remaining 7 tablespoons olive oil.

Serve with bread and a little cheese.

VARIATION

Another classic dish prepared as *yiahni* on Ikaria is made with potatoes. To make potatoes *yiahni*, substitute 2 pounds (1 kg) of Yukon Gold or other potatoes for the peppers. Peel and cut them into quarters or 1-inch (2.5-cm) rounds and proceed with the recipe from step 2, simmering until tender, 25 to 30 minutes.

BRAISED SPRING GREENS WITH FRESH ALMONDS

Horta sto Tetzeri me Tsagala

After my first experience plucking and eating raw green almonds off the trees in our garden in mid-June when they are in season, I've become an enormous fan of these grassy, refreshing treats.

MAKES 4 TO 6 SERVINGS

²/₃ cup Greek extra virgin olive oil

2 leeks, cleaned and coarsely chopped

5 spring onions, coarsely chopped

2 fresh garlic stalks, finely chopped, or 1 garlic clove, minced

1 pound baby spinach, washed and chopped

1 to 2 bunches fresh chervil, chopped

Leaves of 1 bunch fresh mint, chopped

2 bunches sweet sorrel, chopped

1 tablespoon tomato paste

²/₃ cup water

Salt and freshly ground black pepper

²/₃ cup green almonds

In a large, wide pot, heat ½ cup of the olive oil over medium heat. Add the leeks, spring onions, and garlic and cook until wilted and translucent, about 8 minutes. Add the spinach, chervil, mint, and sorrel, in batches if necessary, and stir with a wooden spoon until the greens lose enough volume to fit inside the pot.

Dilute the tomato paste in the water and add to the pot, cover, and simmer over low heat until the greens are very tender, about 20 minutes. Season with salt and pepper to taste. Add the green almonds and continue cooking another 5 minutes. Remove from the heat, pour in the remaining olive oil, stir, and let stand, covered, for 15 to 20 minutes before serving.

GREEN ALMONDS WITH ONIONS AND TOMATOES

Tsagala Yiahni

Older Ikarians remember plucking green almonds off the tree in the spring and relishing them as a snack. They have a slightly acidic, refreshing, lemony flavor. Some cooks pickle green almonds, in the shell. The kernel is also added to tomatoes, apples, green figs, and apricots put up in sugar syrup.

MAKES 2 SERVINGS

½ pound (about 50) green almonds, rinsed

⅓ cup Greek extra virgin olive oil, plus more for drizzling

1 large red onion, finely chopped

1½ cups chopped plum tomatoes

A pinch of sugar

Salt and freshly ground black pepper

Fresh lemon juice, strained

Using a paring knife, scrape around the seams of each almond, but do not remove the outer fuzzy layer. In a medium skillet, heat the olive oil over medium heat. Add the onion and cook until soft, about 8 minutes.

Add the almonds and toss to coat in the oil. Add the tomatoes. Pour in enough water to come about halfway up the contents of the skillet. Season with the sugar and salt and pepper to taste. Cover and simmer over medium heat until the almonds are soft and break apart. Drizzle in additional olive oil and add a spritz of lemon juice if desired.

BRAISED CAULIFLOWER

Kounoupidi Yiahni

In mid-August, Ikarians start to work on their winter gardens and right about then start planting, among other things, cruciferous vegetables such as cauliflower and broccoli. Both are used in simple boiled winter salads, with plenty of olive oil, lemon juice, and crunchy sea salt. Cauliflower, in the Ikarian kitchen and in the Greek country kitchen in general, is also a vegetable that finds its way into the stew pot, with onions, tomatoes, and winter aromatics such as celery and leeks. You can serve this dish together with good whole-grain bread and feta, or with a little cooked rice.

MAKES 4 SERVINGS

⅓ cup Greek extra virgin olive oil, plus more for drizzling

1 large red onion, coarsely chopped (about 1 cup)

2 leeks, cleaned and cut crosswise into 1½-inch (4-cm) cylinders

1 cup finely chopped Chinese celery, with leaves

3 garlic cloves, chopped

1 large head cauliflower, about 2 pounds (1 kg), cut into small florets

1½ cups chopped plum tomatoes or good-quality canned tomatoes

1 cup dry white wine or water

2 tablespoons *petimezi* (grape molasses), optional

Sea salt and freshly ground black pepper

½ cup chopped fresh flat-leaf parsley leaves

In a large, wide pot or deep skillet, heat the olive oil over medium heat. Add the onion, leeks, and celery and cook, stirring occasionally, until soft, about 8 minutes. Add the garlic and stir a few times.

Add the cauliflower to the pot and stir to coat in the oil. Pour in the tomatoes. As soon as the liquid comes to a simmer, add the wine (or water). When it comes to a simmer again, reduce the heat, add the *petimezi* (if using), and season to taste with salt and pepper. Cover and cook gently until the cauliflower is very tender, about 45 minutes.

Stir in the parsley and drizzle with additional olive oil. Serve.

STUFFED TOMATOES AND PEPPERS

Yemista

Stuffed tomatoes and peppers are a classic summer dish all over Greece. One of my favorite renditions is made by my friend Eleni Karimali, who together with her husband, Yiorgo, runs the family winery and B&B. She uses brown rice and a wood-fired oven to bake the vegetables.

MAKES 6 SERVINGS (2 STUFFED VEGETABLES EACH)

6 large firm-ripe tomatoes

6 large green bell peppers

4 tablespoons Greek extra virgin olive oil

4 large onions, finely chopped or grated (see Note)

1 cup long-grain brown rice

2 garlic cloves, chopped

⅓ cup raisins

¾ cup water

Salt and freshly ground black pepper

½ cup chopped fresh flat-leaf parsley

1 cup chopped fresh mint (or half mint and half pennyroyal, if available)

½ cup chopped fresh dill or wild fennel

Slice off the top of each tomato with a very sharp knife; keep each vegetable and cap together. Using a teaspoon, gently scoop out the pulp of each tomato, being careful not to tear the outer skin. Leave a shell thick enough to hold stuffing (about ½ inch [1.3 cm]). Pulse the pulp in a food processor until smooth. Set aside.

Carefully slice off the tops of the peppers, leaving the stems intact. Remove the peppers' seeds with a spoon. If desired, using a paring knife, trim away the inner ribs, which can be tough when cooked.

In a large heavy skillet, heat 2 tablespoons of the oil over medium heat. Add the onions and cook, stirring, until translucent and soft, about 10 minutes. Add the rice and stir frequently for 3 to 4 minutes. Add the tomato pulp, garlic, raisins, and water. Reduce the heat, cover the skillet, and simmer until the rice is softened but not cooked and most of the liquid is absorbed (the mixture should be moist), 15 to 20 minutes. Season the stuffing with salt and pepper and toss in the herbs.

Preheat the oven to 350°F (175°C).

Stuff the vegetables with the rice filling and crown with their own caps. Place in a baking pan. Add a little water to the pan (about ¼ cup), drizzle the remaining 2 tablespoons oil over the vegetables, and bake until the vegetables are soft and blistery and the rice is cooked, 1 hour to 1 hour 30 minutes. Baste with pan juices during baking. Serve hot or cold.

NOTE: *Grating onions on the large holes of a box grater reduces a whole onion to fine pieces. The juice is never discarded but added to the food, caramelizing slightly and adding a subtle sweetness to the final dish.*

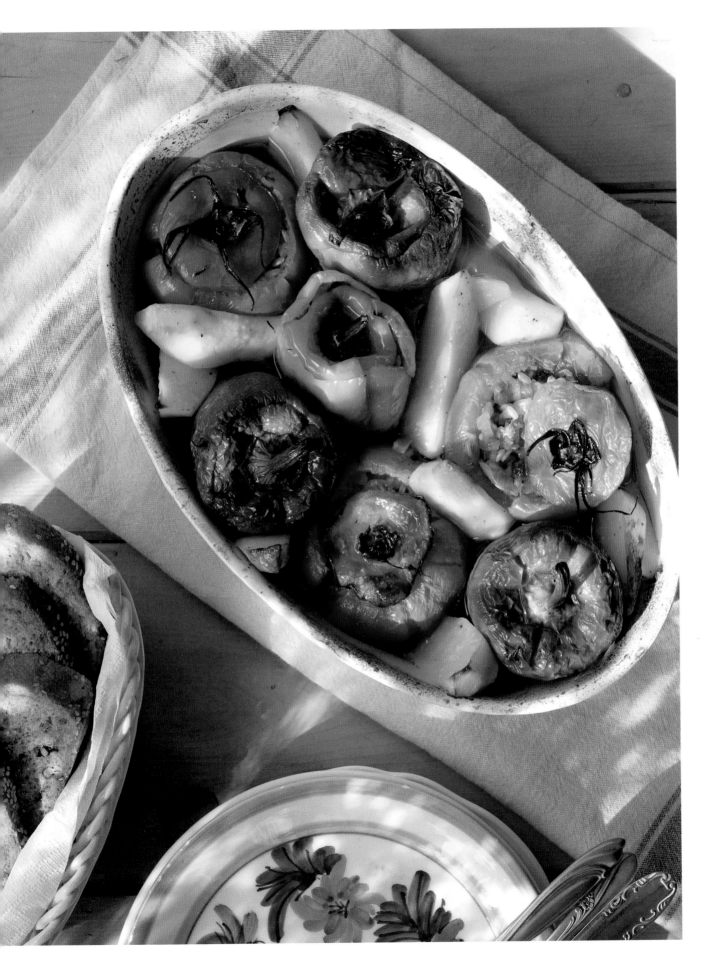

IKARIAN-STYLE STUFFED ZUCCHINI

Kariotika Kolokythakia Yemista

Zucchini, perhaps more than any other summer vegetable, makes for something akin to a seasonal national dish on Ikaria. Large ones, sometimes almost the size of American footballs, are shredded and used in pies; medium zucchini are savored as one of the very best vegetables for stuffing, and the Ikarian touch here is the addition of carrots and mint. Another distinction is that on Ikaria, stuffed zucchini are generally cooked in a pot, not in the oven.

If you can get hold of the small-leafed, rare pennyroyal, *fliskouni* to the locals on Ikaria, chop some up for the filling, too.

MAKES 10 SERVINGS

- 10 zucchini (8 to 10 inches [20 to 25 cm] long and 2½ inches [6.5 cm] in diameter)
- ½ cup Greek extra virgin olive oil
- 3 large red onions, or 2 large onions and 1 fennel bulb, finely chopped (3 to 3½ cups total)
- 2 large carrots, grated
- 2 garlic cloves, minced
- 1 cup medium-grain rice, such as Greek "glacé"
- 1 cup water

- 1 cup finely chopped fresh flat-leaf parsley leaves
- 1 cup finely chopped fresh mint leaves
- 1 cup finely chopped wild fennel or dill
- 3 or 4 zucchini flowers (optional), stamens or pistils removed, cut into very thin strips
- Salt and freshly ground black pepper
- Juice of 2 lemons
- 1 tablespoon all-purpose flour (optional)

Trim the ends of the zucchini and halve the zucchini crosswise to get two barrels. Using a teaspoon or melon baller, remove the pulp inside each of the zucchini halves, being careful not to puncture the shells. Leave about ¼ inch of zucchini shell so that they don't fall apart when cooking. Finely chop the pulp and set aside.

In a large skillet, heat 2 tablespoons of the olive oil over medium heat. Add the onions (or onions and fennel), carrots, and garlic and cook, stirring frequently, until wilted, about 10 minutes.

Add the rice and stir to coat in the oil. Add the water and zucchini pulp. Simmer until the rice has absorbed most of the liquid, about 15 minutes. Remove from the heat and mix in the herbs and zucchini flowers (if using). Season to taste with salt and pepper. Let the filling cool slightly.

When the filling has cooled to warm or tepid, stuff the zucchini. Place the stuffed zucchini snugly next to each other upright in a medium pot. Pour in the remaining 6 tablespoons olive oil and enough water to come about halfway up the zucchini. Place the lid on the pot and simmer the stuffed zucchini over low heat until the zucchini is tender and the rice cooked, about 40 minutes.

About 5 minutes before removing the zucchini, either pour in the lemon juice or whisk together the lemon juice and flour to form a thick batterlike liquid. Pour this into the pot and tilt gently from side to side to thicken the liquid. This combination of lemon and flour, called *alevrolemono*, was a way to achieve the creamy consistency of avgolemono (egg-lemon liaison) without the eggs and it was a common addition to various vegetable dishes, especially during periods of fasting. Serve the stuffed zucchini with plain lemon juice or with its creamier cousin, alevrolemono.

MINT IN IKARIA'S KITCHEN

Mint is always one of the main herbs used to season stuffed summer vegetables on Ikaria, but older cooks on the island traditionally add the once-prevalent *fliskouni*, or pennyroyal, a slim-leaved wild mint sometimes called "Lurk in the Ditch" or "Pudding Grass" in English, after its growing manner and its use. Pennyroyal is one of the many herbs that find their way into the pot and cup on Ikaria, as a seasoning in dishes like stuffed tomatoes, peppers, and zucchini but also dried and sipped as a therapeutic infusion. It is known for its anti-inflammatory properties and is one of the most popular herbal teas on the island, perhaps one of many reasons why the population of spry nonagenarians flourishes on Ikaria!

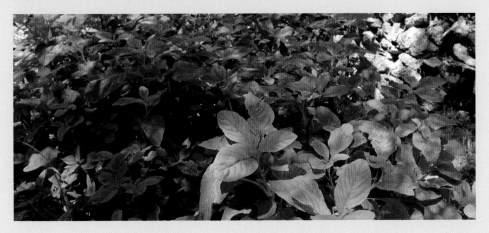

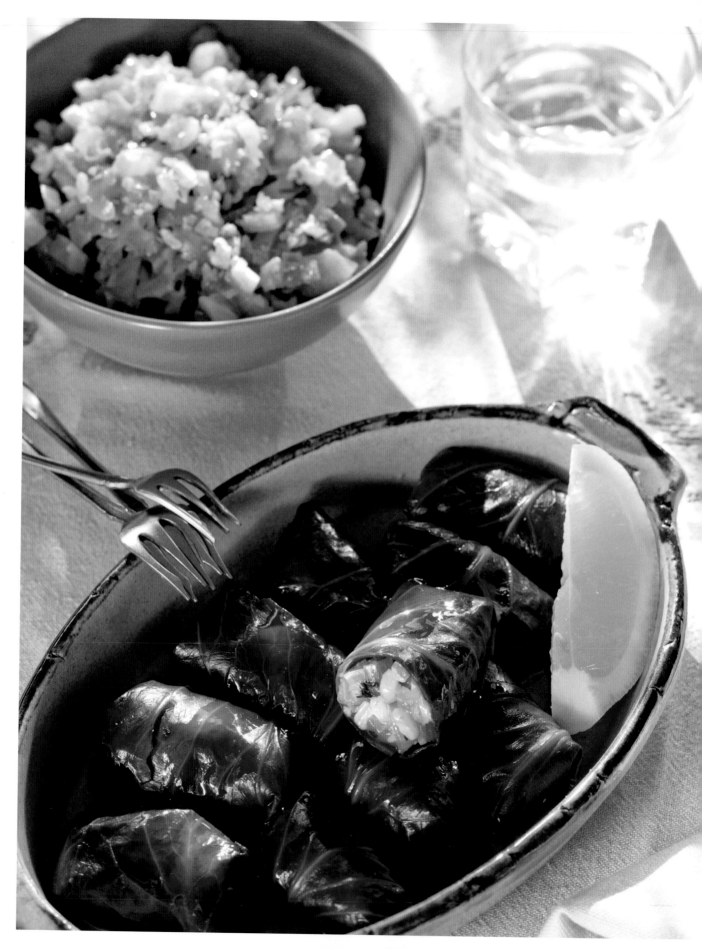

COLLARD GREEN DOLMADES FILLED WITH DRIED CORN AND HERBS

Yiaprakia

The first time I heard about this version of stuffed cabbage I was in the house where my father grew up and where my 95-year-old Aunt Mary still lived. She was a great source of knowledge about old Ikarian dishes and always remembered them with deep-felt nostalgia. Back in the day when she was a girl only well-to-do families in Greece could afford rice. On Ikaria, in its place, people used dried corn, which they grew and dried in the sun, reserving the amberlike little kernels for use in dishes that went hand in hand with the cold, damp months of winter. Trying to replicate the dish was also an adventure until I stumbled upon Amish dried sweet corn, which is easy to source by mail in the United States.

MAKES 6 SERVINGS

2 cups dried sweet corn kernels

24 large fresh collard greens, stems trimmed

½ cup Greek extra virgin olive oil

3 large red onions, finely chopped

1 cup chopped fresh mint leaves

1 cup chopped wild fennel or 1 fennel bulb, finely chopped

½ cup chopped fresh chervil (optional)

1½ cup chopped fresh flat-leaf parsley

Salt and freshly ground black pepper

Soak the corn kernels overnight, refrigerated in cold water. Drain.

Bring a large pot of salted water to a rolling boil and blanch the collard greens for 1 minute, just to soften a bit. Drain into a colander and rinse under cold water. Pat dry and set aside.

In a large skillet, heat 2 tablespoons of the olive oil over low heat. Add the onions and cook until very pale golden, about 10 minutes.

Combine the drained corn, onions, and chopped herbs. Season to taste with salt and pepper.

Place 2 tablespoons of the filling on the bottom center of each collard leaf and roll up into cylinders, folding in the sides to form the dolmades (like spring rolls). Pour 2 tablespoons of the olive oil on the bottom of a large, wide pot and place the collard dolmades seam-side down, one snugly next to the other. Add enough water just to cover. Cover the pot and bring to a simmer over medium heat. Reduce the heat and cook slowly until leaves and filling are tender, about 30 minutes. Remove from the heat, pour in the remaining 4 tablespoons olive oil, and serve.

(continued)

Collard Green Dolmades with Avgolemono: Follow the recipe, opposite, but substitute short-grain rice for the corn. To make the avgolemono, whisk together 2 large egg yolks and the juice of 1 lemon until frothy. Very slowly add two ladlefuls of hot pot juices from the stuffed, cooked leaves, whisking vigorously all the while. Pour the egg-lemon mixture back into the pot, tilt so that it is evenly distributed, and serve immediately.

HOW TO DRY CORN

Corn—real corn, not GMO corn—is, indeed, an amazing grain, if only we consumed it with the wisdom of traditional cultures. For one, corn contains a slew of antioxidants. It contains high amounts of dietary fiber, which is good for our digestion, and proteins, and a bevy of B vitamins (all good for our blood sugar) including folate. It is surprisingly rich in iron.

Drying it is a tradition in many parts of the world, as the crop is only in season a few weeks a year and it has to be preserved. The trick is to dry the corn right after picking, before its sugars start turning to starch. That way, the drying concentrates the corn's natural sugars and lends the final product a subtle, toasty, sweet flavor.

A generation ago, Ikarians used to dry their corn in order to keep it for a variety of uses all winter long. My neighbor Stefanos recalls his mother oven-drying the corn whole on the cob before removing the kernels. The baking at low temperature was a way to stave off worms and other insects.

Corn varieties have changed tremendously over the last decades. We still plant an old variety of corn, one the locals say is "indigenous" (of course it can't be, corn being a New World crop), which is small, white, sweet, and quite tough.

It takes about 6 ears of corn to get 2 cups of dried corn kernels. I have adapted the method of drying the kernels so that this works in a modern kitchen. To make your own dried corn, buy organic, non-GMO, sweet corn. Husk the ears, making sure to remove all the silk. Blanch the corn in a pot of boiling water for 5 minutes. Remove with tongs and plunge into a large basin filled with ice and water.

Dry the ears with paper towels, then cut the corn kernels from the ear. Spread the kernels onto a baking sheet in a single layer. Place in a 140°F (60°C) oven to dry. Turn the corn every couple of hours. Depending upon the moisture in the corn, the drying process will take 4 to 8 hours or more.

Allow the corn to cure on the counter for a couple of days before placing in an airtight container. Store in a cool, dark place until ready to use.

ZUCCHINI BLOSSOMS STUFFED WITH RICE AND HERBS

Anthoi Yemistoi

Admittedly, this is not an easy dish to make if you're not a gardener who happens to grow zucchini and who has access to the freshest flowers, which are always wide-open and glorious first thing in the morning. You could conceivably buy the blossoms from a farmers' market, but the cost would transform this dish from a simple summer treat into a pricey, almost forbidding delicacy. That seems to defeat the purpose of trying to eat well on a mainly vegetarian diet.

If you do have your own flowers, hopefully organic, cut them early in the morning, remove the stamens or pistils, tuck one inside the other so that they remain open, and place on a baking sheet or plate lined with paper towels. Cover with more paper towels and top with one layer of dampened paper towel. Refrigerate up to 48 hours.

Zucchini flowers when cooked are delicate and have a melt-in-your-mouth texture.

MAKES 6 SERVINGS

1½ cups short-grain rice

1 cup chopped wild fennel or ⅔ cup snipped fresh dill

1 cup chopped fresh mint leaves

1 garlic clove, minced

Salt and freshly ground black pepper

6 tablespoons Greek extra virgin olive oil

36 zucchini flowers, pistils or stamens and any small insects removed

In a bowl, combine the rice, fennel (or dill), mint, garlic, and salt and pepper to taste. Stir in 3 tablespoons of the olive oil.

Drizzle about 1 tablespoon of the olive oil on the bottom of a large, wide pot. Using a teaspoon, carefully fill each of the flowers with the rice mixture. Gently twist the ends closed. As you work, carefully place the stuffed flowers side by side in the pot. They should sit snugly next to one another, in a single, or, if necessary, double layer.

Add enough water to barely cover the flowers. Place a plate over them to keep them in place while they cook. Cover the pot and bring to a simmer over medium heat, then reduce the heat and slowly simmer the stuffed blossoms until the filling is cooked and the flowers are opaque, about 20 minutes. Drizzle the remaining 2 tablespoons olive oil into the pot just before serving.

GRAPE LEAVES STUFFED WITH RICE AND HERBS

Dolmadakia

This is a traditional recipe for stuffed grape leaves, with one local touch in the use of fennel fronds, preferably from wild fennel.

If you have access to fresh grape leaves in the spring, by all means collect and use them. You can blanch and freeze the fresh leaves. Trim off the tough stems, blanch in batches, cool in an ice bath, and pack them in stacks of 50 in plastic zip-seal bags, pressing out all the air, then freeze.

As a general rule, *dolmadakia* may be stuffed either with rice and herbs, as in this recipe, in a version often referred to as *yialantzi*, or with a combination of rice and ground beef or lamb. The sweetness of so many onions in the filling counters the innate acidity of the leaves.

MAKES 6 TO 8 SERVINGS

½ pound (220 g) fresh grape leaves, or 1 jar (16 ounces [450 g]) brine-packed grape leaves

½ cup Greek extra virgin olive oil

5 large onions, finely chopped

1 cup finely chopped scallions

2 garlic cloves, finely chopped

1 cup long-grain rice

1 scant teaspoon ground cumin

Salt and freshly ground black pepper

4 to 5 cups water

1 cup finely chopped fennel fronds

½ cup finely chopped fresh dill

½ cup finely chopped fresh flat-leaf parsley

⅓ cup finely chopped fresh mint

Juice of 2 lemons, strained

Plain Greek yogurt (optional)

If using brined grape leaves, rinse them very well and blanch them in scalding water for 2 to 3 minutes to soften. Remove with a slotted spoon, and place in a bowl of ice water. Drain and rinse several times.

If using fresh grape leaves, trim the stem and use directly.

In a large, heavy skillet, heat ¼ cup of the olive oil over medium heat. Add the onions and scallions and cook until completely soft, 8 to 10 minutes. Add the garlic and stir for 1 minute. Add the rice and cook, stirring constantly, for 5 minutes. Add the cumin, salt and pepper to taste, and 1 cup water. Cover and simmer until the rice is softened but not cooked completely and the water absorbed, about 10 minutes. Remove and cool. Toss in the herbs.

Separate the grape leaves that are too small or too irregular to roll. Pour 2 tablespoons olive oil in the bottom of a medium saucepan and spread 4 or 5 of the irregular leaves over the oil.

To assemble the stuffed grape leaves, take one leaf at a time, and snip off any remainder of a hard stem. Place 1 teaspoon of the rice mixture in the center bottom of the leaf. Fold the left and right sides over the filling and roll up, gently but tightly, from bottom to top, until a bite-size log is formed. Place seam-side down in the pot. Repeat with remaining stuffing and leaves. Pour the remaining olive oil, lemon juice, and enough water to cover the leaves by about ¾ inch (2 cm) into the pot. Place a piece of parchment paper then a plate over the grape leaves so they don't loosen while cooking. Cover the pot and cook over low heat until the leaves are tender and the rice is thoroughly cooked, 40 minutes.

Serve warm or cold, with yogurt on the side, if desired.

GRAPE LEAF NUTRITION

Grape leaves, such an iconic Greek ingredient, are surprisingly rich in essential nutrients. Their high fiber content helps us feel sated and slows down digestion so that sugar is released gradually into the bloodstream. They contain vitamins A and K, which help in cell development, skin and eye health, and bloodflow. The calcium and iron inherent in the leaves promote healthy bones, teeth, and circulation.

A meal or meze of three stuffed grape leaves provides us with antioxidants, bone-strengthening minerals, carbohydrates, dietary fiber, protein, and a little fat. Most of the leaf is water though!

SOUFICO ON THE SOUTH SIDE

Soufico Manganitiotiko

Even in a place as small as Ikaria, there are regional differences when it comes to *soufico*, one of the most iconic local specialties. Soufico on the south side is typically prepared by chopping all the vegetables and cooking them together in one large, deep skillet or wide pot.

MAKES 4 TO 6 SERVINGS

6 to 8 tablespoons Greek extra virgin olive oil

3 large onions, chopped (about 3 cups)

2 large green bell peppers, cut into 1-inch (2.5-cm) squares

3 garlic cloves, finely chopped

Salt and freshly ground black pepper

2 medium eggplants, cut into 1-inch (2.5 cm) chunks or cubes

4 medium zucchini, cut into 1-inch (2.5 cm) chunks or cubes

2 large firm-ripe tomatoes, chopped

2 teaspoons dried Greek oregano or savory

In a large, wide pot or deep skillet, heat 2 tablespoons of the olive oil over medium heat. Add the onions, bell peppers, and garlic and cook until wilted, about 7 minutes. Season lightly with salt and pepper.

Pour in another 2 tablespoons olive oil and add the eggplants. Cook until soft, 8 to 10 minutes. Add the zucchini, toss to combine, then add the tomatoes, oregano (or savory), and a little more salt and black pepper.

Cover and cook until the vegetables are soft, about 25 minutes. Remove and pour in the remaining 2 to 4 tablespoons olive oil, to taste. Serve warm or at room temperature.

SMOTHERED SUMMER VEGETABLES FROM IKARIA

Soufico

Soufico is arguably the best-known dish on Ikaria, the one recipe almost everyone on the island cites as being completely unique to the place. And yet, its origins are unclear. It belongs to the general category of Mediterranean dishes, from ratatouille to caponata, where the roster of summer vegetables—eggplants, zucchini, peppers, and tomatoes—works so harmoniously together in one pot. Its name might derive from the Italian *soffocare,* which means "to smother," perhaps because of the way the vegetables are so deliciously smothered in olive oil; local sleuths, however, say it derives from *sou'fika* or *s'afika* in the local dialect, which means "I left you some," as in it is so good, one always leaves a portion for the man in the family should he return home.

To me what is most interesting is that in the 99 square miles that make up Ikaria, there are at least four versions: one from the north side; one from the south (in which the vegetables are cut up into small pieces and fried all together); a third, made in the fall, with pumpkin and peppers; and a very old version that has neither eggplants, zucchini, peppers, nor potatoes but is an unlikely combination of herring, tomatoes, and onions (see page 158).

The version below is from the northern part of the island, with one change by me: I bake the vegetables instead of frying each of them individually, in order to make the dish lighter.

MAKES 6 SERVINGS

Salt and freshly ground black pepper

2 medium eggplants, cut crosswise into rounds ¼ inch (6 mm) thick

2 large green bell peppers, cut into 1-inch (2.5-cm) strips

3 medium zucchini (about 2 inches [5 cm] in diameter), cut crosswise into rounds ¼ inch (6 mm) thick

½ cup Greek extra virgin olive oil, plus more for brushing

3 large onions, finely chopped (about 3 cups)

3 garlic cloves, finely chopped

2 large potatoes, peeled and cut into rounds ¼ inch (6 mm) thick

3 large firm-ripe tomatoes, grated

4 to 5 tablespoons fresh oregano leaves

6 to 12 zucchini blossoms (optional)

In separate colanders, lightly salt the eggplants, peppers, and zucchini. Drain for 1 hour. Wipe dry without washing.

Preheat the broiler. Brush the eggplants, peppers, and zucchini with olive oil and broil lightly, to soften. There should be very little color on the vegetables.

(continued)

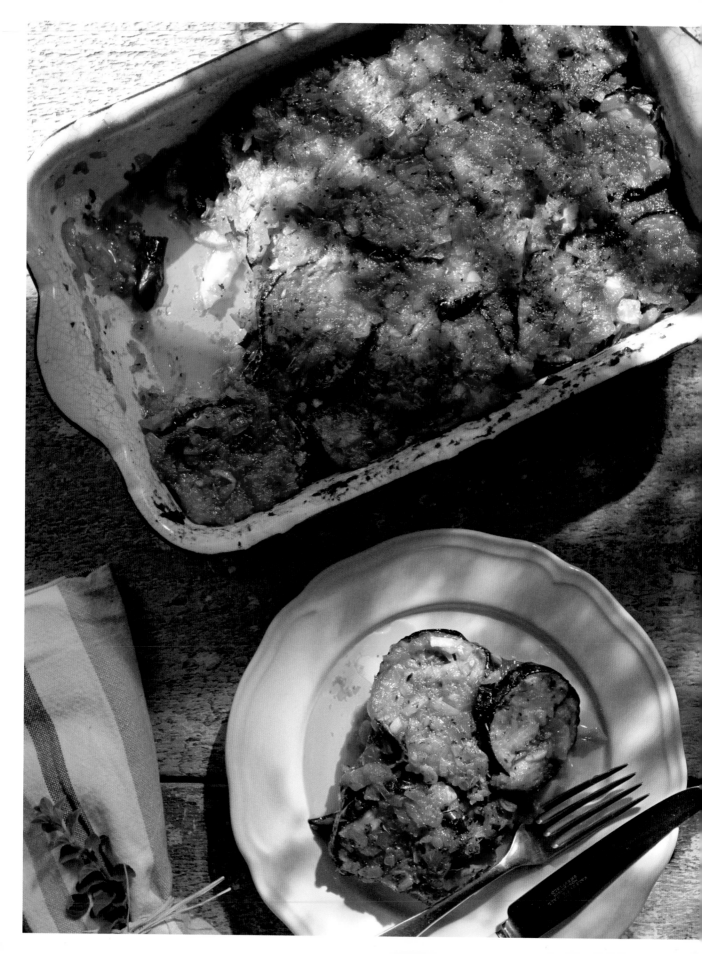

In a large skillet, heat 2 tablespoons of olive oil and lightly cook the onions and garlic, until wilted, 6 to 7 minutes.

Remove with a slotted spoon and set aside. Replenish the oil in the skillet if necessary. Add the potato slices and fry lightly until their edges begin to color.

Oil a 6-quart ovenproof casserole or Dutch oven. Spread 2 tablespoons of the onions and garlic on the bottom. Mix with 2 tablespoons of the grated tomato. Season with a little salt and black pepper. Arrange all of the potatoes in a single overlapping layer on the bottom, over the tomato-onion mixture. Season lightly with salt and black pepper. Next, in this order, spread: bell peppers, more onion-garlic-tomatoes, a little fresh oregano, salt, and black pepper; then eggplant, more onion-garlic-tomatoes, salt, black pepper, and oregano; then zucchini slices, onion-garlic-tomato mixture, salt, and pepper.

Continue layering until all vegetables are used up, saving about ½ cup of the tomatoes and onion mixture for last. As you layer, press down with a spatula so that the vegetables are layered compactly. Spread the zucchini blossoms, if using, decoratively on the surface. Spread the remaining tomato-onion mixture over the top.

At this point you can bake the *soufico*, covered, in a preheated oven at 350°F (175°C) until very soft and almost caramelized, about 35 minutes. Or you can cook it on top of the stove, over low heat, covered, for about 30 minutes, or until the vegetables are very soft and any liquid they let off has evaporated.

WINTER SOUFICO WITH PUMPKIN AND DRIED CHILES

Heimoniatiko Soufico

Pumpkin has long been an important local vegetable and several varieties are grown on the island. In the summer, almost every garden is fringed with pumpkin plants, their long ribbed stems crawling chaotically in and out of other plants, and their big floppy leaves monopolizing ground space.

But once picked, they last all winter and into spring. Local recipes with pumpkin abound: in small skillet pies, floured and fried as a meze, in rice dishes, and in countless one-pot stews.

One of my favorites is this winter rendition of the island's best-known dish, *soufico*. "No tomatoes," Myrsina Roussou, the 80-something mother of our friend Yiannis, advised emphatically. "And don't grate the pumpkin. Cut in chunks." Her other suggestion was to add dried peppers.

MAKES 4 TO 6 SERVINGS

8 dried red or green bell peppers (see Note) or dried ancho chile peppers, seeded

3 pounds fresh pumpkin, peeled and seeded

½ cup Greek extra virgin olive oil

3 red onions, coarsely chopped

3 garlic cloves, minced

1 tablespoon dried mint

2 teaspoons paprika

½ to 1 teaspoon cayenne pepper (optional)

Sea salt and freshly ground black pepper

2 to 3 tablespoons red wine vinegar (to taste)

Place the dried peppers or chiles in a medium bowl and cover with warm water to rehydrate. Let them sit for 30 minutes, or until soft. Reserving the soaking water, drain the peppers. Cut the rehydrated chile peppers into thirds across the width.

Cut the pumpkin into 1½-inch (4 cm) chunks.

In a wide pot, Dutch oven, or deep skillet, heat 3 tablespoons of the olive oil over medium heat. Add the onions, reduce the heat, and cook, stirring occasionally, until the onions are soft and slightly caramelized, 15 to 20 minutes. Stir in the garlic.

Add the pumpkin to the pot and stir to coat in the oil. Add the peppers, mint, paprika, cayenne, and salt and black pepper to taste. Cook, covered, over low heat, until the pumpkin is tender but not mushy, about 25 to 30 minutes. Gently stir in the vinegar, adjust the seasoning with salt and black pepper and serve, drizzled with the remaining 5 tablespoons olive oil.

NOTE: *You can oven-dry your own peppers. If using red or green bell peppers, remove the caps and seeds and quarter the peppers lengthwise. Place on a baking sheet lined with parchment and bake at 250°F (120°C) for about 2 hours, or until dehydrated. Turn once during the drying process.*

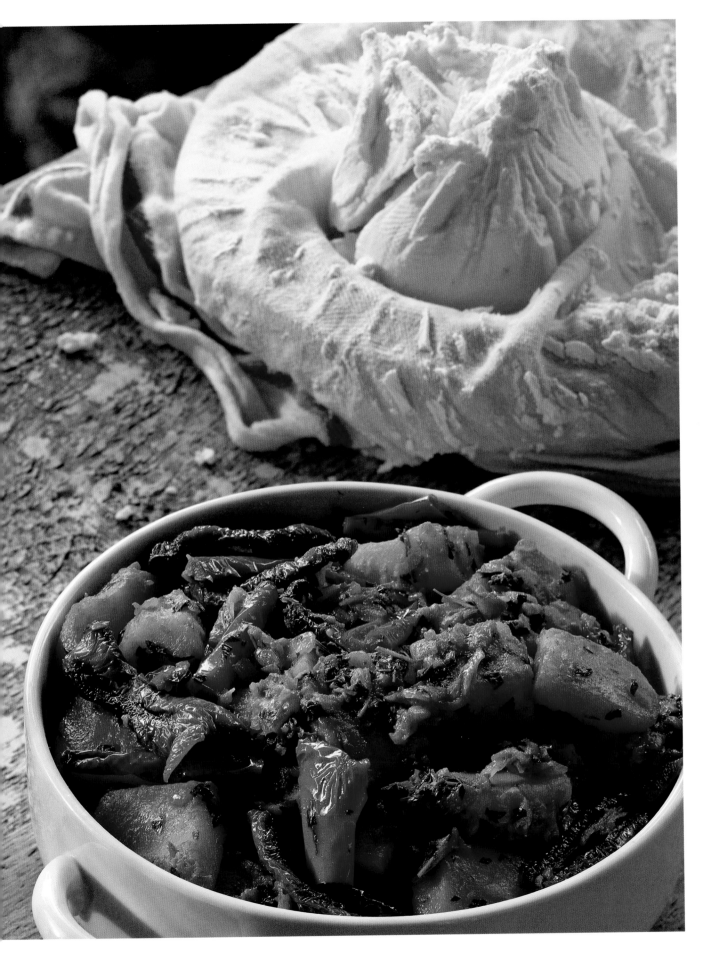

PUMPKIN AND SWEET POTATOES ROASTED WITH LEEKS AND MALLOW

Tabouras, Glykopatates, Prasa kai Moloha ston Fourno

You can taste the change of seasons in this old dish, which is made toward the end of Greek summer, at that time of the year when gardens overflow with the last of the warm-weather vegetables and the first of the winter crops. Mallow, which grows wild, often near stinging nettles, all over the island, flowers in the summer in Ikaria. Serve the dish accompanied, if desired, with a little Greek feta and whole-grain bread.

MAKES 4 TO 6 SERVINGS

⅔ cup Greek extra virgin olive oil

2 leeks, halved lengthwise, cleaned, and sliced crosswise into thin half-moons

1 red onion, finely chopped (about 1 cup)

1½ pounds (750 g) pumpkin, peeled, seeded, and cut into 1½-inch (4-cm) cubes

½ pound sweet potatoes, peeled and cubed like the pumpkin

Salt and freshly ground black pepper

3 cups chopped mallow leaves*

½ cup finely chopped Chinese celery

½ cup snipped fresh dill

1½ cups coarsely chopped canned plum tomatoes

Preheat the oven to 375°F (190°C).

In a large skillet, heat 2 tablespoons of the olive oil over medium heat. Add the leeks and onion and cook until soft, 7 to 8 minutes.

In a large ovenproof clay or ceramic dish or in a baking pan, toss the onion-leek mixture with the pumpkin, sweet potatoes, 2 tablespoons of the olive oil, and salt and pepper to taste. Toss gently to coat. Cover the pan and roast the vegetables until about two-thirds of the way cooked.

Add the mallow, celery, dill, and tomatoes and gently toss. Season to taste with additional salt and pepper. Stir in all but 2 tablespoons of the olive oil. Cover the pan again and continue roasting until the pumpkin and sweet potatoes are very tender and the greens cooked, another 20 minutes.

Remove from the oven, drizzle the reserved 2 tablespoons olive oil over the dish, and serve.

*You can substitute Swiss chard for the mallow.

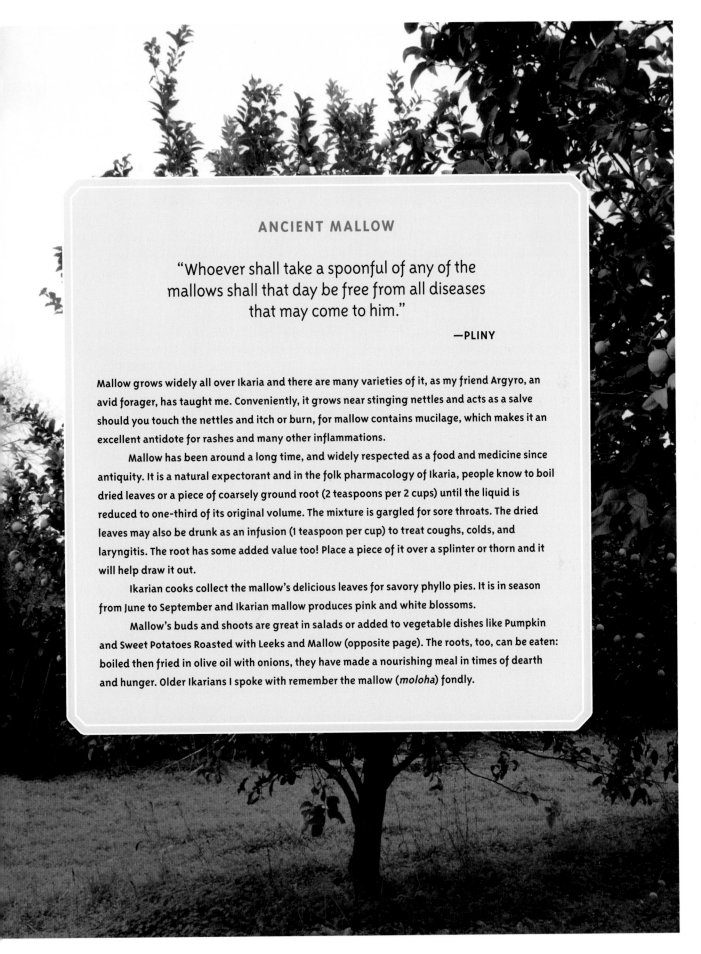

ANCIENT MALLOW

"Whoever shall take a spoonful of any of the mallows shall that day be free from all diseases that may come to him."

—PLINY

Mallow grows widely all over Ikaria and there are many varieties of it, as my friend Argyro, an avid forager, has taught me. Conveniently, it grows near stinging nettles and acts as a salve should you touch the nettles and itch or burn, for mallow contains mucilage, which makes it an excellent antidote for rashes and many other inflammations.

Mallow has been around a long time, and widely respected as a food and medicine since antiquity. It is a natural expectorant and in the folk pharmacology of Ikaria, people know to boil dried leaves or a piece of coarsely ground root (2 teaspoons per 2 cups) until the liquid is reduced to one-third of its original volume. The mixture is gargled for sore throats. The dried leaves may also be drunk as an infusion (1 teaspoon per cup) to treat coughs, colds, and laryngitis. The root has some added value too! Place a piece of it over a splinter or thorn and it will help draw it out.

Ikarian cooks collect the mallow's delicious leaves for savory phyllo pies. It is in season from June to September and Ikarian mallow produces pink and white blossoms.

Mallow's buds and shoots are great in salads or added to vegetable dishes like Pumpkin and Sweet Potatoes Roasted with Leeks and Mallow (opposite page). The roots, too, can be eaten: boiled then fried in olive oil with onions, they have made a nourishing meal in times of dearth and hunger. Older Ikarians I spoke with remember the mallow (*moloha*) fondly.

STEWED FRESH OKRA

Bamiyes Yiahni

Like taro root, which most people in the West associate with the cuisines of Africa and Latin America, so, too, is okra a vegetable not generally associated with the Mediterranean. Okra brings to mind the foods, again, of Africa, and its path west with the slave trade to far-off places like New Orleans. But Greeks love it. On Ikaria many people grow okra and know to use the smallest pods, for once they grow past about 1½ inches they become woody and fibrous. The most popular way to eat it on Ikaria and throughout Greece is stewed, as in the dish below. Okra has a distinct slippery texture, which many people find distasteful. The Greeks sprinkle vinegar over it, which helps firm up the okra and makes it more palatable.

MAKES 4 TO 6 SERVINGS

2 pounds (1 kg) small fresh okra*

1 cup red wine vinegar

8 tablespoons Greek extra virgin olive oil

1 large red onion, finely chopped

3 garlic cloves, minced

2 large firm-ripe tomatoes, grated, or 2 cups good-quality canned chopped plum tomatoes

Salt and freshly ground black pepper

6 medium potatoes, peeled and quartered

½ cup chopped fresh flat-leaf parsley leaves

Trim the okra by cutting away the tough rim at the stem end. Rinse well. Place the okra in a large bowl and toss with the vinegar. This helps firm up its slippery texture. Set aside for 1 hour, then drain.

In a large skillet, heat 3 tablespoons of the olive oil over medium heat and cook the onion, stirring, until wilted, about 8 minutes. Stir in the garlic.

Add the okra and grated tomatoes. Season to taste with salt and pepper. Add enough water just to come about halfway up the okra. Cover and simmer over low heat for 35 minutes. Add the potatoes and a little water if necessary to keep the contents of the pot from burning. Continue cooking until the potatoes and okra are both tender, about 30 minutes longer. About 10 minutes before removing from the heat, add the parsley, and season with pepper and additional salt if necessary.

Just before serving pour in remaining 5 tablespoons olive oil.

*You may also use frozen okra, in which case step 1 won't be necessary. Thaw before cooking.

ONION AND TOMATO STEW WITH HERRING

Soufico me Renga

Herring, like salt cod, is a most uncharacteristic fish for impoverished islanders, as it does not ply local waters. But it was once very cheap and it keeps well and was sold by itinerant merchants and local shopkeepers. To this day, herring has a special place in the Greek food psyche, as a delicious treat. In other parts of the country, herring was the stuff of salads—skinned, filleted, and served with a fistful of parsley, olive oil, and lemon juice—but on Ikaria, other recipes evolved. In the Smoked Herring Rice recipe (page 201), I explain how it was the food of last resort, when there was literally nothing else to eat. The recipe below is something I worked out on my own after reading a rudimentary description of the dish in a three-tome history of the island, *Laografica tis Ikarias*, by the folklorist Alexis Poulianos.

MAKES 4 TO 6 SERVINGS

2 smoked herrings, filleted (see Note)

2 cups milk

²/₃ cup Greek extra virgin olive oil

2 pounds boiling or cippolini onions, whole but peeled

2 cups chopped canned or grated fresh tomatoes

2 tablespoons tomato paste

¼ cup water

Freshly ground black pepper

Brown or white rice, for serving

Steep the herring fillets in the milk for 2 hours to desalt them. Drain and rinse.

In a large heavy pot or Dutch oven, heat ⅓ cup of the olive oil over medium-low heat. Add the onions and cook until they begin to caramelize, 15 to 20 minutes.

Add the chopped tomatoes and bring to a boil. Dilute the tomato paste in the water and add to the pot. Add the smoked herring fillets. Season with pepper and simmer, covered, over low heat until the sauce thickens.

Serve the stew over brown or white rice.

NOTE: *To fillet a smoked herring, heat water to the boiling point in a deep skillet and submerge the herrings. Return to a boil. As soon as the skin begins to crack open, turn the heat off. Remove with a slotted spoon and place on a plate. Peel off the leathery metallic skin and discard. Hold the herring up by its tail and split it by hand down the middle to fillet.*

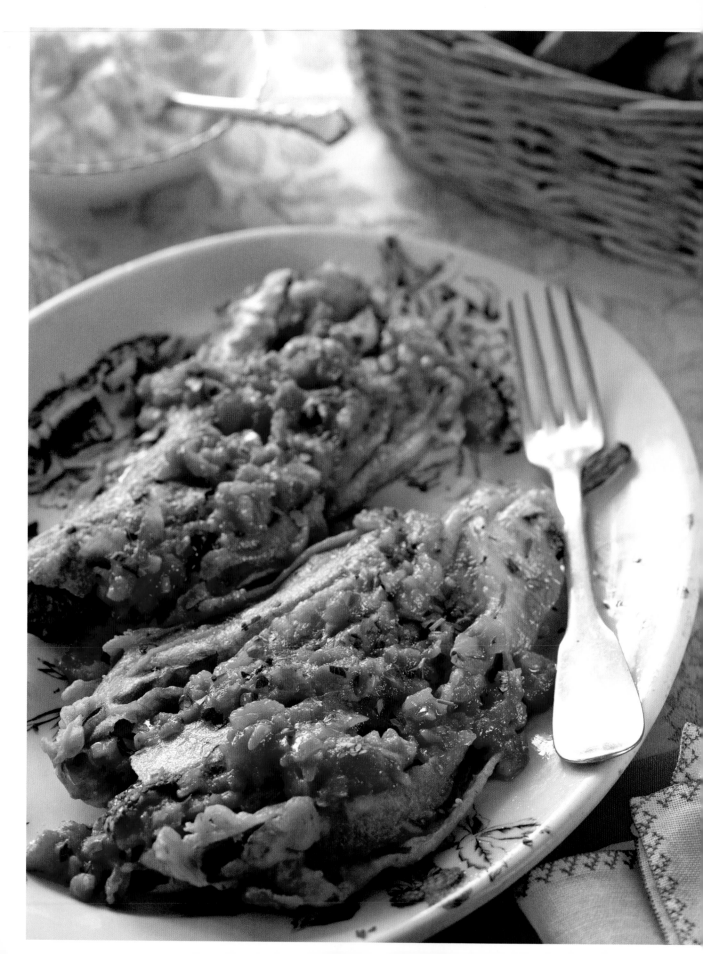

WHOLE BATTER-COOKED EGGPLANTS WITH TOMATOES, ONIONS, AND GARLIC

Melitzanes me Kourkouti kai Tomata

I sat with Myrsina Roussou, 80 or so, in her garden in Manganitis while she recounted numerous recipes and details about the life and food on the island in the 1940s. She mentioned this eggplant dish, which I had heard about from Niki Kohyla-Fakari in Raches, another friend, who recalled her mother making this dish. The eggplants are a bit crunchy thanks to the batter they are fried in, but the tomato sauce is the perfect foil, simple, sweet, and light. You can easily serve this dish as a meze, too, or as local cooks do, with *skordalia* (pages 9 and 11).

MAKES 6 SERVINGS

3 tablespoons Greek extra virgin olive oil

1 large red onion, finely chopped (about 1 cup)

4 garlic cloves, minced

3 cups chopped or pureed tomatoes, preferably fresh

Salt and freshly ground black pepper

Pinch of sugar (optional)

6 Japanese eggplants (long and thin)

1 cup all-purpose flour

1 cup water

Olive oil, for frying

1 small bunch fresh flat-leaf parsley (leaves only), finely chopped

In a medium pot, heat the olive oil over medium heat. Add the onion and cook until wilted, about 8 minutes. Add the garlic and stir to soften. Pour in the tomatoes and season with salt and pepper. If the tomatoes are acidic, add the sugar. Simmer uncovered until thick, about 30 minutes.

Meanwhile, to prepare the eggplants, keep the stems attached and the eggplants whole. With a sharp knife, starting about ½ inch below the stem, cut the eggplants lengthwise to get 3 or 4 slices. The eggplant will look a little like a fan. Season the flesh lightly with salt.

In a wide bowl, whisk together the flour, water, and a little salt.

In a large nonstick skillet, heat about 1 inch of olive oil over medium heat. Press the eggplants into the batter so that both sides of every fanlike slice are covered in batter. Let the excess drip off. Place them, one or two at a time, in the oil. Cook, turning once, until golden brown and soft.

Remove the eggplant with a slotted spoon and drain on paper towels.

To serve, place on a platter, spoon the tomato sauce on top, and sprinkle with parsley.

ONION-AND-TOMATO-STUFFED EGGPLANTS WITH CHOPPED OLIVES AND HERBS

Imam Bayildi

The name of this dish translates as "the imam [priest] fainted." It's both a Turkish and Greek favorite whose name is meant to show just how good it is—so good, in other words, that the priest passed out upon eating it. And no wonder, since *imam bayildi* is the ultimate summer comfort food, luxuriously unctuous, soft, filling, and easy to eat both warm and at room temperature. Indeed, it's even better the next day. The flavors of the vegetables melt together

MAKES 4 TO 8 SERVINGS

FILLING

⅓ cup Greek extra virgin olive oil

6 large red onions, coarsely chopped (about 6 cups)

4 garlic cloves, minced

2 cups coarsely chopped plum tomatoes, with juices

⅓ cup dry red wine

Salt and freshly ground black pepper

1½ cups finely chopped fresh flat-leaf parsley

½ cup chopped Kalamata olives

EGGPLANTS

4 large eggplants, stems removed and halved lengthwise

Olive oil, for brushing

Salt and freshly ground black pepper

For the filling: In a large heavy skillet, heat the olive oil over medium heat. Add the onions and garlic. Cover, reduce the heat to low, and let the mixture steam in the oil, stirring occasionally, until soft and lightly colored, 12 to 15 minutes.

Add the tomatoes, increase the heat, and bring to a simmer. Pour in the wine. As soon as it steams off, reduce the heat and simmer the filling partially covered until there is no longer any liquid in the pan from the tomatoes. Five minutes before removing, season to taste with salt and pepper. Remove and cool slightly. Stir in the parsley and olives.

Meanwhile, for the eggplants: Position a rack 8 inches (20 cm) from the heat and preheat the broiler. Lightly oil a shallow baking pan.

Brush both sides of the eggplants generously with olive oil (the eggplants should glisten from the oil) and place cut-side up on the baking pan. Broil the eggplants until the flesh is softened, 10 to 12 minutes. Turn and repeat on the other side until softened, about 5 minutes longer. The eggplant should not be fully cooked. Take care, too, not to char the eggplants (this is why they are being cooked 8 inches from the heat). Remove and cool slightly. Turn the oven to 350°F (175°C). (Traditionally, the eggplant halves are fried but this makes for a much heavier end result.)

Scrape out as much of the pulp as possible without puncturing the eggplant. Chop the pulp and mix it in with the onion mixture. Taste and season with additional salt and pepper as needed. Fill the eggplants with the onion mixture, forming a rounded mound in each half. Place in a lightly oiled ovenproof glass or ceramic baking pan and bake until the eggplant is completely soft and all the flavors have melded together, about 30 minutes.

THE MEDITERRANEAN DIET BRINGS INNER PEACE

By now, the world knows that the Mediterranean diet is one of the best diets on the planet for preserving physical well-being and preventing chronic disease. Ikarians know instinctively, empirically, and now, thanks to Western science, quantitatively, that their way of eating promotes not only physical health but emotional and spiritual health, too. Perhaps the renowned French food anthropologist Igor de Garine, in his essay "Alimentation méditerranéenne et réalité" (published by the University of Seville in 1997), notes it most eloquently: "What is confirmed, in my view, is the existence of a Mediterranean Model, which, conceived in its totality, excludes anxiety and a sense of guilt, and rehabilitates a way of eating that is innocent, joyous and impregnated with authentic culture." This is Ikaria, circa 2014—a living philosophy, a way of experiencing time, life, and food that weaves our most visceral emotional and physical experiences together intrinsically, instinctively.

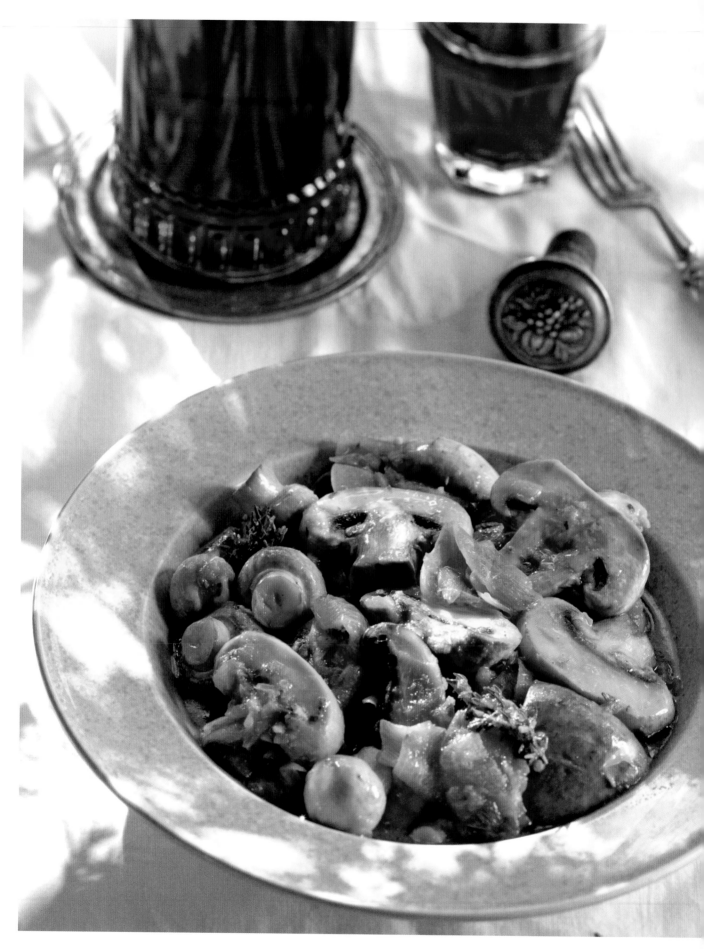

MUSHROOM STEW

Manitaria Yiahni

Ikaria, as I mention in "Mushrooming in the Mountains" (page 27), is a mycologist's paradise. But despite the great variety of wild mushrooms on the island, they are cooked up rather simply, either on the grill, or pickled, or stewed, as below. The mushroom *yiahni* is excellent over pasta or rice or with good country sourdough. It's also excellent with mashed potatoes.

MAKES 4 SERVINGS

1½ pounds (750 g) mixed mushrooms, such as oyster mushrooms, boletus, porcini, chanterelles, portobellos (see Note)

¼ cup Greek extra virgin olive oil

2 large red onions, coarsely chopped (about 2 cups)

2 garlic cloves, finely chopped

½ cup dry red wine

¾ cup chopped canned tomatoes

3 tablespoons red wine vinegar

2 bay leaves

Pinch of ground allspice

3 or 4 sprigs fresh or dried oregano

3 sprigs fresh or dried thyme

Salt and freshly ground black pepper

For large mushrooms such as portobellos and boletus, cut into thick strips or halve, respectively.

In a large, wide pot or Dutch oven, heat the olive oil over medium heat. Add the onions and cook until wilted, about 8 minutes. Stir in the garlic and swirl it around for about a minute.

Add the mushrooms. Cook in the oil for a few minutes, stirring gently. Add the red wine. As soon as it boils off, add the tomatoes, red wine vinegar, bay leaves, allspice, oregano, thyme, and salt and pepper to taste. Cover the pot and simmer over medium-low heat until everything is very tender, 30 to 40 minutes. Serve.

NOTE: *To make this with dried mushrooms, such as dried porcini or chanterelles, reconstitute them in warm water until soft. Drain and strain the soaking liquid. Use in the stew, pouring it in with the wine.*

VARIATION

You can make mushroom and greens stew by adding a pound or two of sweet greens such as chard, spinach, sweet dandelions, sweet sorrel, and/or wild fennel to the stew, right after step 2, before you add the mushrooms. Cook the greens for 10 minutes before adding the mushrooms.

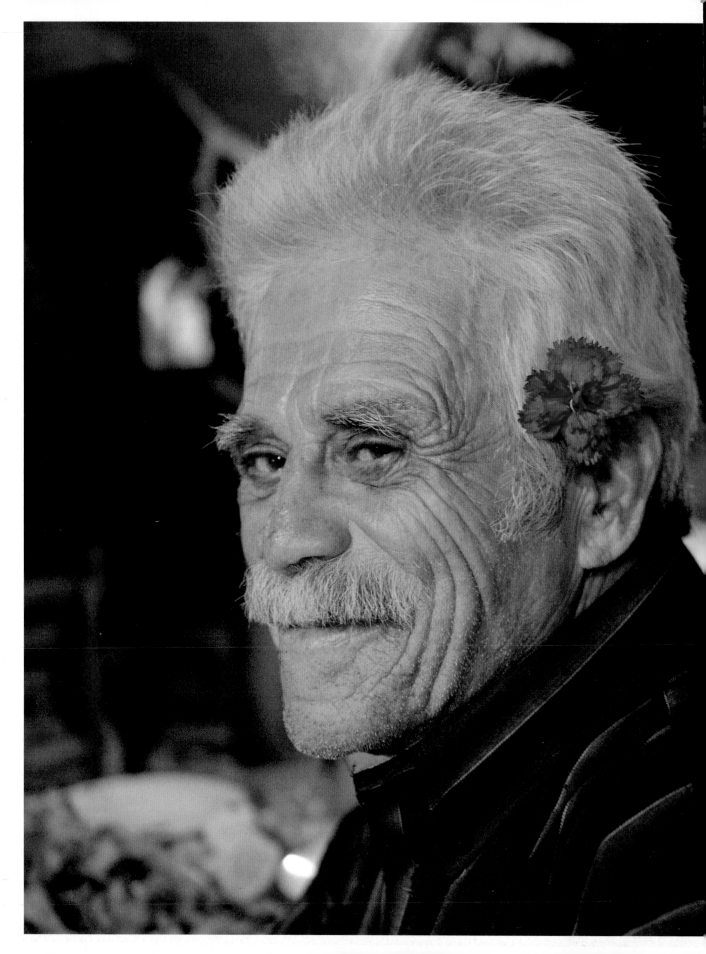

BEANS AND LEGUMES

A LEGACY

OF HEALTH

BEANS AND PULSES ARE ONE OF THE MOST important components of the Mediterranean diet, and continue to provide a great source of protein and balanced nutrition in the local Ikarian diet. People grow beans, and at least one species of legume, the ancient lupine, grows wild all over Ikaria, its bright periwinkle blue flowers sparkling in the forest thicket near our home and elsewhere.

One of the most popular legumes on Ikaria is the black-eyed pea, which is eaten both fresh, pod and all, a summer delight, and then dried and saved for winter. Navy beans, chickpeas, and white beans are all savored in a wide variety of dishes. So are lentils, a pulse, and one of the main staple crops grown on the island until the 1960s, as important for Ikarians' sustenance as barley and wild greens. They are still consumed readily, but not grown any longer.

Beans and pulses are a terrific source of nutrients. They are naturally gluten-free, low in fat, and a great source of cholesterol-free protein. Eating beans also makes us feel sated, explains nutritionist Maria Byron Panayidou. They are a powerhouse of antioxidants, phytochemicals, and important vitamins such as folate. They are exceedingly rich in minerals such as manganese, potassium, iron, phosphorus, copper, and magnesium. The complex carbohydrates they contain, providing a sustained energy source, are digested slowly and are low on the glycemic index.

Fava or broad beans (*koukia* in Greek), chickpeas, black-eyed peas, and lentils are probably the most important legumes in the traditional Ikarian diet. Each one provides stores of health benefits at very low cost. Favas, for example, are rich in protein but also laden with dietary fiber, so much so that one serving provides 66% of the daily recommended allowance, according to the USDA. What that means in practical terms is that they protect the mucous membrane in the colon, thus decreasing our bodies' exposure to toxic substances. Fava beans are also rich in the phytochemical isoflavone, which could help protect against breast cancer.

Chickpeas are also valued for their fiber content and, perhaps more than any other legume, make us feel sated easily. They also carry a unique supply of antioxidants and phytochemicals, including vitamin C, vitamin E, beta-carotene, quercetin, kaempferol, and myricetin, substances that fight disease, such as heart disease and diabetes.

Black-eyed peas, which are actually beans, not peas, contain high amounts of complex carbohydrates, fiber, and protein while being really low in fat. They have an abundance of vitamin K, which is essential in blood clotting; they have a bevy of B vitamins, vitamin A, and lots of potassium, which helps with heart function, as well as good stores of magnesium, calcium, and iron.

Today, beans, legumes, and pulses don't play as major a role on the table as they did 40 and 50 years ago, but there are still plenty of islanders who follow a traditional diet, cooking and eating them at least once and often twice a week.

There is an innate wisdom, too, in the way most Ikarian bean dishes are cooked, that is, almost always in combination with another vegetable, green, or grain. Beans are an "incomplete" protein, a term that refers to foods that contain either low levels of protein or only a few of the nine amino acids our bodies need daily. (Amino acids are the building blocks of protein.) We couldn't function without protein, which comes from the Greek word, protos, or first. Without them our cells and organs, muscles, connective tissue, and even our bones could not hold together. many of our most important hormones, such as insulin, are proteins, as are all the enzymes that help trigger chemical reactions in us. So, when a food contains an incomplete protein, it must be coupled with another incomplete protein to make it complete. Plant-based foods, such as beans, vegetables, and grains are all incomplete proteins, but when eaten together become whole.

The traditional Ikarian recipes in this chapter, such as black-eyed beans with greens, spicy oven-braised beans and pumpkin, Eleni's chickpeas and more, result in dishes chock full of complete protein, food that is healthy, satisfying, and delicious, and totally plant-based.

FRESH OR DRIED FAVA BEAN PUREE

Pourés apo Koukia

Several of the Ikarians over 90 to whom I spoke when researching this book mentioned fava beans as one of the staples in the diets of their youth. They cooked both the fresh and dried beans in the same ways, as stews and puréed with potatoes and garlic.

MAKES ABOUT 4 CUPS

---

2 pounds (1 kg) shelled fresh or frozen fava beans or 1 pound (450 g) split dried fava beans (see Note)

1 russet (baking) or Yukon Gold potato, peeled and cut into 1-inch (2.5-cm) chunks

Sea salt

4 to 6 garlic cloves, minced

²⁄₃ to 1 cup Greek extra virgin olive oil, or more, as needed

¹⁄₃ cup red wine vinegar

FOR FRESH FAVA PUREE: Bring a large pot of salted water to a rolling boil and blanch the fava beans until the skins puff up, about 3 minutes. Remove and drain. Press each fava between your thumb and index finger and squeeze out the bean and discard the membranes.

Place the potato in a pot and cover with cold water. Season with 1 scant teaspoon salt. Simmer over medium heat for 10 minutes, or until about halfway cooked. Add the favas and a little more water if necessary to keep covered. Cook until the beans and potatoes are very tender, about another 10 minutes. Remove and drain, reserving the cooking liquid. Transfer the solids to a food processor or to a large mortar, to be mashed by hand with a pestle.

Pulse or mash the fava-potato mixture with the garlic. Continue either pulsing or mashing and, in alternating doses, drizzle in the olive oil, a little of the reserved cooking liquid, and vinegar until the mixture is smooth and creamy. Season to taste with salt.

FOR DRIED FAVA PUREE: Place the split in a large pot, add enough water to cover by 1 inch (2.5 cm), and bring to a boil. Skim any foam that rises to the top. Cook the favas for about 15 minutes, or until tender but al dente. Add the potatoes and 1 teaspoon salt. Simmer until the favas and potatoes are soft and almost all the liquid has been absorbed, about 20 more minutes.

Reserving the cooking liquid, drain the favas and potatoes. Process or hand-mash as for the fresh fava version.

NOTE: *You can find both whole dried favas and split dried favas in Greek and Middle Eastern grocery stores. The former require overnight soaking, peeling, and then removal of the black eye on the side of the beans; the split dried favas, on the other hand, are easier to use and cook up in a fraction of the time.*

CRANBERRY BEANS COOKED WITH COLLARD GREENS

Karofasola me Lahanides

My friend Eleni Karimali, an excellent cook and farmer in the village of Pygi, taught me to cook onions over low flame in their own juices. She never sautés them at the start of a dish. I follow her rule in this recipe below, and add the oil once the onions have softened—the dish is lighter this way—and then again at the end, when the beans and greens are cooked. Collards and mottled beans create a very earthy final casserole. Both beans and greens should be soft and comforting, then enlivened by the addition of lemon juice.

MAKES 4 SERVINGS

- 1 pound (450 g) dried borlotti or cranberry beans, soaked overnight
- 3 large red onions, chopped
- ½ cup extra Greek virgin olive oil, plus more for serving
- 2 garlic cloves, chopped
- 2 pounds collard greens
- Salt
- Fresh lemon juice, for serving

Drain the beans.

Place the onions in a large, heavy pot. Cover and cook over very low heat until the onions soften and exude their own juices, 6 to 8 minutes, checking occasionally to be sure they don't burn. Add ½ cup of water if necessary.

Add 1 tablespoon of the olive oil and the garlic. Stir a few times to soften, then add the drained beans. Add the remaining 7 tablespoons olive oil and enough water to cover the beans by about 1 inch (2.5 cm). Bring to a simmer, reduce the heat, skim any foam off the surface, and let the beans cook until tender but al dente, about 1 hour. Check now and then for water content and replenish if necessary to keep the beans from burning.

In the meantime, as the beans cook, trim, chop and rinse the collard greens. Add them to the beans. Season to taste with salt. Simmer until beans and collards are tender, another 15 to 20 minutes.

Serve hot, warm, or at room temperature. Drizzle with olive oil and lemon juice to taste.

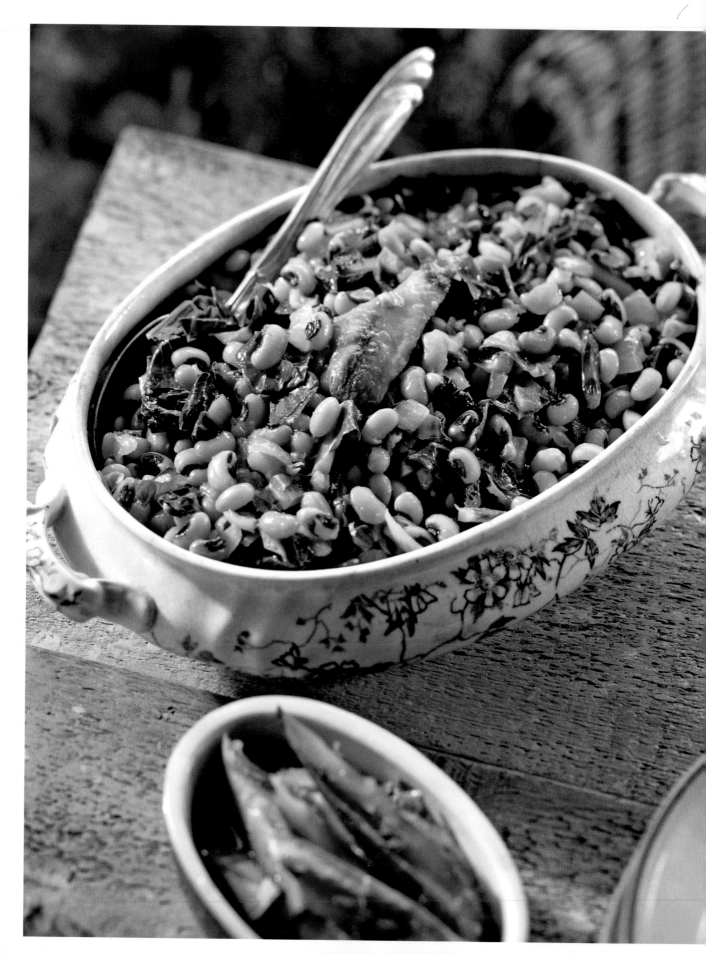

SPICY BLACK-EYED PEAS AND GREENS WITH SMOKED HERRING

Pikantika Mavromatika me Horta kai Renga

Smoked herring, although not native to the Aegean, always seemed to be on hand in the larders and pantries of Ikarian cooks a generation or two ago. It was cheap and easy to keep and it was the classic poor man's *meze*, especially for ouzo, all over Greece. There are a handful of recipes that call for smoked herring in the old island repertoire. This one is robust and spicy; Ikarian cooks often throw a hot pepper or two into bean stews and casseroles.

MAKES 4 TO 6 SERVINGS

- 1 pound (450 g) dried black-eyed peas, rinsed
- 2 large red onions, finely chopped
- 1 or 2 fresh or dried chile peppers
- 2 pounds (1 kg) collard greens or kale, trimmed and coarsely chopped
- 1 cup Greek extra virgin olive oil
- Salt and freshly ground black pepper
- 3 ounces (85 g) smoked herring fillets, Greek lakerda (salted mackerel in olive oil), or salted anchovies or sardines, rinsed

Place the black-eyed peas in a large pot with ample cold water and bring to a boil. Remove, drain, and return to the pot with enough fresh water to cover by 1 inch (2.5 cm). Bring to a boil, reduce the heat to a simmer, and cook until the black-eyed peas are tender but al dente and the liquid has reduced by at least half, about 30 minutes.

Add the onions, chile(s), collards (or kale), ½ cup of the olive oil, and salt and pepper to taste. Cover and cook until all the vegetables are tender and there is almost no liquid left in the pot, another 30 minutes or so.

Remove from the heat to cool slightly, then mix in the remaining ½ cup olive oil. Serve either with the fish on top or on the side.

GREENS AND BEANS, IRON, AND VITAMIN C

Beans are rich in iron, but in a form that our bodies cannot absorb easily. Greens are a rich source of vitamin C, which is necessary for helping our bodies absorb iron. It isn't by accident that so many bean and greens combinations exist in the 'poor man's' diet of Ikaria.

BLACK-EYED PEAS WITH SUN-DRIED TOMATOES AND WILD FENNEL

Mavromatika me Liasti Tomata kai Maratho

My neighbor Titika transforms a good portion of her summer garden bounty into sun-dried vegetables, which she adds to bean dishes in the winter. Black-eyed peas are a popular legume on Ikaria; wild fennel is the herb of choice for so many dishes, since it grows wild everywhere; and the tomatoes lend tang and color. If you can access other sun-dried vegetables such as zucchini, peppers, and eggplant, you may also add them to this fragrant, brightly colored stew.

MAKES 6 SERVINGS

8 sun-dried tomatoes, preferably organic and preferably not in olive oil

2 large red onions, finely chopped

2 garlic cloves, minced

1 pound (450 g) dried black-eyed peas, rinsed

2 cups chopped fennel fronds or wild fennel

Salt and freshly ground black pepper

½ cup Greek extra virgin olive oil

Soak the tomatoes in a little warm water for about 30 minutes to rehydrate.

Meanwhile, in a heavy-bottomed pot, cook the onions over low heat, covered, until soft, about 10 minutes. Check every few minutes and add either a few tablespoons of water or olive oil to keep from burning. Stir in the garlic.

Add the black-eyed peas to the pot. Stir to combine with the onion-garlic mixture. Add enough water to cover the peas by 1 inch (2.5 cm). Cover, bring to a simmer over medium heat, and cook for 30 minutes.

Drain the sun-dried tomatoes and pour their soaking liquid into the pot. Chop them coarsely. Add the tomatoes and fennel to the pot. Season to taste with salt and pepper. Add a little water if necessary to keep the beans moist, and continue simmering until the peas are tender, about another 25 minutes. Remove from the heat and stir in the olive oil. Serve.

SPICY OVEN-BRAISED BEANS AND PUMPKIN

Fasolia me Taboura ston Fourno

I take some liberties with the dish below, a wartime recipe for sustenance that Ikarians ate during the long, hard years of the German occupation and ensuing Greek Civil War. Ikarian pumpkin, *tabouras* in the local dialect, is a variety similar to the long, ribbed calabaza squash. It is planted and grows in gardens all over the island. The combination of pumpkin, beans, tomatoes, and olive oil is a nutritional powerhouse, despite this recipe's humble origins. The original recipe is a one-pot stew. I opted to bake this instead, in order to achieve an almost caramelized, slightly charred end result, and I tinkered a bit with the flavor palette, by tossing in a small fistful of sage leaves and thyme. As a variation, you can also add 2 to 3 tablespoons of balsamic vinegar mixed with 2 tablespoons of Ikarian or other Greek honey 15 minutes before removing from the oven.

MAKES 4 TO 6 SERVINGS

- 1 pound dried navy beans, soaked overnight
- 3 pounds (1.5 kg) pumpkin or butternut or calabaza squash
- 3 large red onions, coarsely chopped
- 3 garlic cloves, minced
- 1 cup chopped plum tomatoes
- 2 fresh or dried chile peppers (optional)
- 4 sage leaves
- 6 to 8 sprigs fresh thyme
- ⅔ cup Greek extra virgin olive oil
- Salt and freshly ground black pepper

Drain the beans and place in a large pot with fresh cold water to cover by 1 inch (2.5 cm). Bring to a boil and simmer until al dente, about 40 minutes, skimming the foam off the surface of the pot. Drain the beans and reserve the cooking liquid.

Preheat the oven to 350°F (175°C).

Peel and seed the pumpkin (or squash). Cut into 1½-inch (4-cm) chunks.

Place the drained beans, pumpkin chunks, onions, garlic, tomatoes, chile peppers (if using), sage, thyme, olive oil, and salt and pepper to taste in an ovenproof glass or ceramic baking dish. Pour in enough of the reserved bean liquid to come about one-third of the way up the contents of the baking dish.

Cover the dish with its lid (or with parchment paper, then foil) and bake for 35 to 40 minutes. Uncover and continue baking until there is no liquid left in the baking dish and the pumpkin and beans begin to char lightly on top, about 15 to 20 minutes.

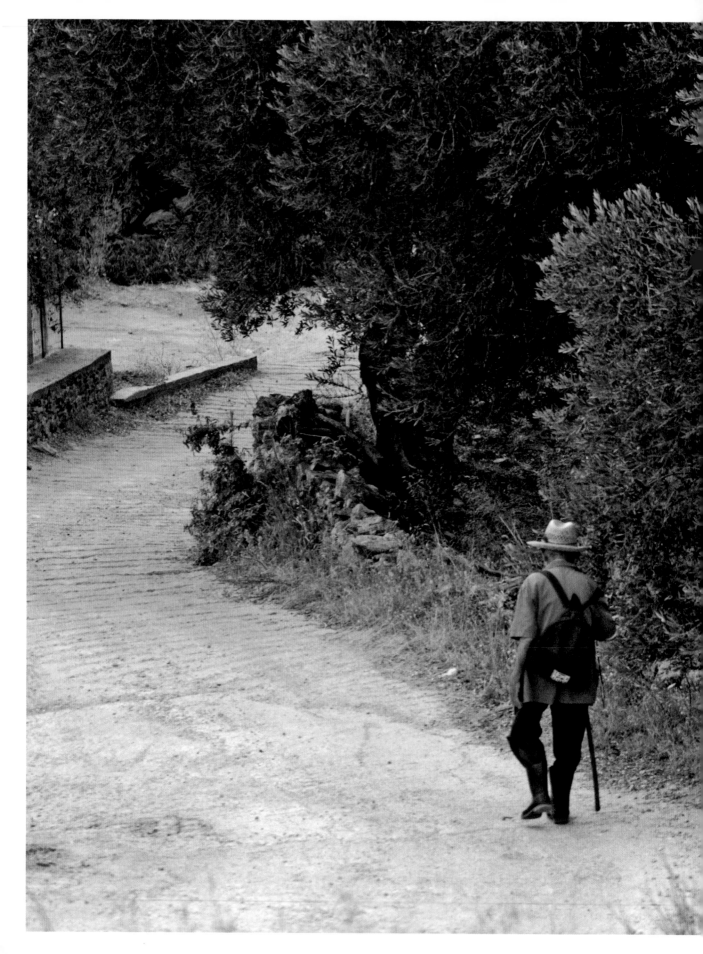

LEMONY FAVA BEANS WITH PICKLED BULBS

Koukia Lemonata me Volvous

This dish calls for one of the most sought-after Ikarian ingredients: *volvoi* (see "Pickled Wild Hyacinth Bulbs," page 33). The wild hyacinth bulbs are blanched in order to rid them of their inherent bitterness, then put up in either salt or vinegar brine. The Sicilians know them as *lampascione*, and you can find them in jars on the shelves of Greek, Middle Eastern, and Italian grocery stores. A not-so-close approximation, but workable nonetheless, would be pickled pearl onions or shallots. If you like sharp, acidic flavors, then this is a dish you will love. The mint, of course, softens the briny intensity of the bulbs. Fava beans are by nature mild and very earthy. Sweetness, acidity, and the comforting subtleness of the beans work together to make this a complex layering of flavors.

MAKES 6 SERVINGS

1 pound (450 g) dried fava beans, soaked overnight

²/₃ cup Greek extra virgin olive oil

1 large red onion, finely chopped (about 1 cup)

4 garlic cloves, minced

1 cup chopped fresh mint

2 teaspoons dried Greek oregano or 2 tablespoons chopped fresh oregano

2 cups rinsed, drained *volvoi* or pickled onions or shallots

Salt and freshly ground black pepper

Juice of 2 lemons, strained

Rinse the beans in a colander and place them in a large pot with enough water to cover. Bring to a boil, reduce the heat, and simmer, uncovered, for 10 minutes. Remove from the heat and drain. The water will be gray and murky.

Return the beans to the pot and add fresh water to cover by 2 inches (5 cm). Bring to a boil, then reduce to a simmer and cook, uncovered, until the beans are al dente, 50 minutes to 1 hour. Remove from the heat and drain. Cool slightly and, using a sharp paring knife, remove the leathery membrane and the dark "eye" on one side of each bean.

In a large wide pot, heat 2 tablespoons of the olive oil over low heat. Add the onion and garlic, cover, and cook until soft, 8 to 10 minutes. Add the beans, herbs, and *volvoi*. Season with a little salt and pepper. Add enough water to come about two-thirds of the way up the beans. Cover and simmer over medium heat until the beans are completely tender, another 20 to 25 minutes.

Remove from the heat, and pour in the remaining olive oil and the lemon juice. Adjust the seasoning with salt and pepper and serve immediately.

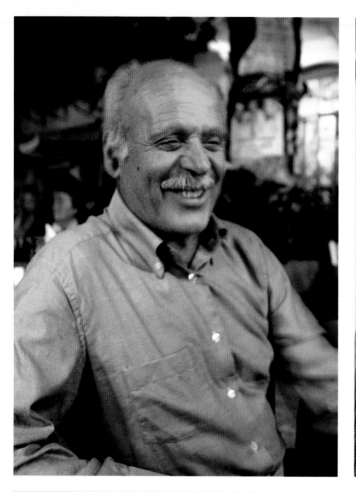
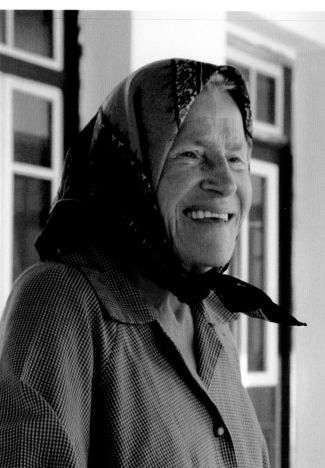
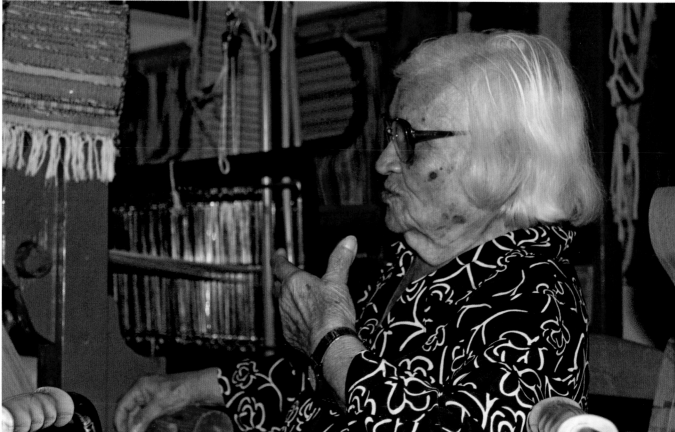

KNOWING AND LOVING THE OLD

When *The Blue Zones* author Dan Buettner and his team contacted me in the early spring of 2009 asking for insights into the healthy, life-giving foods of Ikaria, I, like most other Ikarians, had never given a second thought to longevity. But it was all around me, on and off the island.

My husband's maternal grandmother, for example, from Ikaria, lived to 100; my own Brooklyn-born mother, also of Ikarian descent, thin her whole life despite a diet of Entenmann's crumb cake and peanut-butter-and-jelly sandwiches, died at the age of 95, pretty much well until the end; my paternal Aunt Mary, who taught me so much about how to be close to nature, both through the foods we eat and the rhythms we keep, survived several wars on two continents, family deaths, and much hardship, and returned to Ikaria in 1970 to live out the rest of her years. They turned out to be many. She passed away at 95, after breaking a hip and surviving, releasing herself from the island's old-age home to go back to her humble, one-room home, and living out the rest of her days still active, gardening and knowing everything from village gossip to world news.

Her neighbor and our good friend, Combos, aka Kostas Kohylas, nearing 90, still seems very much in love with Lambrini, his wife of 60-plus years; dances at village celebrations; and drives an hour and back several times a week to Proispera, along the northwestern coast, where he keeps his goats, tends his olive and fruit groves, and tills his extended gardens.

My good friend and fellow Ikarian-American, Basil Safos, has an extended family worthy of study, for all his aunts and uncles on his father's side are still alive or lived well into their nineties, in the United States, active, spry, and alert. His dad Costas, a lovely, gentle man, is 95 as of this writing and still takes his daily stroll in New York City, covering several miles a day to keep fit. Not all of the reasons for Ikarians' legendary longevity are surely environmental; some, indeed, must be genetic.

Longevity was all around me and always had been on Ikaria, but the old are part of the fabric of life in the village and in our communi-

ties off the island. My mother lived with my sister and her family until the very last day of her life, and it gave her purpose and a sense of belonging.

I set out to meet other nonagenarians and centenarians on my native island while researching this book, and by far was most impressed with a sweet but iron-willed lady named Ioanna Prois, whose 101st birthday party I finagled an invitation to—not a hard thing to do in a village on the island. I met her in the summer of 2013. Her narrow garden just outside the village of Christos was filled with friends from 3 to 95 and she was clearly basking in her celebrity, even getting up with her walker to dance a few steps of the *kariotiko*, or island dance. I had never met a woman quite like her, widowed for nearly 40 years and still working as a weaver, both in Athens where she lives half the year and on Ikaria, where she spends the warmer months, helped by her grandchildren. Her daughter, whom I met at her birthday celebration,

(continued)

passed away a few months later, sadly from an aneurysm.

Ioanna is petite and stooped over but her skin is smooth and almost wrinkle-free. Her white hair is neatly cropped. Her mind and wit are razor-sharp. On Ikaria, it's common to ask someone his lineage, with the simple question "Who do you belong to?" meaning, for women, who is your father and/or husband; for men, the question refers to paternal bloodlines. So, of course, she asked me, and to my surprise and hers it turned out that she was a schoolmate, in the one-room schoolhouse just up the road from her home, of my father, who, like her, was born in 1912. She remembered everything about him, his red hair and blue eyes and mischievous humor, his stint as an altar boy and his nickname, "little bishop." But unlike so many of the very old, she didn't only remember the remote past; indeed, I had gone up to see her a few days later and I was about 10 minutes late. I found her at her loom and she reprimanded me, having remembered very solidly the time of our appointment and the nature of our rendezvous: not to learn to weave, of course, although she still teaches, but to ask her about her diet and life on Ikaria when she was a girl.

"We didn't have very much to eat. Mostly *horta* [greens]," was her de facto reply. Then I asked her the obvious question that begged to be asked, about her secret to longevity. "I have always worked and I get great satisfaction from my loom, from creating; I always wake up positive; and I never give up hope and I don't eat very much."

She told me the story of her rocks, a whole collection of local rocks she's picked up and painted over the years and had even gathered into a collection of published photos, one of several books of her work. "I became interested in rocks many years ago because I started to notice how unique each one is. Every rock has its own story to tell, so long as we take the time to look. Just like people, so long as we take time."

Ioanna is one of many centenarians on Ikaria. Another, Grigoris Tsahas, on the south side of the island, is 101. He smokes, drinks about half a liter of wine every day, and walks to the village café and back daily, about a mile and a half in total. He's been an avid smoker for 70 years. But he radiates happiness, health, and stealth, with a crushing handshake and a Frank Sinatra smile.

Then there is our good friend Yiorgos Stenos, nowhere near 100 but robust and vigorous at 83, the legs and charm of Fred Astaire. What I've seen in Yiorgos is something I've noticed in almost everyone on the island well up there in years: a joyful heart, an active body, and no small supply of discipline, perhaps rooted in childhoods marked by poverty and dearth. "If I eat a lot in the afternoon, I never eat at night. But I always drink two and a half cups of wine every day with lunch, never more. In the summer, I add ice," he says matter-of-factly, then explains his theory about the local wine: "It is good because not all the grape juice ever turns to alcohol." He is up at about 7 every day, heads to his bees, and then to his warehouse and general store, and is back for a nap around 3, emerging sometime in the evening, and by that I mean after 10, to take part in village life, at the *cafeneion* mostly. In countless conversations with him over the years, I have been surprised to learn that there are many parts of the island he's never been to. "I am happy right here, right now." Perhaps that attitude is the real secret to longevity.

LEMONY CHICKPEAS BRAISED WITH CHARD AND DILL

Revithia me Seskoula kai Anitho

Legumes and vegetables or greens go hand in hand in so many Greek and local Ikarian recipes. The combination is soothing. Ikarian cooks often add carrots, which add color and sweetness to the final dish. Like all of the bean and vegetable combinations, this stands alone as a perfect vegetarian main course. Serve it with a little goat's milk cheese or feta, good bread, and a drizzling of great olive oil. You won't believe how satisfying it is.

MAKES 4 TO 6 SERVINGS

½ pound (225 g) dried chickpeas, soaked overnight

1 cup Greek extra virgin olive oil

1 large red onion, coarsely chopped (about 1 cup)

2 carrots, finely chopped

3 garlic cloves, thinly sliced

1½ pounds (750 g) green Swiss chard, coarsely chopped

Juice of 2 lemons

1 cup snipped fresh dill

Salt and freshly ground black pepper

Drain the chickpeas and transfer to a pot with enough fresh water to cover by 2 inches (5 cm). Bring to a boil over medium heat, reduce to a simmer, and cook the chickpeas until they are tender but not mushy, about 1 hour 30 minutes. Reserving the cooking liquid, drain the chickpeas and set aside, covered.

Preheat the oven to 375°F (190°C).

In a large, deep skillet or wide pot, heat 3 tablespoons of the olive oil over medium heat. Add the onion and carrots and cook, stirring, until glistening and softened, about 10 minutes. Add the garlic and stir everything together for a few minutes. Add the chard to the pot and cook just until wilted.

Transfer the chickpea and vegetable mixture to an ovenproof glass or ceramic baking dish. Pour half of the remaining olive oil, half the lemon juice, and enough of the reserved cooking liquid to come just below the surface of the chickpeas. Stir in the dill and season to taste with salt and pepper.

Cover with the lid (or parchment paper and then foil) and bake until the whole mixture is dense and creamy, almost like porridge, but with the chickpeas still holding their shape, 35 to 40 minutes.

Add the remaining oil and juice. Adjust the seasoning. Serve hot, warm, or at room temperature.

ELENI'S BAKED CHICKPEAS

Ta Revithia tis Elenis

I just love this dish. For one, it's beautiful when cooked: The peppers and onions that top the chickpeas char slightly, and the simple combination of herbs, chickpeas, and vegetables is brilliant. It is my friend Eleni Karimali's recipe. She makes this for us and her pension guests every summer and she presents it dramatically, parading it from her wood-burning oven to our table in a large clay baking dish. We literally ooh and aah when she presents it. This is served on its own, as a main course, with good bread, a little feta cheese, maybe a dish of boiled greens or a salad. You can serve it right out of the oven or at room temperature.

MAKES 6 SERVINGS

1 pound dried chickpeas, soaked overnight

6 sprigs fresh thyme

2 sprigs fresh rosemary

3 bay leaves

Salt and freshly ground black pepper

3 large red onions, halved and sliced

3 garlic cloves, cut into slivers

1 red bell pepper, cut into ¼-inch (6-mm) rings

1 green bell pepper, cut into ¼-inch (6-mm) rings

1 yellow bell pepper, cut into ¼-inch (6-mm) rings

1 small carrot, halved lengthwise and cut lengthwise into thin (⅛-inch [3-mm]) strips

2 large firm-ripe tomatoes, cut crosswise into 6 slices

⅔ cup Greek extra virgin olive oil

Drain the chickpeas and place back in a large pot with enough fresh cold water to cover by 2 inches. Bring to a boil, then reduce to a simmer and cook until halfway to tender, about 1 hour. Reserving the cooking liquid, drain the chickpeas.

Meanwhile, preheat the oven to 325°F (160°C).

Place the drained chickpeas in an ovenproof clay or ceramic baking dish with a lid. Pour in enough of the reserved cooking liquid to come about two-thirds of the way up the beans. Add the herbs to the pan. Season with salt and black pepper.

Layering them in the following order, arrange the onions, garlic, bell peppers, carrot, and tomatoes over the chickpeas. Drizzle ⅓ cup of the olive oil over the contents of the baking dish. Cover the pan with its lid (or with parchment paper, then foil) and bake the chickpeas for 2 hours 30 minutes. Remove the cover and bake until very tender and the liquid is almost all gone and the vegetables on top are almost charred, another 30 minutes. Serve hot, warm, or at room temperature.

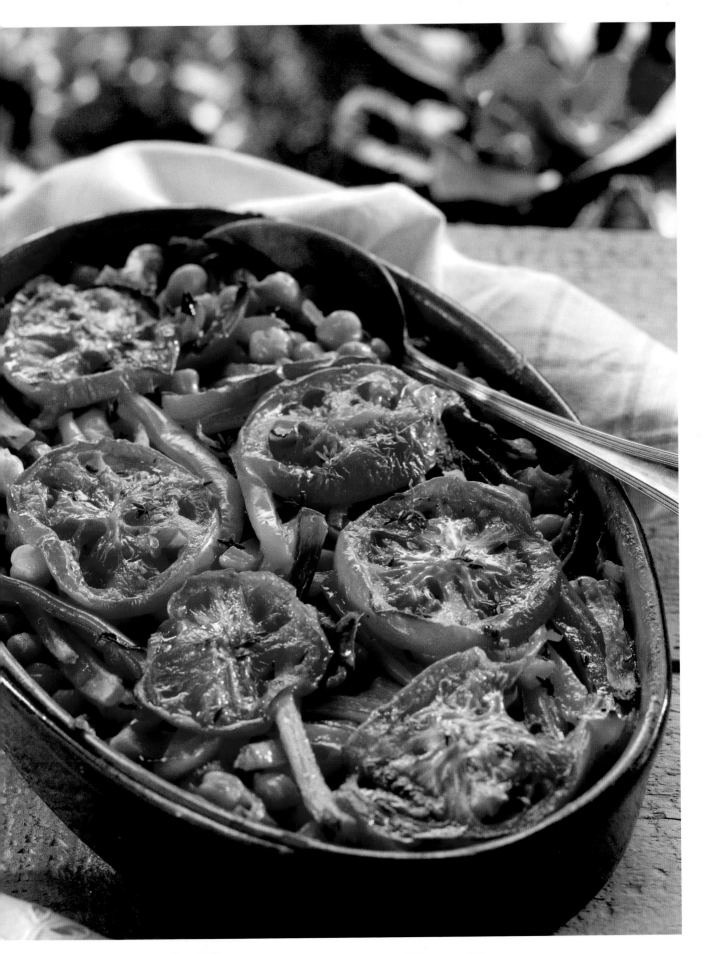

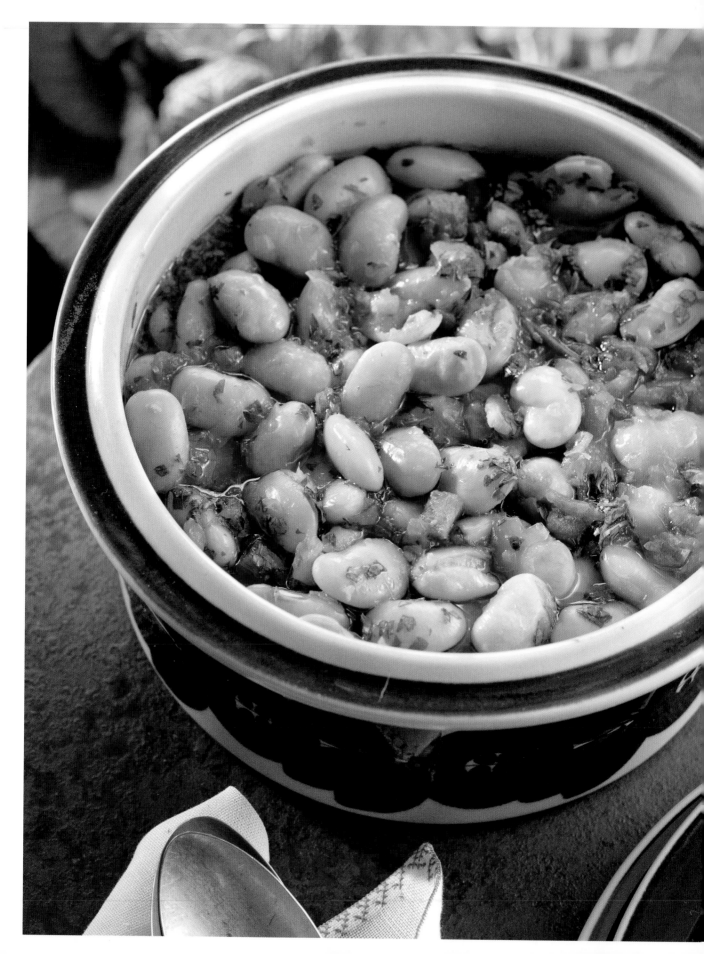

GIANT BEANS BAKED WITH GRAPE MOLASSES AND HERBS

Gigantes me Petimezi kai Myrodika

I have made this dish in other versions, with my favorite Ikarian pine honey and fresh orange juice. *Petimezi*, the subtle, sweet syrup made by cooking down clarified grape must, is one of the world's oldest natural sweeteners. In this dish, it lends balance to the already earthy beans and it pairs beautifully with the tomatoes and herbs.

Greek giant beans (called *gigantes*) are unique for their quality and their ability to cook up into creamy beans that still hold their shape. The best come from northern Greece and may be found in Greek and some gourmet shops around the country. You can substitute butter beans or lima beans, but they will need less cooking time.

MAKES 6 TO 8 SERVINGS

- 1 pound (450 g) dried Greek giant beans (gigantes), soaked overnight
- 2 large red onions, chopped (about 2 cups)
- 2 large garlic cloves, chopped
- 2 bay leaves
- 2 cups chopped fresh or canned plum tomatoes
- ⅔ cup Greek extra virgin olive oil
- 3 tablespoons *petimezi*
- 2 to 3 tablespoons red wine vinegar (to taste)
- Sea salt and freshly ground black pepper
- 1 cup chopped fresh flat-leaf parsley
- ½ cup chopped fresh oregano leaves

Drain the beans and place them in a large pot with enough fresh cold water to cover by about 2½ inches (6 cm). Bring to a boil over medium heat, reduce to a simmer, and cook uncovered until the beans are slightly undercooked, about 1 hour. As they simmer, skim off the foam that forms on the surface of the water.

Preheat the oven to 375°F (190°C).

Reserving the cooking liquid, drain the beans and transfer to a large baking dish. Add the onions, garlic, bay leaves, tomatoes, ⅓ cup of the olive oil, the *petimezi*, and vinegar and salt and pepper to taste and stir to combine thoroughly with the beans.

Add enough of the reserved cooking liquid to come up just below the surface of the beans. Cover with parchment paper, then foil, and bake until just tender, about 1 hour. Uncover, stir in the herbs, and continue baking until almost all the liquid has been absorbed and the beans still hold their shape but are very soft and buttery on the inside, another 20 to 30 minutes.

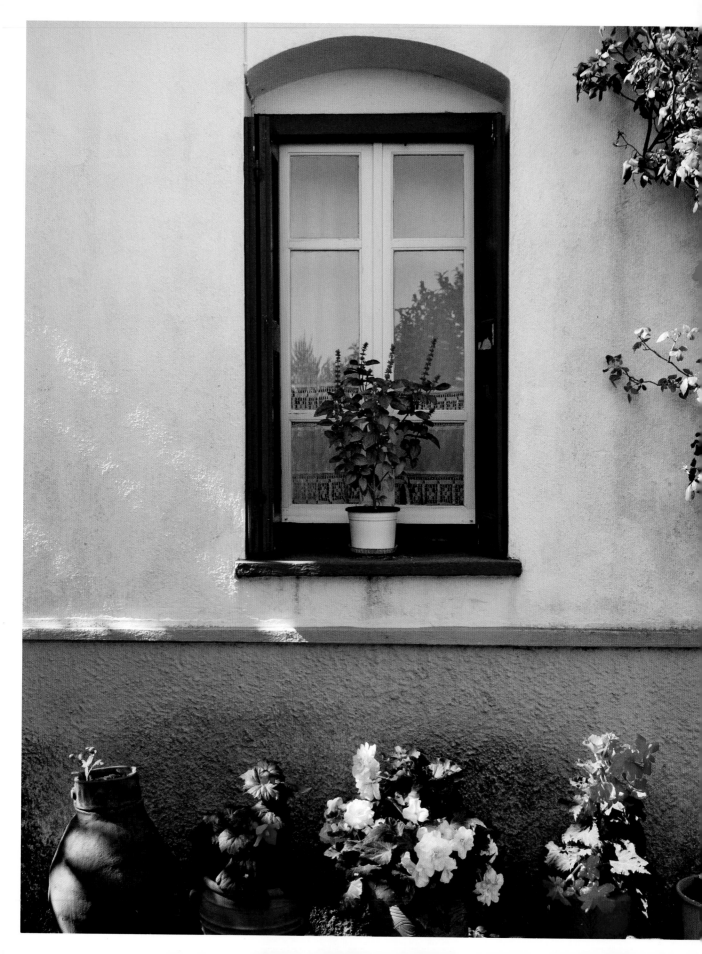

PASTA AND RICE

PASTA AND RELATED WHEAT PRODUCTS HAVE LONG been staples on Ikaria and throughout Greece. Indeed, one of the things few people even realize about Greek cuisine is the long history of pasta in the diet, dating to the stone-grilled strips of batter the ancients called *laganum*, by some accounts a precursor to flat, wide noodles, and the tremendous variety of shapes that exist from region to region to this day.

On Ikaria, the main local pasta shape is called *matsi*, and it can be either a flat strand similar to, but shorter than, fettuccine, or curled, or a small square. A few devoted traditionalists still make it by hand.

Yet the story of pasta on Ikaria is a little ironic, because wheat, such a Mediterranean diet staple, never really flourished on the island. Old varieties like dinkel and spelt grew for eons, but only in a few places since there is so little arable land. In the early part of the 20th century, an Ikarian emigrant to Australia, on one of his intermittent trips back to the island to visit his wife and children, planted a strain of wheat that took hold on the north side of the island. The locals nicknamed it Canberra! But mostly, wheat used in Ikarian homes was actually grown by the Ikarian charcoal makers, who worked across the water on the coast of Asia Minor (Turkey) and owned and tilled fields there. They'd leave in the spring to sow and work, and return in the late fall with the harvest and enough money to see their families through the winter.

The traditional pasta dishes, still made on the island, are very simple, typically with nothing more than the pasta itself, plain cooked tomatoes, and olive oil, or layered with home-brined goat's milk cheese and hot olive oil—dishes, in other words, that evolved from the need to fill bellies with what was on hand.

Today, home cooks still make pasta, and at least one artisanal cooperative on the island produces local shapes for sale. But mostly, pasta now is packaged and dried and recipes run the gamut from classic pastitsio to the Ikarian fare mentioned above.

Despite the fact that wheat was a difficult crop to grow on Ikaria, it was still a part of the traditional diet in all the manifestations just mentioned. Rice, however, was not a mainstream grain until fairly recently in both the Ikarian and overall Greek diet.

It wasn't grown commercially in Greece until after the 1950s, when the country, decimated by World War II and then by a bloody civil war, began to rebuild itself, in large part with moneys from the Marshall Plan. American agronomists headed to northern Greece and taught local farmers how to cultivate what would become one of the most important Greek crops. Rice used to be the grain of feasts and illness: a rarity saved for wedding meals, Christmas, New Year's, and Easter dishes, or, in the form of simple soups and puddings, for family members who were under the weather. Bulgur and dried corn kernels (see page 146) were much more common in pilafs, stuffed vegetables, and soups.

Today, despite Ikaria's relative isolation and rural lifestyle, limitations in the food supply have all but disappeared. Almost no one grows his own wheat anymore and one would be hard-pressed to find someone under 60 who remembers the time when rice was a rare, expensive grain. Dishes typically associated with rice—pilafs, certain soups, stuffed grape leaves, and stuffed vegetables—on Ikaria were more commonly made with bulgur and dried corn.

But other grain preparations are still part of the living tradition. Many people, for example, still make their own *trahana* (page 98) with milk from their own goats or bought from neighbors. Home cooks still make their own pasta, if not regularly then at least on special occasions like "Cheese Sunday," the Sunday before Lent starts, when tradition dictates one indulge in a steaming bowl of fresh pasta with lots of cheese and butter. Generally, now, common Greek dishes like pastitsio (thick spaghetti layered with ground meat and béchamel) and *yiouvetsi* (orzo baked with chicken or lamb) are everyday recipes even on Ikaria. As for rice, just the fact that dishes like summer vegetables stuffed with rice and herbs have become everyday fare speaks tomes for how common now is rice, the once-exotic grain reserved for celebrations and convalescence. Most local recipes for both are still simple, characterized by fresh herbs, easy techniques, and seasonal ingredients.

ELENI KARIMALI'S NOODLES WITH YOGURT AND HERBS

Oi Hilopites tis Elenis me Yiaourti kai Myrodika

The local homemade pasta variety, a flat, longish shape a little like fettuccine, is called *matsi*, perhaps after the Semitic matzoh. *Matsi*, either as a flat, eggless noodle or a square-shaped one, is found all over the eastern Aegean.

Our friend Eleni makes this delicious dish at the pension and winery she and her husband run in the village of Pygi. She makes all of her own pasta, and her small, cozy kitchen filled with wooden bowls, jars of preserves, and racks of dowels where strands of her fresh pasta hang to dry is one of my favorite places on the island. The herbs that she cuts for this dish come from the garden that surrounds her home. Use the freshest possible herbs for the best possible flavor, and try to source Greek yogurt from small producers (page 299).

MAKES 4 TO 6 SERVINGS

6 tablespoons Greek extra virgin olive oil

1 large red onion, finely chopped

2 garlic cloves, minced or very thinly sliced

2 cups finely chopped mixed fresh herbs: marjoram, mint, oregano, wild fennel, parsley, thyme

Salt and freshly ground black pepper

1 pound fettuccine or tagliatelle, preferably fresh

2 cups plain Greek yogurt

1 teaspoon grated lemon peel

In a medium skillet, heat 2 tablespoons of the olive oil over medium heat. Add the onion and garlic and cook until soft, about 8 minutes.

In a small bowl, combine the herbs, onion-garlic mixture, and salt and pepper to taste.

Bring a large pot of well-salted water to a rolling boil and cook the pasta to desired doneness. Before draining, ladle out 2 cups of the pasta cooking water and whisk them into the yogurt, together with the remaining 4 tablespoons of olive oil and the lemon peel.

Drain the pasta and toss it together with the yogurt mixture and herbs. Season to taste with additional salt and pepper and serve hot.

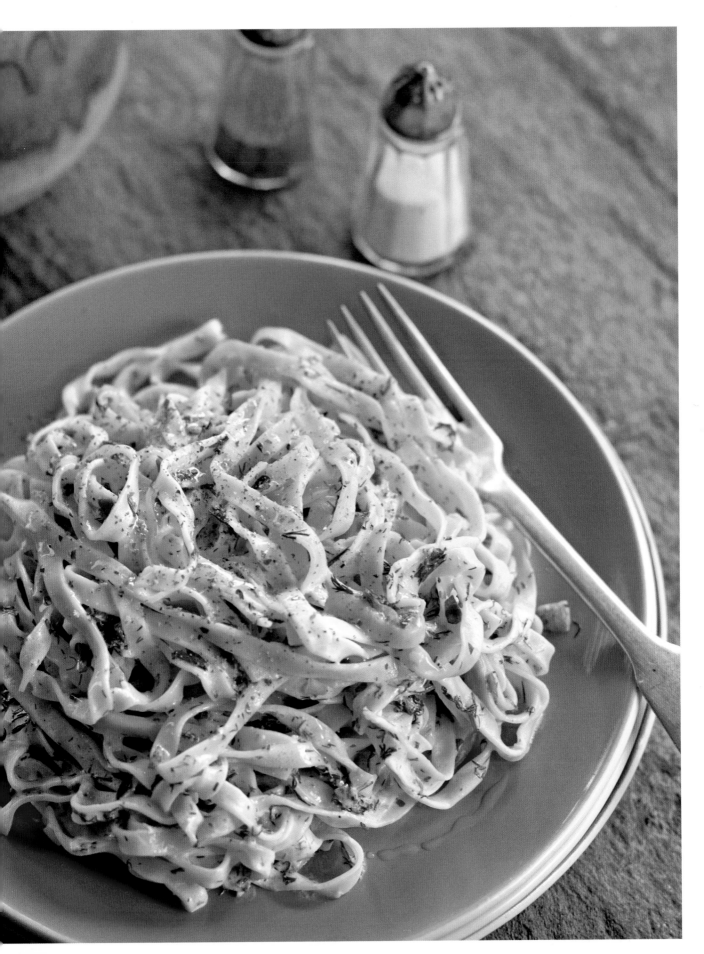

SIMPLE PASTA AND TOMATOES, IKARIA-STYLE

Y Pio Apli Kariotiki Makaronada

This is the simplest of meals, prepared with homemade pasta that Ikarian kids almost always helped roll, or with store-bought thick, tubular spaghetti and a very simple tomato sauce made from grated fresh summer tomatoes. (You can make this dish without the tomatoes, too.) Preserved goat's milk cheese is in the larder of every home, too, the family goat or goats usually tied to a tree outside the house.

MAKES 4 TO 6 SERVINGS

---

1 pound thick tubular spaghetti

8 tablespoons Greek extra virgin olive oil

6 firm-ripe tomatoes, grated on the large holes of a box grater

Salt and freshly ground black pepper

Pinch of sugar (optional)

2 cups coarsely grated dried goat's milk cheese, such as Greek Myzithra or Ikarian *kathoura*, or sharp sheep's milk cheese such as pecorino or aged Ikarian *kathoura*

Bring a large pot of well-salted water to a rolling boil and cook the pasta to desired doneness.

Meanwhile, in a deep skillet, heat 2 tablespoons of the olive oil over medium heat. Add the tomatoes, season with salt and pepper to taste, and simmer just long enough to cook off the excess liquid from the tomatoes, 10 to 15 minutes. If the tomatoes are acidic, add a pinch of sugar.

Drain the pasta and toss with 2 tablespoons of the olive oil.

Place one-third of the pasta on a serving platter and sprinkle with one-third of the cheese and one-third of the tomatoes. Repeat two more times.

In a small saucepan, heat the remaining 6 tablespoons olive oil and pour over the pasta. Toss to combine and to soften and melt the cheese with the hot oil. Serve immediately.

RED GOAT AND PASTA

Katsikaki Kokkinisto me Zymarika

Goat is by far the "national dish" on Ikaria, and it's easy to understand why. As of this writing, there are about 8,000 permanent inhabitants on the island and about 40,000 goats. But even before the ruminant population swelled to uncontrollable numbers—the result of pay-per-goat EU subsidies that encouraged shepherds to increase their herds—*really, truly*, wild goats called *rasko* were still the traditional source of protein, providing everything from milk to meat.

Goat is savored young, milk-fed or just a little older, and roasted whole right around Easter. It's also carved up into pieces whose destination is either the grill (goat chops), the oven, the stew pot, or the cauldron. Lemons, garlic, and oregano are one trio of seasonings for Ikaria's goats, but so are tomato, garlic, and herbs, as in this recipe, which is a traditional Sunday dish on the island.

MAKES 6 TO 8 SERVINGS

½ cup Greek extra virgin olive oil

4 pounds (2 kg) bone-in goat shoulder, cut into serving pieces

2 large onions, quartered

4 garlic cloves, minced

Salt and freshly ground black pepper

2 cups chopped fresh or canned plum tomatoes

1 tablespoon tomato paste

1 tablespoon dried Greek oregano

2 bay leaves

4 allspice berries

1 pound Greek noodles (*hilopittes* or *matsi*), tagliatelle, fettucine, or egg noodles

1 cup grated Greek Myzithra cheese, aged Ikarian *kathoura*, or pecorino

In a large, wide pot, heat the olive oil over medium heat. Add the meat in batches if necessary and sear until browned. Add the quartered onions and stir until softened, 10 to 15 minutes. Stir in the garlic. Season to taste with salt and pepper.

Pour in the tomatoes, tomato paste, herbs, allspice berries, and enough water to cover the contents of the pot. Bring to a boil. Reduce the heat, cover, and simmer until the goat is very tender and falling off the bone and the sauce thick, about 2 hours. Remove the goat from the pot and transfer to a platter. Tent the goat with foil to keep warm. Remove the herbs and allspice berries from the sauce with a slotted spoon and discard.

Dilute the sauce with enough water to come about two-thirds of the way up the pot. Bring to a boil. Add the pasta and simmer until it becomes softer than al dente and the sauce thickens slightly.

Serve the pasta and sauce on a platter, place the goat meat on top, and sprinkle both with grated cheese.

SOUP-STEW WITH BULGUR AND LAMB

Tsorvas me Pligouri

Here's an old Ikarian recipe for a hearty winter dish that's not quite a soup and not quite a stew. I doctored it up a little by adding vegetables to the broth for flavor. You can also add a bit of tomato paste and even some mushrooms to the pot to achieve an earthier aroma. I've been tempted to throw in a dash of sheep's-milk butter for extra flavor, but this is not something any country cook on Ikaria would probably ever do! I suggest serving the soup-stew with bread and one of the *kopanisti* (cheese spread) recipes (pages 6 and 7).

MAKES 6 TO 8 SERVINGS

2 pounds (1 kg) bone-in lamb, goat, or pork shoulder, cut into serving pieces

1 large onion, peeled and whole, plus 1 onion, finely chopped

2 celery stalks, halved

1 carrot, peeled and whole

2 bay leaves

3 or 4 sprigs fresh thyme

2 quarts water

Salt and freshly ground black pepper

½ cup Greek extra virgin olive oil

1½ cups coarse bulgur wheat

Juice of 1 to 2 lemons (to taste), strained

Rinse and pat the meat dry. Place the meat, whole onion, celery, carrot, bay leaves, thyme, and water in a large pot. Bring to a boil, reduce the heat, season generously with salt and pepper, and simmer, skimming the foam off the top, until the meat is so tender it is falling off the bone, about 2 hours.

Remove the meat with a slotted spoon and set aside to cool. Pull the meat off the bone and shred. Strain and reserve the meat broth, discarding the vegetables and herbs.

In a large, wide pot or Dutch oven, heat ¼ cup of the olive oil over medium heat. Add the chopped onion and cook, stirring occasionally, until soft, 8 to 10 minutes. Add the bulgur and toss to coat in the oil. Add 4 cups of the meat broth to the bulgur, cover, and bring to a boil. Reduce the heat to low. Add the shredded meat to the bulgur and simmer, stirring occasionally, until the bulgur is soft and swollen and the mixture thicker than porridge, 10 to 12 minutes.

Remove from the heat, and stir in the remaining ¼ cup olive oil and lemon juice. Adjust the seasoning with more salt and pepper, if desired. Serve.

PERIWINKLE PILAF

Pilafi me to Salingari tis Thalassas

Periwinkles, beautiful, tiny mollusks, are one of the great gratis treats on Ikaria, so long as one is willing to dive for them. This is an old recipe, which I have modified a little to suit modern palates. If you can't find periwinkles, you can just as easily use small clams or small, fresh sea whelks, which do require time to clean and shell. Canned whelks are also available. This dish, when eaten on the island, is saturated with the briny, iodine-tinged flavor of the sea.

MAKES 4 SERVINGS

6 cups live periwinkles (see Note)

6 cups water

1 tablespoon coarse sea salt

½ cup Greek extra virgin olive oil

1 large red onion, grated (on the large holes of a box grater) or minced, with juices

1 cup long-grain rice

1 cup grated fresh tomato or chopped canned plum tomatoes

½ cup dry white wine

1 fresh or dried chile pepper (optional)

Salt and freshly ground black pepper

2 tablespoons chopped fresh flat-leaf parsley

Lemon wedges, for serving

Rinse the periwinkles under cold running water.

In a pot, bring the water and the coarse salt to a rolling boil. Add the periwinkles and cook for 5 minutes. Remove the periwinkles with a slotted spoon. Reserve the cooking liquid and ,when it has cooled a little, filter it through a fine-mesh sieve lined with a coffee filter or a double thickness of cheesecloth.

In a large, deep skillet or shallow, wide pot or Dutch oven, heat ¼ cup of the olive oil over medium heat. Add the onion and cook, stirring, until soft, 8 to 10 minutes.

Add the rice and toss to coat. Stir in the tomatoes, 1 cup of the filtered broth, ½ cup tap water, the wine, and the chile pepper (if using), and season with salt and black pepper. Simmer, covered, until the rice is almost cooked, about 15 minutes.

Toss the periwinkles into the rice mixture. Cook together until the rice is completely done. Sprinkle with the parsley and serve with lemon wedges.

NOTE: *You can also make the dish with small clams. First rinse the clams well and steep them in a bucket or basin of cold water, swishing around to dislodge any sand. Do this three or four times, emptying and replenishing the water each time. Place the clams in a steamer basket inside a large, wide pot filled with 6 cups of water. Cover and steam until the clam shells have opened, about 5 minutes. Discard any that have not opened. Toss the clams with the rice when you would have added the periwinkles.*

LIMPET OR CLAM PILAF

Pilafi me Petalides

Limpets are small gastropods that cling tenaciously to the rocky coast of Ikaria. They used to be very plentiful and their shells almost alabaster white. But nowadays, their numbers are dwindling and rogue tar deposits sometimes turn their grayish white shells charcoal black. But Ikarians know how to distinguish the good ones from lesser-quality limpets and seek them out, scraping them off rocks when weather permits.

Sometimes they're blanched and served almost like a salad, with olive oil, lemon juice, and parsley, or they are cooked, as in this old recipe. If limpets are not available, you can substitute small clams.

MAKES 4 TO 6 SERVINGS

2 pounds (1 kg) fresh (live) limpets or small clams

2 cups water

2 garlic cloves, peeled and whole

3 tablespoons Greek extra virgin olive oil

1 large red onion, finely chopped

1 cup long-grain rice

Salt and freshly ground black pepper

1 tomato, grated

2 tablespoons chopped fresh oregano

2 teaspoons red wine vinegar

Soak the limpets or clams in a large basin of cold water, changing the water every hour or so, for about 3 hours, to rid them of their grit and sand.

In a large pot, combine the water and the garlic. If using limpets, blanch for 2 to 3 minutes in the garlic-flavored water and drain. Scrape the limpets out of their shells with a small spoon and set aside. If using clams, cover and steam in the garlic-flavored water over high heat until their shells open, about 5 minutes. Remove. Drain and discard any whose shells have not opened. Set aside the opened ones.

Pour the steaming liquid through a fine-mesh sieve lined with a coffee filter or a double thickness of cheesecloth and reserve it.

In a large, wide pot, heat the olive oil over medium heat. Add the onion, reduce the heat to low, cover, and cook, stirring occasionally, until soft, about 10 minutes. Add the rice and stir to coat.

Pour in 1½ cups of the reserved limpet/clam cooking liquid and a little salt and pepper. Add the tomato and oregano and cook, stirring, until about half the liquid is absorbed, about 5 minutes.

Add the limpets (or clams) and the vinegar. Cook all together for a few more minutes, until the rice is done. Cover the pilaf with a clean kitchen towel and let stand for 10 to 15 minutes before serving.

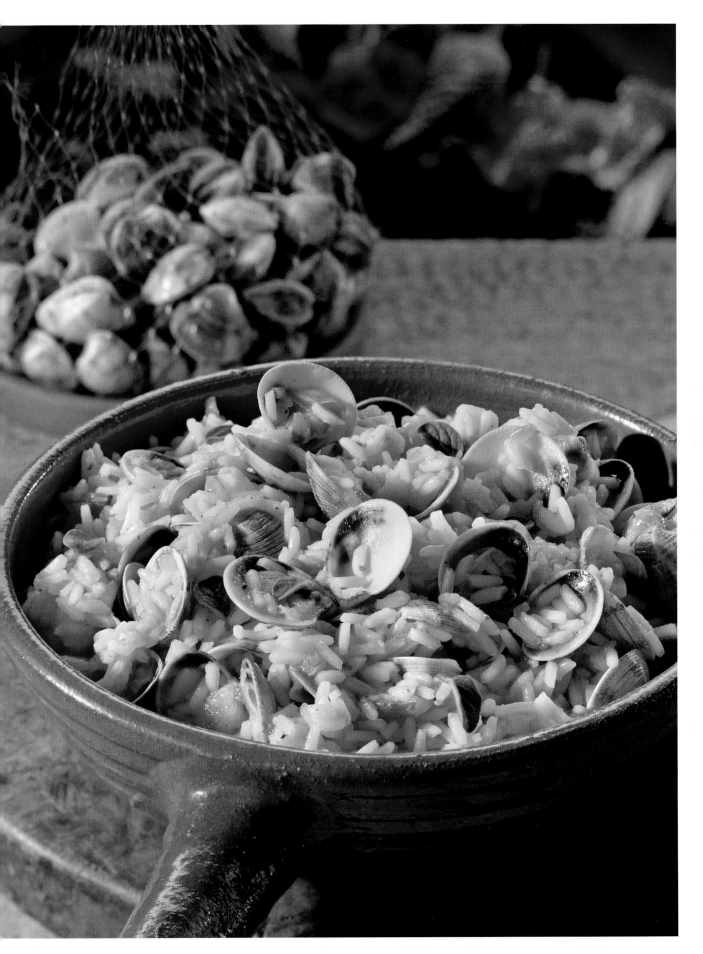

SEA URCHIN AND FRESH TOMATO PILAF

Pilafi me Ahino

Islanders on Ikaria, inured to the easy reach of sea urchins, not only savor them raw, but also pour them into a steaming pilaf with fresh tomatoes and a little black pepper.

If you have access to fresh (live) sea urchins, opening them is easy. Take scissors and cut into the little hole and then around it, like cutting a circle. Dislodge the cut piece of shell with the scissors. Pour out the juice, which may contain sand. Squeeze a bit of lemon into the open sea urchin and, using a spoon, scoop out and slurp up its flesh. Or simply empty its flesh into a small bowl filled with a little salted water, without squeezing lemon into it, if you want to use the sea urchin for a dish such as the pilaf that follows. Drain and use. When you buy sea urchin, it usually is packed in a little salt water. Sea urchins are a great source of protein, fiber, and vitamins C, A, and E. They contain minerals such as zinc, iodine, and calcium. Greeks consider them aphrodisiac, perhaps with good reason: Vitamin E helps circulation and zinc recharges our libidos. Combined with rice, they provide a balanced meal.

MAKES 4 SERVINGS

4 tablespoons Greek extra virgin olive oil

1 medium red onion, finely chopped or grated (about $2/3$ cup), with juices

1 garlic clove, minced

1 cup long-grain rice

1 cup grated fresh tomatoes

3 or 4 sprigs fresh marjoram

3 cups water or fish stock

$2/3$ cup dry sherry or Ikarian red or white table wine

$1\frac{1}{2}$ cups sea urchin flesh and juices

Sea salt and freshly ground black pepper

Finely grated peel of 1 lemon

In a wide, shallow pot or deep skillet, heat 2 tablespoons of the olive oil over medium heat. Add the onion and cook until soft, 8 to 10 minutes. Add the garlic, and give it a few swirls to coat it in the oil. Add the rice and stir to coat in the olive oil.

Stir in the tomatoes and marjoram. As the juices are absorbed, add 1 cup of the water (or stock) and stir. Cover, reduce the heat to low, and cook until the liquid is almost absorbed. Add the sherry and stir. Add another 1 cup of the water (or stock), stir, cover, and simmer until almost completely absorbed.

Add the sea urchin and its juices and remaining 1 cup water (or stock). Season to taste with salt and pepper and simmer, covered, until the pilaf is soft, almost like risotto. Stir in the lemon peel. Remove from the heat, remove and discard the marjoram, and stir in the remaining 2 tablespoons olive oil. Serve immediately.

LEEK RICE

Prasorizo

Like spinach rice, leek rice is one of the simple, country dishes on Ikaria (and elsewhere) that are easy, nutritious, and prepared from simple, available ingredients. Although all the vegetable rice dishes in this chapter and, indeed, in the Greek kitchen, are meant traditionally to be eaten as main courses, especially but not exclusively during periods of fasting, I often use them as accompaniments to fish and other protein. A pinch of saffron, while not Ikarian in any way, also adds great flavor to this dish. In all of these vegetable rice dishes, the rice is cooked for more time than most American cooks are used to, until *very* tender. Greeks love their rice dishes soft and creamy.

MAKES 4 SERVINGS

½ cup Greek extra virgin olive oil, plus more for serving

3 leeks, trimmed of the toughest part of the greens, cleaned, and coarsely chopped

1 garlic clove, chopped

1 cup long-grain rice

1 cup chopped fresh or canned plum tomatoes

2 cups water

Salt and freshly ground black pepper

In a large, wide pot or deep skillet, heat the olive oil over low heat. Add the leeks and cook until wilted, 8 to 10 minutes. Add the garlic and stir to coat in the olive oil.

Add the rice and stir to coat. Stir in the tomatoes, water, and salt and pepper to taste. Reduce the heat, cover, and cook until the liquid is absorbed and the rice very tender, about 25 minutes.

Serve drizzled with olive oil.

VARIATION

Cabbage Rice: Follow the directions above, but substitute 1 large onion for the leeks, and add 4 cups shredded green cabbage to the pot when you cook the onion and garlic. You can omit the tomato if desired, but 2½ cups of water if you do so. The cabbage will release a little liquid.

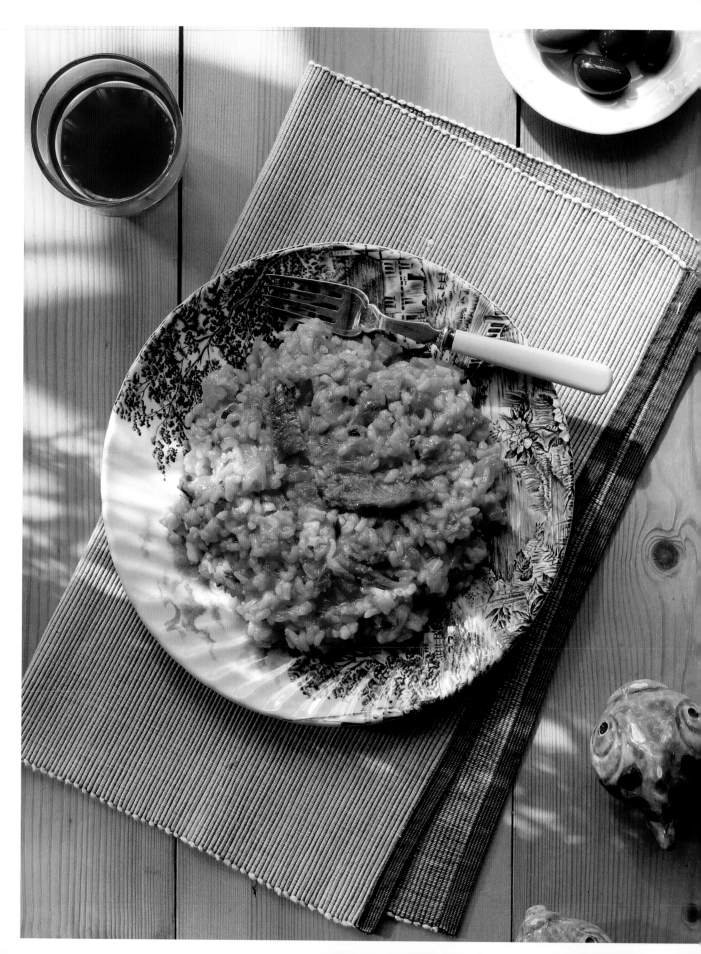

SMOKED HERRING RICE

Pilafi me Renga

This is one of the most interesting and unusual recipes I found in my talks with older people on Ikaria. It's a dish they remember from the Occupation, one that helped stave off hunger. "We ate this when there was nothing else to eat!" says Yiorgos Stenos, my source for much information on old Ikarian ways. "There were always salted herrings and salt cod in the shops and pantries before the War," he adds. "With some onions, tomatoes, and olive oil we made this a meal." Actually, it's quite a delicious and ingenious dish.

And, it's full of good, sound nutrition. Herring, like other fish, contains high levels of omega-3 fatty acids, protein, and vitamins, especially D and B_{12}. It's a good source of minerals like zinc and calcium. It's at the bottom of the food chain, which means it's relatively clean and free of contaminants like mercury, which is more prevalent in larger, predatory fish.

You can find whole smoked herring in Greek, Middle Eastern, Caribbean, and other ethnic markets.

MAKES 4 SERVINGS

2 whole smoked herrings or 10 ounces (285 g) herring fillets

½ cup Greek extra virgin olive oil

1 onion, minced

1 cup long-grain rice

1 cup grated or pureed fresh tomatoes or chopped canned tomatoes

Salt and freshly ground black pepper

1 cup chopped fresh flat-leaf parsley

If using whole smoked herrings: Fill a wide pot or deep skillet with 6 cups of water and bring to a boil. Add the whole herrings, poach for 2 to 3 minutes, and carefully remove with a slotted spoon. Transfer to a plate. Let the fish cool. Remove its skin, which will have puffed up. Carefully remove the fillets and discard the head, bones, and skin. Shred the flesh into small pieces. Reserve the cooking liquid.

If using fillets: Poach for 3 minutes in 2½ cups unsalted boiling water. Remove, cool, and shred as above. Reserve the cooking liquid, measure out 2 cups, and set aside.

In a large, wide pot or deep skillet, heat ¼ cup of the olive oil over medium heat. Add the onion and cook until soft, 8 to 10 minutes. Add the rice, tomatoes, and reserved cooking liquid. Simmer the rice until half cooked. Add the shredded herring and stir gently. Cook over low heat until the rice is tender, 8 to 10 more minutes. Taste and adjust the seasoning with salt, if needed, and pepper. Stir in the chopped parsley. Mix in the remaining ¼ cup olive oil just before serving.

WEDDING MEALS

Catering for a wedding on Ikaria is a sight. At both weddings and local feasts, 2,000 or 3,000 people attend, all hungry! The cooking takes place at various times and in various kitchens. At my wedding on the island, 30 years ago as of this writing, my mother-in-law and her cousins rolled and fried 2,000 meatballs. The women on both sides of the family always help with the food, especially the individual things, like Ikarian *pitarakia* (Small Herb and Greens Pies, page 116), dips, and pastries.

But the men handle the big stuff—namely the roasted goats and the *gamopilafo*, which is rice cooked in goat broth, a necessary item on the table and a salve for the wine that flows and flows.

Salads, dips, little pies, hand-rolled grape leaves, meatballs, rice, boiled goat, and roasted goat are on the traditional menu. For the small stuff, the women might start weeks ahead, or even months, as for dolmades, anticipating that the grape leaves are only in season in the spring. They roll, and freeze, and then cook off the day of the event.

For the big stuff, the cooking starts on the night before the wedding. At the village center, where most cooking facilities are, the aroma of country goat poaching in huge copper pots, usually outdoors under a small protective roof, pervades everything. The rice is cooked in that broth, which is seasoned with spices, herbs, tomatoes, and sometimes wine.

Then, the day of the wedding or christening, all the friends of the couple volunteer in the kitchen, plating the first few rounds of *mezedes*, then the boiled meat and rice and, finally, the roast. They set about 40 portions at a time on large planks and bear them shoulder to shoulder, delivering them in sections across the village square or churchyard. It is a surprisingly effective and fast way to get so much food out to so many people.

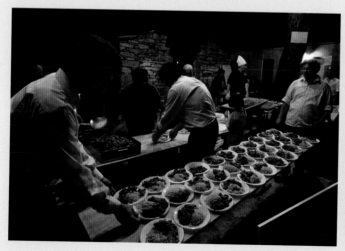
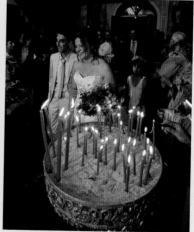

WEDDING RICE

Gamopilafo

Here's a recipe for wedding rice, a delicious combination of meat broth and spices toned down, not in flavor but in quantity, for the needs of an average family dinner. The pilaf rice, a short-grain variety, is available in Greek and Middle Eastern food stores.

MAKES 8 SERVINGS

- ⅔ cup Greek extra virgin olive oil
- 3 pounds (1.5 kg) bone-in goat or lamb, leg or shoulder, cut into large serving pieces
- 2 large red onions, finely chopped
- ½ teaspoon ground allspice
- 1 scant teaspoon ground cinnamon
- 2 cups white wine

- 3 cups chopped canned plum tomatoes or grated fresh tomatoes
- 3 bay leaves
- 5 or 6 allspice berries
- 1 cinnamon stick
- Salt and freshly ground black pepper
- 1½ cups short-grain rice (for pilafs)

In a large, wide pot, heat the olive oil over high heat. Add the meat, in batches if necessary, and sear until browned on all sides. Remove the meat and set aside, tented with foil.

Add the onions to the pot, reduce the heat, and cook until soft, 10 to 12 minutes. Stir the ground allspice and cinnamon into the wilted onions.

Return the meat to the pot. Pour in the wine and as soon as it steams up, add the tomatoes, bay leaves, allspice berries, cinnamon stick, and salt and pepper to taste. Add enough water to come just below the surface of the meat. Cover, reduce the heat to low, and simmer until the meat is so tender it falls off the bone, about 2 hours 30 minutes.

Using a slotted spoon, remove the meat, cinnamon stick, and allspice berries. Set the meat aside on a plate, tented with foil to keep it warm. Discard the spices.

Measure the liquid in the pot and add enough water to make 4 cups total. Bring to a boil. Stir the rice into the broth and cook over low heat until the rice is tender.

Serve immediately, with the warm meat on top.

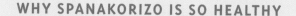

WHY SPANAKORIZO IS SO HEALTHY

The calcium in the rice combined with the inulin in the spinach gives spanakorizo bone-strengthening deliciousness. The duet of olive oil, with its monounsaturated fat, and the vitamin K in the spinach helps prevent blood clotting and lowers bad (LDL) cholesterol. The beta-carotene in the spinach in combination with great extra virgin olive oil also gives our complexions a healthy glow. Add to the spanakorizo a squeeze of lemon, and you also help your body to easily absorb the iron in the spinach.

Spanakorizo is stereotypical on the Ikarian table and on the wider Greek table, too. It is something home cooks make as a fairly quick, cheap, easy meal. It is also an excellent example of the mantra of this book and of the Mediterranean Diet as a whole: that the simple, delicious, seasonal, real food from this part of the world carries innate nutritional wisdom in almost every bite.

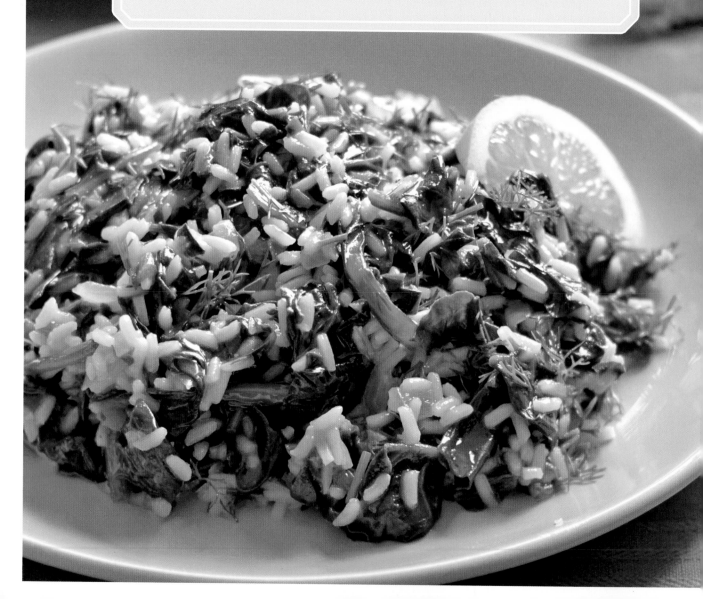

SPINACH RICE

Spanakorizo

Spinach rice is still one of the classics of the Greek table, on Ikaria and all over the country. But rice was not always plentiful. Older recipes for this dish call for bulgur instead, which may be substituted in this and other pilafs.

MAKES 4 SERVINGS

4 tablespoons Greek extra virgin olive oil

1 cup finely chopped red onion

1 garlic clove, minced

1 cup long-grain rice

8 cups chopped fresh spinach, about 1 pound (450 g), stems removed, cleaned well

½ cup water

½ cup chopped wild fennel fronds or dill

Sea salt and freshly ground black pepper

Juice of 2 lemons, strained

In a large heavy skillet, heat 2 tablespoons of the olive oil over medium heat. Add the onion and cook stirring frequently, until soft, 2 to 3 minutes. Stir in the garlic. Add the rice and stir with a wooden spoon over medium-low heat for 3 minutes.

Add the spinach, cover, and cook until the spinach loses most of its volume. Add the water, fennel (or dill), and salt and pepper to taste. Simmer, covered, stirring occasionally until all the liquid is absorbed and the rice is cooked and very tender, 25 to 30 minutes. Add more water as needed if you think it is necessary to achieve a creamy consistency. You can do so about halfway into cooking the mixture. Add the lemon juice 3 minutes before the end.

VARIATION

Spinach-Bulgur Pilaf: A generation ago, bulgur wheat was less expensive and more prevalent than rice and many of the vegetable pilafs we know today were made, in fact, with bulgur. For this pilaf, just substitute the same quantity coarsely milled bulgur for the rice and cook in exactly the same way. You can substitute coarse bulgur in any of the vegetable pilafs.

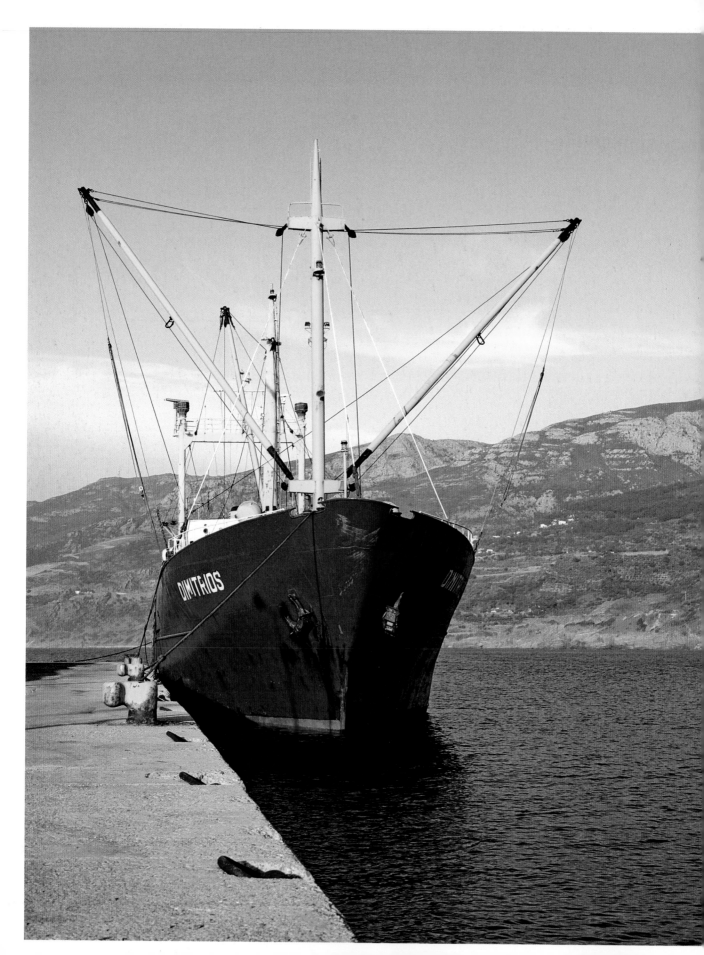

SEA LIFE

ON AND OFF
THE TABLE

THE SEA SURROUNDS US ON IKARIA, AND IS VISI-
ble from almost every angle, every height. It's a provider of sustenance, employment, excitement, pleasure, and memories; it's a force to be reckoned with. I've feasted from it and feared it, I've been calmed by it and frustrated by it, especially in August when the northerly *meltemia* winds blow. But mostly, I've been in awe of it, of how it changes from second to second, of its secret life and its role as shaper of Ikarian history and cuisine.

The sea is why Ikaria remained so isolated for so many centuries (thus preserving local customs, even now) and the reason why the island has been a place of exile throughout almost all its history. Ikarian waters are the roughest sailing ground in the Aegean. Once you reach the island it is hard to leave, even today, if the Beaufort scale, which measures wind strength and wave height, goes past 8, which means a very choppy Aegean. The island was earmarked from the Hellenistic period to the military dictatorships of the 20th century as a place to send political undesirables; once they were on the island, there really was no viable way for them to get off. That the islanders made them feel welcome is part of the sense of solidarity and hospitality that still runs deep on Ikaria. And the sea is still fierce. Even today, one rarely sees sailboats plying local waters because the winds are too strong.

The sea is why Ikaria's earliest villages were inland and camouflaged, lookouts where locals could see pirates and other threats approaching, without themselves being seen.

But the sea is also Ikaria's lifeline and siren call. Without it, so many generations of Ikarian men would have had no livelihood, some as fishermen but most as sailors. Tourism might have developed more quickly had the island's waters been easier to ply, but today its beaches are one reason why people do flock here in the summer. I knew the murky Atlantic before I ever dipped a toe in the Aegean, but I remember the feeling of floating in the water at Messakti Beach in the early '70s and seeing the sea floor with my naked eye, for the first time at the age of 12. It was and still is pure joy.

But the sea is also flavor. It's octopus fresh, chewy, and intensely salty; it's Ikarian lobster grilled at Karakas' taverna in Karkinagri on the south side and served with island lemons and rustic local olive oil; it's red mullets and the sweet, delicate flesh of 6-inch-long *ballades*, which are one of Ikaria's most prized local fish, members of the bream family.

For Ikarians most of the sea's bounty is cooked in the simplest ways: fried, like sand-smelts; poached or boiled for soup; grilled or sometimes—rarely—baked. When fish is so fresh it practically jumps out of the water, all you really need or want to do is to cook it as simply and as close to the time it was caught as possible.

Greek seafood aficionados think about fish in several terms: Beyond differentiating between species, they categorize fish by perceived or inherent quality, and they think about fish by size and fleshiness to know which cooking method is best.

"Ah, grouper? That's an A category fish. Wild bream—a B class fish," Niko, a good friend and a once-avid fisherman stated matter-of-factly to me on one of many days his wife, Argyro, had made one of her soothing fish soups with his catch of gelatinous grouper, scorpion fish, and a score of other, smaller fish. It's a feast we have repeated many times at his home in Raches.

Neither boniness, nor size, nor fleshiness necessarily determines the categories that fish fall into; it's all about flavor. Ultimately, it is the sweetness of the flesh that determines which category people consider a fish to be in, and that flavor is directly related to the fishes' own diet and environment.

Ikaria is still blessed, despite the ever-encroaching dangers of pollution and overfishing, with a rich marine life. Indeed, one of its ancient names was Icthyoessa, which means "plentiful of fish." Deepwater and surface fish still abound, as do octopus, squid, flying squid, a few mollusks, crabs, and several varieties of lobster. There are about 100 miles of coastline around the island, and Ikarian waters boast both rich biodiversity and large areas of seagrass beds, which provide food and shelter for many species of fish.

FISH IN THE IKARIAN KITCHEN

Fish is integral to the diet on Ikaria and a general rule applies: Small fish are fried, and large fish are grilled, baked, or made into soup.

Smaller species that abound in local waters include sand-smelts (eaten whole, bones and all, for plenty of phosphorous), bogue, and several varieties of bream, among them what is known locally as *sargos* and another, much-loved bream species, *kefalades* or *balades*, which we devour in the summer. Red mullets, *barbounia*, also abound and are great pan-fried. So are the webbed fins of small stingrays, or *salahia*. And yet another favorite is hake, or *bakaliaraki*, as well as *galeos*, dogfish. A lot of pan-fried fish is served with *skordalia*, the garlic puree made throughout Greece; on Ikaria, it is most commonly made with a base of stale bread.

Small oily fish, such as sardines, don't abound in Ikaria's deep waters, but several other, larger, species of oily fish do, among them amberjack, or *mayiatiko*, literally "May fish," alluding to its season. Mackerel and chub mackerel migrate through Ikarian waters, too. Local cooks grill or bake them. Large tuna—both the rare yellowfin and more abundant bluefin—as well as swordfish, also migrate past Ikarian waters, and you can sometimes find them in local fish markets. Wrasse or parrotfish are both esteemed, but the latter is unique. Because it's an herbivore, people eat it viscera and all, generally grilled.

If there were such a thing as fish royalty, the grouper would be king, but right up there in high esteem is also the wild gilt-head bream and swordfish, both excellent on the grill. Some of the best fish are the rockfish, such as *skorpina*, or scorpion fish, and grouper, *rofos*. Grouper head, which is very gelatinous, makes thick, delicious soup and scorpion fish, when large, taste like lobsters on the grill; smaller ones are excellent in soup. Stargazers, or *lihnos* in Greek, which as my husband, an avid fisherman, points out "has a jaw that juts out, like the Spanish kings that Goya painted," are also delicious grilled or in soup. One of the tastiest soup fish is the weever, or *drakena*, which needs to be cleaned with care because of its poisonous spines.

This isn't by any means a definitive list of all the fish that swim in and around Ikarian waters. It is just a sampling of the most popular species.

How to Pan-Fry Fish

Small fish like bogue and smelts as well as slightly larger fish, such as red mullets, grey mullets, and various species of bream, are all well suited for frying.

Scale and gut the fish. Keep the heads on. Dredge lightly in flour. Heat about ½ inch (1.5 cm) olive oil in a large, heavy skillet until just below the smoke point, about 325°F (162°C). Slip a few pieces of fish at a time into the oil and fry, leaving to crisp and turn golden on one side before carefully flipping with a spatula to the other side. Remove, drain on paper towels, and serve with lemon wedges.

STOVETOP SALT COD WITH TOMATOES AND ONIONS

Plaki me Bakaliaro sto sto Tsoukali

This dish, called *plaki* all over Greece, is usually prepared in the oven. But on Ikaria, *plaki* is almost always a stovetop preparation, because until a generation ago very few homes had electric ovens.

In this recipe, I'm taking the liberty of adding a little bit of grape molasses, called *petimezi*, to the sauce. The grape molasses has a very subtle sweetness that balances the acidity of the tomatoes.

MAKES 4 TO 6 SERVINGS

- ½ cup Greek extra virgin olive oil, plus more for garnish
- 2 large red onions, cut into ¼-inch (6 mm) rounds
- 3 garlic cloves, finely chopped
- 1 pound (450 g) large firm-ripe fresh tomatoes, chopped, or 2 cups canned plum tomatoes with juice
- ½ cup dry red wine

- 3 tablespoons *petimezi* (grape molasses) or sweet wine, such as Mavrodafni or port
- 2 bay leaves
- Salt and freshly ground black pepper
- 2¼ pounds (1 kg) salt cod, soaked and softened (see Note)
- 4 to 5 tablespoons chopped fresh flat-leaf parsley

In a large, wide pot, heat ¼ cup of the olive oil over medium heat. Add the onions and garlic and cook until soft, about 10 minutes.

Add the tomatoes, red wine, *petimezi* (or sweet wine), and bay leaves. Season lightly to taste with salt and pepper. Cover and simmer over low heat until the sauce is thick, 20 to 25 minutes.

Place the fish on top. Spoon a little sauce over it in the pot. Continue to cook over low heat, covered, until the fish is fork-tender, about 15 minutes. Sprinkle with parsley, pour in the remaining ¼ cup olive oil, and serve.

NOTE: *Cut the salt cod into serving pieces and soak them in cold water for 2 to 3 days, refrigerated, changing the water every 4 to 5 hours.*

VARIATION

Use hake or swordfish, cut into steaks about 1½ inches (4 cm) thick, in place of salt cod.

HAKE BAKED WITH OKRA

Bakaliarakia me Bamiyes

Okra and small hake—*bakaliarakia* in Greek—are both plentiful in the summer. Hake, like its relatives cod, haddock, and pollock, is fleshy white fish with a clean texture and a mild flavor. Okra in many ways is the opposite, slippery in texture and very earthy in flavor. The acidity in the tomato that goes into this dish, too, brings it all together.

This dish, and others like it, where fish and vegetables are married, is nutritionally complete. Hake, a deep-sea member of the cod family, is a powerhouse of omega-3 fatty acids, protein, and vitamins B_1, B_2, and B_3, and a good source of phosphorous. Okra, on the other hand, is known for its high levels of vitamins C, K, and B_6. It is rich in fiber, which helps us digest better and stabilizes blood sugar. One ingredient deals with our arteries and the fat deposits in them and the other with sugar levels, digestion, and kidney health," as Maria Byron Panayidou, the resident nutritionist for this book says.

MAKES 4 SERVINGS

- 1 pound (450 g) baby okra
- Salt and freshly ground black pepper
- ⅓ cup red wine vinegar
- 2¼ pounds (1 kg) whole hakes, head on, gutted and scaled
- Juice of 1 lemon, strained
- ⅔ cup Greek extra virgin olive oil

- 2 large red onions, finely chopped (about 2 cups)
- 2 garlic cloves, minced
- 3 large firm-ripe tomatoes, grated or pureed
- Pinch of sugar
- ½ cup finely chopped fresh flat-leaf parsley

Trim the okra: Using a small, sharp paring knife, trim around the base of the stem. Place the okra in a shallow bowl and toss with 1 teaspoon of salt and the vinegar. Let stand, preferably in the sun, for an hour. (This helps the okra attain a firmer, less mucilaginous texture.)

Meanwhile, season the hake with salt and freshly ground black pepper and sprinkle with the lemon juice. Cover and refrigerate for 1 hour.

In a large, wide pot or deep skillet, heat ⅓ cup of the olive oil over medium heat. Reduce the heat, add the onions and garlic, and cook, stirring, until soft, 10 to 12 minutes.

Add the okra, turning gently to coat in the olive oil. Add the tomatoes, sugar, and additional salt and pepper. Cover and cook over low heat until slightly thickened, about 10 minutes.

Gently place the hake over the okra, in one layer if possible. Cook until fork-tender, about 20 minutes. Approximately 5 minutes before removing from the heat, sprinkle in the parsley.

FISH COOKED OVER WINTER GREENS

Psari sto Tsoukali me Horta

This is an old recipe, one that calls for several rare greens, namely milkweed (*galatsida*) and Mediterranean hartwort (*kafkalida*). On Ikaria, these grow in the winter and early spring and people collect them avidly (see "A Whole World of Greens and Herbs," page 48). In the States, the options are a bit different, since many edible weeds are considered pests and have been killed off by the extensive use of pesticides. But you can buy seeds and cultivate them or scour specialty produce companies for some. For the recipe below, you can also replace the rare stuff with Swiss chard, spinach, or sweet dandelions. Please note, too, that milkweed, which is very common and used in many recipes on Ikaria, can be bitter and toxic when raw. Boiling milkweed, as in the dish below, removes any toxicity.

As with Hake Baked with Okra (opposite), so does this dish cover many of our nutritional needs, with the fish providing a healthy protein and low fat and the greens providing vitamin C.

MAKES 4 TO 6 SERVINGS

2¼ pounds (1 kg) salt cod, cut into serving pieces, soaked, and desalted (see Note, page 80), or other white fish, cut into steaks

⅔ cup Greek extra virgin olive oil

2 large red onions, chopped

1 bunch Chinese celery, with leaves, chopped

3 garlic cloves, chopped

4 large potatoes, peeled and cut into ½-inch (1.5-cm) rounds

1 bunch flat-leaf parsley, chopped

4 cups mixed aromatic greens and herbs, which may include chervil, milkweed, sweet sorrel, sweet dandelion, spinach, chard, wild fennel, and dill

Salt and freshly ground black pepper

Rinse and drain the salt cod, if using, and set aside.

In a large, wide pot, heat ⅓ cup of the olive oil over low heat. Add the onions, celery, and garlic and cook, stirring occasionally, until soft, about 12 minutes.

Place the potatoes, parsley, and greens in alternating layers in the pot, seasoning each layer lightly with salt and pepper. Cover the pot, reduce the heat to low, and simmer until the potatoes are about halfway cooked, 12 to 15 minutes.

If using fresh fish, season with salt and pepper. Place the fish on top. Cover and cook until the fish is fork-tender, about 20 minutes. Remove from the heat, pour in the remaining ⅓ cup olive oil, and serve.

THE FISHERMEN OF IKARIA

Fishermen spend their days untangling and cleaning debris, shells, and flotsam from mountains of canary-yellow nets, or methodically stringing the long line, called *paragadi*, with its 100-odd hooks, around the lip of big plastic wash basins that they've outfitted with cork along the rim, the better to float. My image of them is a composite: Kapetan Dano, a friend, on the edge of Armenistis, the small fishing-village-turned-tourist-town near our home, copper-skinned and squinting in the sun; Karacas, with his droopy face, a yard of thick, ripply flesh stretched over a few inches of bones, such a contrast to his hands, which are powerful and muscular; Kollia, with the aquiline, sculpted profile of an ancient Greek, angles sweetened by a windswept head of long curly hair and dimples. These are some of the faces that bring us fresh summer fish, and to do so, it takes patience, hard but slow work, and knowledge.

Fishermen are generally a taciturn lot. The ones I know use their hands to express most things. The size of a catch is what they show by opening their palms to various lengths; a red mullet is delicious when it's "this big," as Karakas, who also owns a small fish tavern in Karkinagri, on the south side, said once, showing me his index finger, as thick as a cigar.

The fishing methods on Ikaria are still traditional and, thankfully, regulated. Sport fishermen cannot bring in more than 6 kilos (about 13 pounds) at a time.

When they fish with nets, there are two types. One, with bigger holes, is dropped "like a curtain," explains Karakas, that has little lead weights on the bottom; fine-holed nets float on the surface to catch smaller fish. The long line drops several hundred feet, each hook baited. These are jobs they do at night, then head out in the morning, having left floaters, to see what they've caught. A hundred hooks might yield four or five fish in total. The *katheti*, another long line, has fewer hooks but requires attention. It's something they drop if they're on board, to tug and pull at whatever may get snagged. It takes hours at sea.

On Ikaria, the fishing is good but erratic, especially on the north side, which can get rough. Fishermen are devoted to it and totally present, knowing the winds, the clouds, the moon, and, not least of all, the seabeds where prized fish like mullets or bream cavort.

This is life in the moment. Aware. Alert. Full. And for fish lovers like me, it's the moment, too, that matters, when the catch is but an hour or two out of the water, sputtering on a grill, and brimming with all the life, lore, and flavor of the magical Aegean.

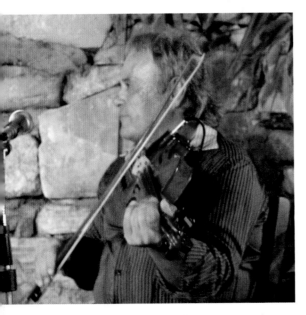

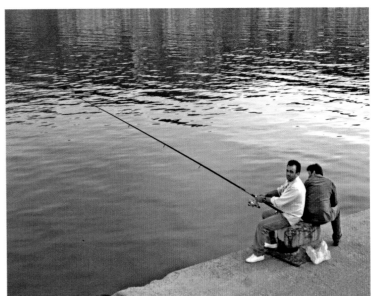

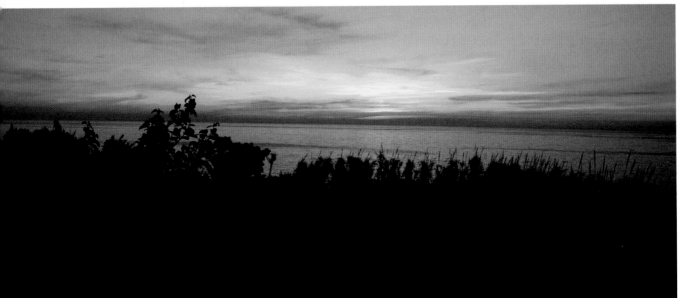

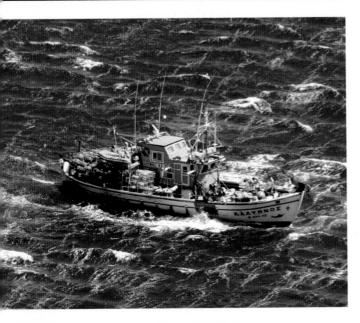

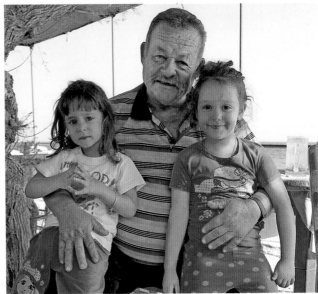

BOGUE IN THE SKILLET WITH OREGANO AND OLIVE OIL

Gopes Ladorigani

Myrsina Roussou shared this recipe with me one summer day in 2013 as we sat in the shade of her terrace in Manganitis. "It doesn't take but 10 minutes," she added, right after describing the whole dish. Bogue is one of the easiest fish to catch—kids do it all summer long with nets from the shallow piers all over Ikaria.

Any small fry, such as smelts or whiting, may also be substituted. The only herb in this dish is dried oregano, which in other parts of the world tends to be deemed too strong to pair with fish. In Greece, oregano is virtually the only herb used to season fish.

MAKES 4 TO 6 SERVINGS

½ cup Greek extra virgin olive oil

1 pound (450 g) whole bogue, gutted and scaled

Salt and freshly ground black pepper

Juice of 1 to 2 lemons (to taste)

2 garlic cloves, thinly sliced

1 tablespoon dried Greek oregano

¼ cup water

Pour the olive oil into a large, deep skillet. Place the fish snugly one next to the other in a single layer inside the skillet. Season the fish with salt and pepper and sprinkle with the juice of 1 lemon. Sprinkle with the garlic and oregano. Pour the water into the skillet. Cook over medium-high heat, shaking the pan back and forth a little every few minutes, until the fish is fork-tender, about 12 to 15 minutes.

Remove and serve. Sprinkle with additional lemon juice, if desired.

GROUPER IN NATURAL ASPIC

Ziladia

I have encountered this unusual dish, which is basically fish gelatin with bits of shredded fish, vegetables, and citrus juice, in several other Greek islands, Samos and Tinos among them. On Ikaria, this old dish is almost always made with grouper, while elsewhere in the Aegean it is sometimes made with conger eel. Grouper is delicate and also excellent in soups and on the grill. You can use lemon juice or, if available, a bit of the juice of Seville oranges, *nerantzia* to the Greeks, to flavor the gelatin.

This recipe is interesting from a nutritional standpoint, too, as Maria Byron Panayidou explains, because the natural fish gelatin is essentially fat free but provides that smooth, velvety, satisfying mouthfeel that less salutary products like butter and cream achieve.

MAKES 6 TO 8 SERVINGS

1 whole grouper, about 3 pounds (1.4 kg), gutted and scaled

2 red onions, finely chopped

3 carrots, finely chopped

2 celery stalks, diced

Sea salt and cracked black pepper

½ cup Greek extra virgin olive oil

Juice of 2 lemons,* strained

Cut the fish into large pieces, about 2 inches thick. Wrap the fish in a large piece of cheesecloth. Keep the head separate.

Place the fish pieces, fish head, and vegetables in a large pot and pour in enough water to cover by about 1 inch. Bring to a boil, reduce the heat, and season with salt and pepper. Pour in the olive oil. Simmer until the vegetables and fish are very soft, 35 to 40 minutes.

Strain the broth and reserve it. Place the vegetables in a 13 x 9 inch (33 x 23 cm) glass or ceramic dish. Shred the fish into small pieces and spread evenly among the vegetables.

Mix the lemon juice with the reserved fish broth. Taste and adjust the seasoning with additional salt and pepper or lemon juice. Pour over the fish and vegetables. Cover with plastic wrap and refrigerate until set, about 6 hours.

To serve, cut into square or diamond-shaped pieces.

*You could substitute the strained juice of 1 lemon and 1 Seville orange for the juice of 2 lemons.

PAN-FRIED FISH IN VINEGAR AND ROSEMARY SAUCE

Psari Marinato

In many parts of Greece, a combination of vinegar and rosemary (sometimes with other ingredients such as garlic and raisins) was poured on leftover fried fish to help preserve it for a second day. You can certainly do that if you have leftover fried fish, reserving the oil and replenishing and reheating it, then making the sauce as described here. This recipe explains how to prepare the whole dish, including fried fish, from scratch.

Adding this particular sauce to leftover fried fish is an example of the innate wisdom of Greek and Mediterranean cooks. "Vinegar contains 5% acetic acid, which kills bacteria and other micro-organisms. Thus, these two ingredients work synergistically to preserve the pan-fried cold fish," according to Maria Byron Panayidou, this book's nutritionist. The rosemary in the sauce has the added benefit of working "as an antioxidant, which preserves the flavor and the appearance of food by preventing oxidation, which is the key component of decomposition of foods." Rosemary is also a good source of iron, calcium, vitamin B_6, and A.

MAKES 4 TO 6 SERVINGS

Olive oil, for frying

2¼ pounds (1 kg) whole bogue, red mullet, or other small fish, gutted and scaled

1 tablespoon all-purpose flour, plus more for dredging

2 garlic cloves, chopped

1 cup white wine vinegar

½ cup water

2 sprigs fresh rosemary

Salt and freshly ground black pepper

Lightly dredge the fish in flour.

In a large, heavy skillet, heat 1 inch (2.5 cm) of olive oil until the oil ripples. Add the dredged fish a few pieces at a time and pan-fry until golden, turning once, about 7 to 10 minutes per side, depending on the size of the fish. Remove and drain on paper towels. Continue until the fish is all cooked.

At this point, you can serve the fish hot or let it cool and continue to make the sauce.

Strain the cooking oil through a fine-mesh sieve. Wipe the skillet dry and pour the oil back in the skillet. Add the garlic and cook for a few seconds over low heat to soften. Add 1 tablespoon flour and whisk to thicken and keep from lumping. Add the vinegar, water, and rosemary. Cook the sauce for a few minutes until it becomes creamy and thick. Season to taste with salt and pepper. Pour over the fish and serve. Alternatively, reserve the sauce for leftover cold, fried fish.

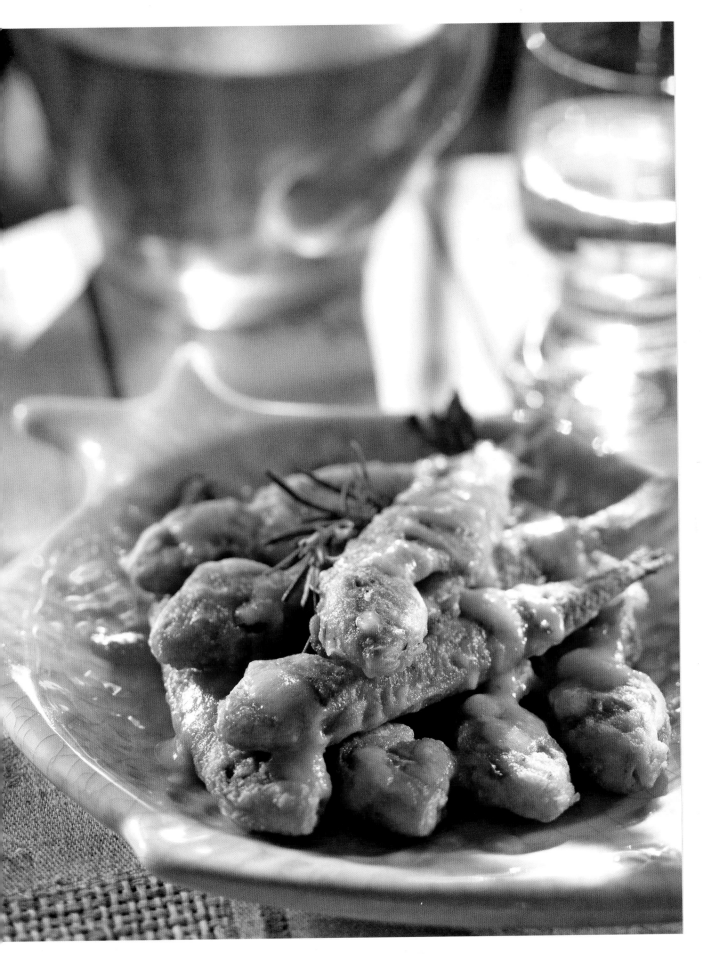

SERIOUS SALT

I got a lesson in salt harvesting from my friend Andreas, a 50-something Philadelphian of Ikarian descent (first generation) who, despite the fact that he was born in the most seminal of American cities, walks, talks (Greek), and lives leanly like an Ikarian from a hundred years ago. To hear him describe the "serious salt" he collects every summer from the easternmost tip of Ikaria, just like generations of islanders had done up until the 1960s, was, to me, an invitation to join him. And so I did, late in the afternoon on an August day, after we had settled on the time (after coffee, around 6) and the place (Niki's bar in Faro). "Wear pants and sneakers," he advised. "Bring a plastic bag and a slotted spoon." (The slotted spoon helps the salt to drain; old timers know to carry the salt off in baskets for the same reason. This I learned after my first salt expedition.)

Collecting serious salt, which has great flavor because it's naturally rich in calcium, magnesium, and potassium as well as dozens of trace minerals—the stuff you might spend a small fortune for were it labeled "fleur de sel du Cailly"—is, well, pretty serious business. We drove to the easternmost tip of the island, within close range of the Hellenistic fortress known as Drakano, walked down a scruffy goat path for about 20 minutes, past a tiny church and across two pristine beaches to our ultimate destination: two small peninsulas of lacerated grayish white granite sculpted into nooks and crannies, and small, flat basins in which our serious salt is found. Climbing over the knife-sharp rocks does indeed require long pants, limber legs, and no small amount of sangfroid. I almost lost my balance several times in the pursuit of serious salt.

At first I was looking in all the wrong places, scraping up the thin, incredibly hard layer of fine salt that settles over everything, mud, sand, and seaweed clumps included. Then I noticed Andreas way off in the distance, much closer to the edge, stooped and very focused. He was seriously busy catching the sea's saline deposits from small, shallow pools naturally formed within this maze of rocks. I can only describe what I at first erroneously collected as salt sludge: wet, white, and/or gray or blond crystals, bigger than oatmeal flakes, that I indiscriminately scooped up, catching some sand and debris in the process. Andreas knew to rake his spoon gently over the surface of the deposits, collecting only the top layer. The whiter the crystals, the cleaner the salt.

Seawater on average is 4% salt, which means that 1 liter contains 40 grams of salt. Every day, with the push and pull of the waves, more seawater is left in these little basins; it evaporates under the hot summer sun, increasing the overall salt content even more. But once the water reaches its saturation point, the salt can no longer dissolve and crystallizes out. This is why you can collect it.

Once harvested, the salt needs to be dried and cleaned. Some people wash it by placing it in a basin and filling the basin with regular tap water. Impurities sink to the bottom, then the salt is spooned out and set in shallow nonreactive (glass or stainless steel) pans to dry in the sun. (Salt is always collected in summer to facilitate this process.) One doesn't have to wash it—that's optional. The drying process pushes any impurities to the surface anyway, which you can just pick off by hand.

My serious Ikarian salt is flaky and very flavorful. I opt to keep it in large crystals. A generation ago, women would crush it by rolling bottles over it.

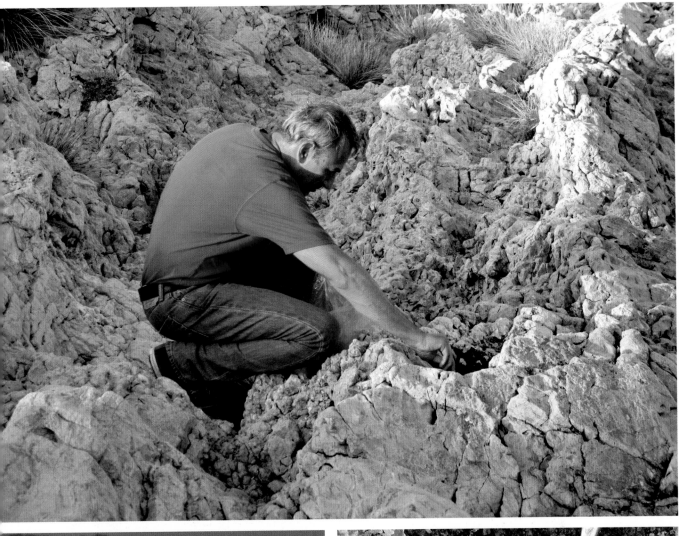

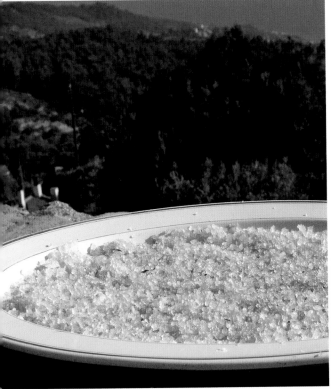

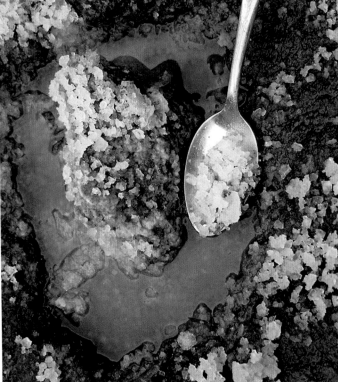

SNAILS SIMMERED WITH TOMATOES, ONIONS, AND SPICES

Karyvolia Stifado tis Athinas

After the first thunderstorms of the fall, Ikarians say it pours water and snails. Snails have been important in the Ikarian and wider Greek diet forever and it's no mystery why. Their small, slithery bodies are nutritional powerhouses. Snails were one of the main sources of protein, too, during the long periods of fasting in the winter and spring and, indeed, their meat is a lot healthier for us than red meat. Snail protein is comprised of the essential amino acids that the human body needs, and contains much less bacteria than other animal proteins. An average snail is 80% water, 15% protein, and 2.4% primarily healthy fat. Snails contain omega-3 fatty acids, which have long been known for their anti-inflammatory qualities, other essential fatty acids (linoleic and linolenic acids), calcium, iron, selenium, copper, zinc, potassium, and magnesium, but also vitamins E, A, K, and B_{12}.

Ikarians used to collect them on the island by the bucket. They are everywhere after it rains, on the edge of every road, on the low-lying rock walls that form the terraced gardens carved into every slope on the island, over piles of wet leaves. They have always been plentiful, so much so that it's the habit to ignore the small ones and go after the larger, meatier kind with grayish white shells.

Ikarians generally cook snails in a *stifado*, that is, with a lot of onions, tomatoes, and herbs. This recipe comes from Athina Moraiti, the aunt of a very good friend of ours, also from Ikaria.

MAKES 6 TO 8 SERVINGS

2¼ pounds (1 kg) snails in the shell, purged (see Note on next page)

1 cup red wine vinegar

Salt and freshly ground black pepper

½ cup Greek extra virgin olive oil

3 large red or yellow onions, finely chopped (about 3 cups)

1 cup chopped tomatoes, with their juices

2 cups water

2 bay leaves

6 or 7 allspice berries

2 or 3 sprigs fresh thyme

1 scant teaspoon sugar

Place the snails in a pot filled with cold water, the vinegar, and a scant tablespoon of salt. Bring to a boil over medium heat. As soon as it comes to a boil, reduce the heat, and simmer for 10 minutes. Skim the foam off the top of the pot. Drain and rinse several times.

In a large, wide pot, heat ¼ cup of the olive oil over medium-low heat. Add the onions and cook until they are very soft and lightly golden, 10 to 12 minutes.

Add the snails and stir. Add the tomatoes with their juices, water, remaining ¼ cup olive oil, bay leaves, allspice, thyme and sugar. Season to taste with salt and pepper. Cover and simmer until the sauce is thick, about 30 minutes. Serve the snails hot or at room temperature, in their shells.

NOTE: *Prior to cooking, snails have to be fed and purged to rid them of impurities. On Ikaria, the tradition is to leave them on a bed of lentiscus leaves, the tough, aromatic plant that grows everywhere on the island. You can also use bulgur. To clean, place the snails in a large basin with uncooked bulgur, or lentiscus leaves if you can find them. Cover the basin with a large kitchen towel. The snails will feed on the bulgur or leaves over 2 to 3 days and purge, at which point they are ready to cook.*

If you collect snails during times of the year when they hibernate, their bodies sealed behind a papery membrane, you have to remove the membrane and purge the snails, as above.

Then, before cooking, check for any that might not be alive by placing them in a basin filled with cold water. The ones that move are alive! Discard the ones that don't wiggle around.

CHEWING THE SEA

Ikaria's coast is not like that of many other islands, which are laced with small shallow coves. The coast around the island is rocky, rich in a large variety of fish, especially deepwater fish, but relatively limited in terms of shellfish and mollusks. There are lobsters, both the Mediterranean (langoustines) variety and the Atlantic type (having been given as a gift to many Mediterranean countries as part of the Marshall Plan), as well as the cylindrical, delicious *koloktypa*, aka Mediterranean slipper lobster.

I remember gathering tiny shrimp off the *nysaki* (tiny island) near the small old port of Yialiskari, with a beautiful little church named after the patron saint of sailors, Aghios Nikolaos. Now the islet is connected to the port artificially, with landfill and breakers, and these tiny shrimp have disappeared.

Spear fishermen emerge with an occasional fan mussel and people still dive for sea urchins, which dot the coast all around the island with their needle-sharp black shells. They aren't as plentiful as they once were, pollution having taken a toll even on pristine Ikaria.

Ditto for the two types of shellfish that provided both nourishment (free, since one just dove for them and still does) and great flavor: *petalides*, or limpets, single-shelled mollusks that cling to the island's rocky coast and are savored in every month of the year except the ones that do not have an "r" in them; and sea snails—periwinkles. My friend Argyro Kohyla-Kouvdou, a fount of knowledge for all things wild and edible, regardless of whether they derive from the land or the sea, recounts her recollection of when she was young and the special treat that sea snails provided. "We'd break a hole in the shell and cook the snails, either as salad or in pilaf— my mother used to add hot peppers. But the best part was sucking the snail out of its shell, a sweet piece of meat, it was like chewing the sea."

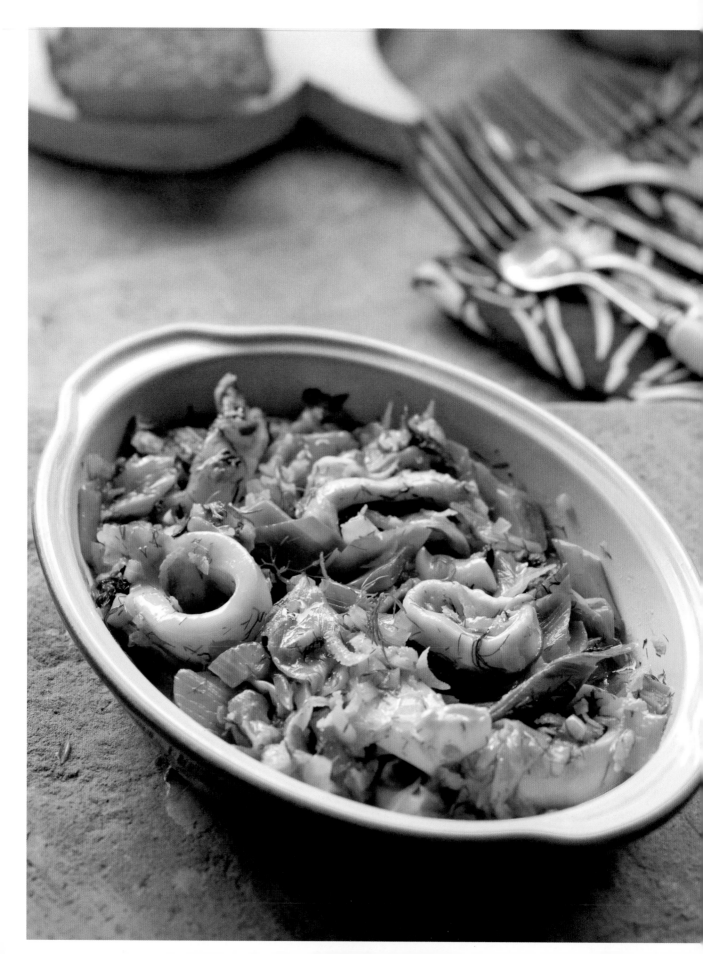

CUTTLEFISH OR SQUID BRAISED WITH FENNEL

Soupia me Maratho

Cuttlefish, sometimes known as sepia, is a popular seafood in Ikaria and Greece, where it is usually sold with its ink intact. In the United States, you can find it cleaned and primed for American tastebuds, no black ink. It is often sold precut and frozen, which is perfectly fine for this recipe, too. This dish is usually made with the local wine, which is semisweet, almost like sherry, which is what I suggest using instead.

This is a recipe that islanders enjoy in the spring, during Lent, when the first wild fennel sprouts. The perky, aromatic, licorice-like flavor of fennel is a beautiful match for the fleshy cuttlefish. You can use large squid in place of the cuttlefish.

MAKES 4 TO 6 SERVINGS

2¼ pounds (1 kg) cuttlefish (sepia),
    preferably fresh,* or squid (see Note)

½ cup Greek extra virgin olive oil

1 leek, cleaned and chopped

1 large red onion, chopped

1 fennel bulb with fronds, chopped

1 garlic clove, minced

1½ cups medium sherry

Sea salt and freshly ground black pepper

1 large bunch wild fennel or dill snipped

Grated peel and juice of 1 lemon

If using fresh cuttlefish, use gloves to clean it because the ink will turn your hands black. To clean: Gently pull away the tentacles. Using your fingers, scoop out the viscera and discard. If the ink sac is intact, set it aside. Pull out the cartilaginous bone on the inside of the cuttlefish and discard. Rinse the cuttlefish gently under cold water. If they are large, cut them into strips 1 inch (2 cm) thick. If using small cuttlefish, leave intact, frozen cuttlefish is already cut into rings. If using squid, clean and cut into large rings.

To prepare the ink, place a coffee filter in a small fine-mesh sieve over a small bowl and press the ink sac with gloved fingers so that it breaks and a few drops of ink drip into the bowl.

In a large, wide pot, heat the olive oil over medium heat. Add leek, onion, and fennel bulb, and cook, stirring, until soft, about 10 minutes. Add the garlic and stir for a minute or two, to soften.

Place the cuttlefish in the pot and stir gently. Pour in the sherry, ink (if using), and salt and pepper. Simmer, covered, until the cuttlefish is almost cooked and tender, about 45 minutes. Add the wild fennel and continue cooking for another 15 minutes or so. Right before the end, stir in the lemon peel and juice. Serve.

NOTE: *To use squid, look for large, fresh squid or large frozen squid, either whole or precut into rings. For fresh squid, remove the tentacles, head, and viscera. Cut the tentacles away from the head just below the eyes. Scoop out the thin strip of cartilage on the inside and discard. Rinse the squid and tentacles well. Frozen squid is already cleaned. It should be thawed overnight in the refrigerator.*

CUTTLEFISH OR SQUID IN WINE

Soupia Krasato

When seafood and meat are cooked in wine, they are often seasoned with a combination of warm spices, such as cinnamon, and sharp herbs like rosemary. The flavor palette is slightly sweet and sour, as in the *stifado* recipe on page 259. These are classic combinations. I like to cook with honey, which I have added in the following recipe, although this is not a local tradition.

MAKES 4 TO 6 SERVINGS

3 pounds (1.4 kg) cuttlefish (sepia), preferably fresh,* or squid (see Note)

½ cup Greek extra virgin olive oil

1 large red onion, finely chopped (about 1 cup)

2 garlic cloves, minced

1½ cups peeled, seeded, chopped tomatoes

1 cup dry red wine

2 tablespoons honey, preferably Ikarian pine or any Greek honey

1 sprig fresh rosemary

2 bay leaves

1 cinnamon stick

4 to 6 allspice berries

Sea salt and freshly ground black pepper

2 tablespoons balsamic vinegar

If using fresh cuttlefish, use gloves to clean it because the ink will turn your hands black. To clean: Gently pull away the tentacles. Cut the tentacles just below the eyes. Using your fingers, scoop out the viscera and discard. If the ink sac is intact, set it aside in the refrigerator or discard. Pull out the cartilaginous bone on the inside of the cuttlefish and discard. Rinse the cuttlefish gently under cold water. If they are large, cut them into strips or rings 1 inch (2 cm) thick. If using small cuttlefish, leave intact. For fresh squid, remove the tentacles, head, and viscera. Cut the tentacles away from the head just below the eyes. Scoop out the thin strip of cartilage on the inside and discard. Rinse the squid and tentacles well. Cut the squid tubes into rings. Frozen squid is already cleaned.

In a heavy, wide pot, or Dutch oven, heat the olive oil over medium heat. Add the onion and cook, stirring, until wilted, about 10 minutes. Add the cuttlefish or squid and stir to coat in the oil. Add the garlic and stir for a minute.

Add the tomatoes, wine, honey, rosemary, bay leaves, cinnamon stick, and allspice berries. Cover and bring to a boil over medium heat. Season lightly with salt and pepper. Reduce the heat and simmer, covered, until the cuttlefish or squid is tender, about 1 hour, or longer if necessary. Add a little water during cooking if necessary to keep the contents of the pot liquid. About 5 minutes before removing from the heat, add the vinegar. Adjust the seasoning with additional salt and pepper, to taste. Remove the rosemary, cool slightly, and serve.

*You can use frozen cuttlefish, which is sold either whole or in thick strips or rings. Thaw overnight in the refrigerator before using.

OCTOPUS LOVE

"Ela, ela ("Come here, Come here"), Yiannis Roussos beckoned, as he kneaded two large octopi under running water in the sink. "Know how to tell the male from the female?"

Admittedly, I didn't.

"Look. The suckers. Here's the female. See how they are side by side, parallel? And look. The male. Zeeg zag [sic] suckers. That's how you know."

So began the lesson in octopus anatomy and cookery from Yiannis Roussos, the suntanned, stocky silver-haired friend of a friend from Manganiti, on the southwestern coast of the island.

Yiannis was dirt-poor as a kid. He spent most of his adult life as a house painter in Chicago. But in the mid-1990s he returned to pursue more artistic endeavors: He plays the fiddle to some local renown at the feasts called *panygyria*. His approach to octopus cookery is the same as his approach to the violin: filled with gusto and an unerring feel for detail.

"I wash, I rub, wash, rub, wash, rub," he explained over the sink. "That's how you get rid of the slime." Next, with a sharp midsize knife he slit open the hood. That surprised me, as I have always known to cut it off under the eyes and, for the most part, to discard it. But no, he cut it up.

That was the last time he used the knife. Setting it aside, he proceeded to tear apart the octopus by hand along the tentacles. "Never a knife here. Never. It makes the octopus tough."

"I'm crafty with octopus because of my childhood," he explained matter-of-factly. "When I was a kid, I almost got a beating over one of these little creatures. Too poor we were for fish. Octopus? Forget it. We lived on *horta* (greens). My father worked in a quarry. He broke apart rocks by hand all day long and usually got paid months later for his work. We always owed the grocer. Then once, I had a taste of octopus, a little bit, at the *cafeneion*. They offered me a chunk this big," he says, pointing to his knuckle. "*Mana mou*, I couldn't believe such a thing existed for us to taste. It was the best thing I had ever eaten.

"Then, once, a few days later, I got a job rowing for a local fisherman. He sent me to his house to get something and there on the table was the family meal: salad, bread, and, under a layer of vegetables one whole cooked octopus, tentacle by tentacle. I had to, had to, had to have this again. So I took one piece. Just one. I swallowed it so fast I didn't even chew. But it wasn't enough. I took a little more, then a little more. So fast, it just slipped down my throat. Before I knew it, I had eaten the whole thing and panicked. So I ran to the boat, and insisted to start working right then and there. I rowed and rowed as fast as I could, but that's what did me in because all the motion made me belch, not once or twice but many times, enough for the captain to sniff octopus on me! He asked me where I had some. I just looked at him. I couldn't lie. He knew. I had eaten his dinner!"

"Fantastic creatures. If you see them in the sea you can't help but feel awe."

"I use no spices. Spices can confuse your tongue. They take too much credit away from the octopus," Yianni says. "And most of the time, anyway, it's the simplest dishes that really make you wonder, because no one believes something so delicious can be made with so few ingredients."

YIANNIS ROUSSOS' CRAFTY OCTOPUS

To Poniro Ktapodi tou Yianni Roussou

2 whole octopi, about 3 pounds (1.4 kg) each (see Note), fresh or frozen (thawed overnight in the refrigerator)

1 cup Greek extra virgin olive oil

$^2/_3$ cup good red wine vinegar

Wash and rub 1 octopus under cold running water, kneading as you go, for about 8 minutes.

Grasp 1 tentacle in one hand and another, adjoining tentacle in the other and pull apart the octopus until you get 8 pieces. Repeat with second octopus.

Place the octopi in a wide, shallow pot or deep skillet. Cover with water and heat over very high heat. As the juices boil, skim the foam off the top. Cook at a rolling boil for about 25 minutes, or until about two-thirds of the juices have cooked off. Add another cup or two of water. Bring back to a boil over medium heat and keep skimming off the foam.

Be attentive, as Yiannis advises: The thinner ends of the tentacles will need less time to cook, so they don't have to be submerged in the liquid once they are tender; they curl up anyway and tend to pop out of the liquid. Using a wooden spoon or fork, submerge the thicker parts so that they cook.

After about 35 minutes, as the octopi nears completion (press a finger into one's flesh to test it; it should be tender), push them to one side and boil the juices, which will foam up on one side of the skillet, until reduced by about half. All in all the octopi should need 40 to 45 minutes of boiling. They will turn deep blackish pink.

When the octopi are tender (but not mushy), very slowly drizzle in the olive oil, pouring it in a slow, steady stream all over the surface of the octopi. Yiannis says the heat should be very high and that "if it catches fire, it's a success!"—I prefer medium heat and the caveat to be careful.

With a wooden spoon or fork, gently stir and dislodge the octopi should they begin to stick to the bottom. The olive oil and pan juices will emulsify and within a few minutes will result in a thick deep reddish brown gravylike liquid. Add the vinegar, cook another 5 minutes, remove from the heat, and serve hot.

NOTE: *Most octopus in the United States comes already cleaned. However, if you are using an octopus that needs to be cleaned, see "How to Clean an Octopus," page 231.*

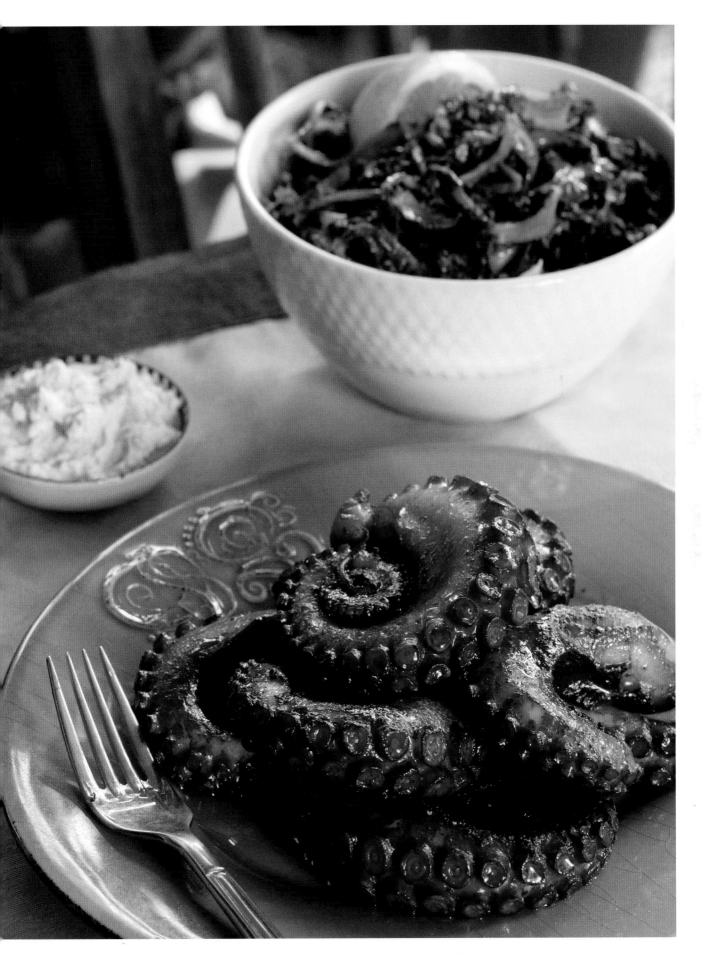

SWEET AND SOUR BRAISED OCTOPUS

Ktapodi Stifado

Stifado is the name given to many different dishes, some with seafood and others with game, chicken, or beef, but all defined by the abundance of small whole onions and a heady sweet and sour flavor thanks to the combination of spices and vinegar. These flavor combinations are all Greek classics, savored on Ikaria, too.

Octopus *stifado* is usually served with potatoes fried in olive oil, boiled Greek noodles, called *hilopites*, which you can find in Greek food stores, or plain boiled rice.

MAKES 4 TO 8 SERVINGS

6 tablespoons Greek extra virgin olive oil

1 large red onion, finely chopped

2 garlic cloves, minced

1 large octopus, about 4 pounds (2 kg) (see Note)

1½ cups canned plum tomatoes, with juice

1 bay leaf

1 sprig fresh rosemary

1 cinnamon stick

5 allspice berries

½ cup dry white wine

2 to 3 tablespoons red wine vinegar (to taste)

16 boiling onions, peeled and whole

In a large, wide pot or deep skillet, heat 2 tablespoons of the olive oil over low heat. Add the red onion and cook, stirring, until very soft, about 10 minutes. Add the garlic and stir a few times until softened. Add the octopus to the pan, cover, and cook over very low heat until it exudes its own liquid and has turned deep pink, about 25 minutes.

Add the plum tomatoes and juice, the bay leaf, rosemary, cinnamon stick, and allspice. As soon as the mixture comes to a boil, add the wine and vinegar. Cover and simmer until the octopus is tender, another 30 minutes or so, depending on the octopus's size.

Meanwhile, in a separate skillet, heat 2 tablespoons of the olive oil over low heat. Add the whole onions and cook, shaking the pan back and forth now and then, until golden, about 25 minutes.

Five to 10 minutes before removing the octopus from the stove, add the whole onions. Let everything simmer together for at least 10 minutes before serving.

Pour in the remaining 2 tablespoons olive oil and serve.

NOTE: *Most octopus in the United States comes already cleaned. However, if you are using an octopus that needs to be cleaned, see "How to Clean an Octopus," opposite.*

SEDUCED BY CEPHALOPODS

Octopus, squid, flying squid, and cuttlefish—all cephalopods and all much beloved by Ikarians and Greeks in general—swim in local waters and provide a great source of protein and omega-3 fatty acids, without too much fat. These ink-expelling, intelligent creatures are chock-full of vitamins, especially vitamins A, D, and several in the B complex, and provide us with a great source of iron, calcium, potassium, phosphorus, copper, zinc, and selenium. Each of those vitamins and minerals in turn helps our bodies in specific ways. Copper helps us absorb iron; selenium helps protect us against arthritis; vitamin B_{12} helps keep migraines at bay; calcium and phosphorous build bones and teeth; vitamin B_3 regulates blood sugar; zinc boosts the immune system; and potassium helps reduce blood pressure levels. Cephalopods also contain taurine, an organic acid that acts as an antioxidant.

HOW TO CLEAN AN OCTOPUS

Most of the octopus sold in American retail markets comes already cleaned, that is, the hood and viscera have been discarded. Often, the purple membrane that clings to the octopus has also been removed. In restaurant kitchens and in the Greek and Middle Eastern markets where I shop in this country, however, I usually encounter octopus in all its natural glory.

To clean it, the method is the same whether fresh or frozen. If using frozen octopus, however, let it stand overnight in the refrigerator to thaw.

Wash the octopus under cold running water. Using a sharp knife or a chef's knife, cut away its hood. You can discard it, or clean out the viscera and chop it up for use in any of the octopus recipes in this book.

Turn the octopus over and, using your hand or a small paring knife, squeeze or cut out the beaklike mouth and two stubby eye sockets on the other side. If desired, peel away the purple membrane. I like it and leave it intact.

OCTOPUS BRAISED WITH TWO WINES

Ktapodi Krasato

The red wine on Ikaria often has a semisweet flavor, almost like sherry, which I approximate in the recipe below by suggesting a combination of sweet and dry vintages. This is a stew not unlike the *stifado* (page 259), but with finely chopped onions instead of whole ones and slightly different spices. Like *stifado*, wine-braised octopus is served either with rice, noodles, or short pasta like ditali.

MAKES 4 TO 8 SERVINGS

½ cup Greek extra virgin olive oil

2 large red onions, grated and with juices (about 2 cups)

3 garlic cloves, minced

1 large octopus, about 4 pounds (2 kg) (see Note)

¾ cup dry red wine

½ cup sweet white wine, such as Samos Muscat

2 tablespoons *petimezi* (grape molasses), optional

2 bay leaves

3 or 4 sprigs fresh thyme

4 or 5 allspice berries

1 heaping tablespoon tomato paste

Salt and freshly ground black pepper

In a large, wide pot or deep skillet, heat the olive oil over medium heat. Add the onions, stir, reduce the heat, and cook until tender and translucent, about 10 minutes. Stir in the garlic.

Place the octopus in the pot. Add the wines, *petimezi* (if using), bay leaves, thyme, and allspice berries. Cover and simmer over low heat for about 40 to 50 minutes, until tenderized but not thoroughly cooked.

Add the tomato paste, stirring gently in the pot until it dissolves. Simmer until tender, about 20 to 30 more minutes, uncovered or partially covered if there is more than two cups of liquid in the pot.

Remove the bay leaves, thyme, and allspice and serve.

NOTE: *Most octopus in the United States comes already cleaned. However, if you are using an octopus that needs to be cleaned, see "How to Clean an Octopus," page 231.*

THE HUNTER'S OCTOPUS . . .

Ikarians are weavers of tales tall and taller . . . and Scoudrano, pictured below, was a guy who liked to tell stories. His real name was Stamatis Kohylas. He died a few years back, having reached somewhere near a three-digit old age. His wife, Vasilia, 101, is still alive and still sits outside in the summers at the family taverna at Armenistis, which was the only place I, or anyone my age, ever remembered Scoudranos being. He was a sometime fisherman. No one ever knew why they called Stamatis Scoudranos. The word doesn't mean anything. The story goes that it was the name of a *cafeneion* somewhere in Asia Minor back then.

Scoudrano never smiled. His expression was like stone and you never knew if he was happy, sad, angry, bored. But he had a wry wit and liked to tell stories, especially from the 1920s and '30s.

His octopus tale goes like this: One day the sea was very rough and he and his brothers couldn't go fishing as planned. The brothers decided to go hunting instead and set out on foot up the mountain. Stamatis opted to go off for limpets, in a nearby cove. The family dog followed him.

He tried to shoo it away toward his brothers' direction, but the dog refused to leave Scoudrano's side. Bent over scraping limpets off the rocks, he happened to notice a huge octopus within arm's reach.

So he grabbed for it. It was something like 12 to 15 pounds (6 to 7 kilos). A monster. He tried to pull it out, but the octopus clung to the rock with all its strength. Scoudranos finally tugged so hard that he unhinged the thing. But as he swung it away from the sea, it slipped out of his arms and down onto the dog's back. The dog went wild, running and howling.

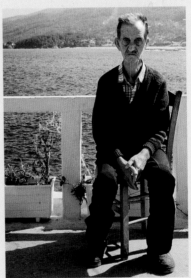

In the meantime, the brothers who had gone hunting had stopped for a smoke about a kilometer up the road from where the octopus flew out of the water. All of a sudden they heard what sounded like thunder, rocks falling, noise all around them, general mayhem coming their way. One of the brothers, Dimitris, turned to see what was happening.

Later that night, settled and calm, Dimitris recounted the tale of how his dog had followed him up the road, and instead of coming back with a fallen bird or two, he arrived with an octopus clenched in his teeth!

And that's the famous story of the hunter's octopus, a tale spun almost a hundred years ago, and still whispering its way around the island and beyond, generations later.

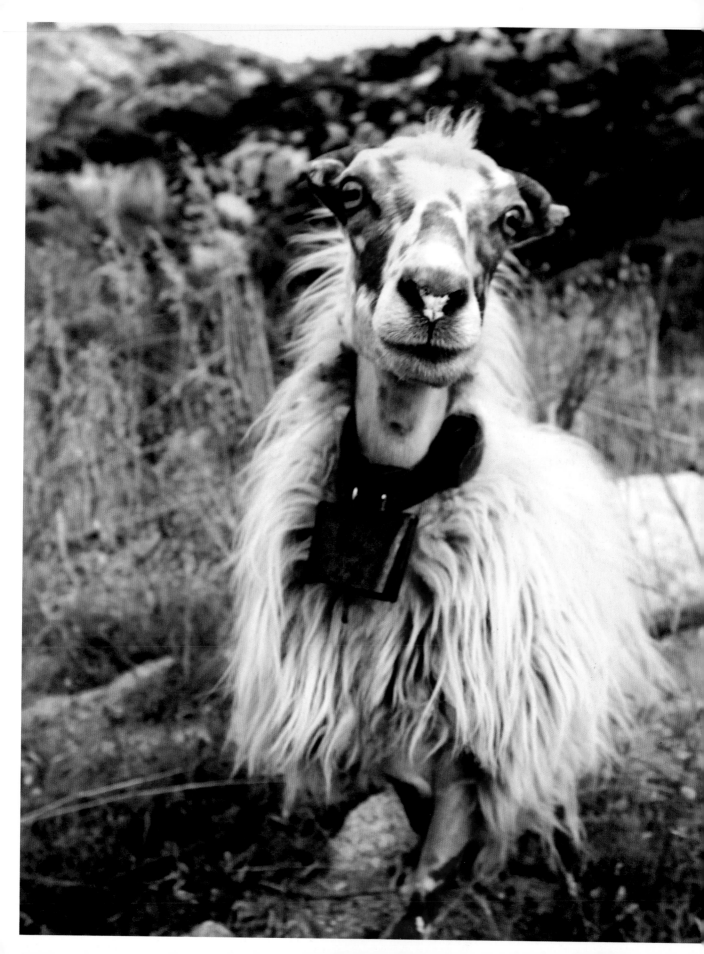

MEAT

ON THE ISLAND OF LONGEVITY

THE MOST TELLING ASPECTS OF THE MEAT CUISINE on Ikaria are that most meat was prepared as a festive or Sunday meal or consumed regularly but sparingly, more as a condiment than as a main-course protein.

Indeed, a 1975 account of how "important" meat was in the diet, from an article written in a local historical magazine called *Ikariaka*, speaks almost exclusively of one meat preparation, a kind of goat meat jerky called *pasturma* (nothing to do with the Armenian and Turkish *bastirma*), which "was never absent" from any Ikarian home but was consumed more as a flavoring agent, a few slices here and there, in bean and vegetable stews and soups.

In my conversations about food with people in their eighties, nineties, and older, most waxed nostalgic about the goat *pasturma* and also made a point of saying how little of it they actually ate, or anything else for that matter.

The dearth of food, the special treat that meat was, even in minuscule quantities, and the reliance on foraged, wild food were basic facts of life during the childhoods of Ikaria's spry and limber aged. The animal proteins that were traditionally available to Ikarians were goat and some lamb, pork, poultry, and some game.

Today, the amount of meat that Greeks consume—and Ikarians are no different—never ceases to amaze me. The latest statistics available, from the journal *The Food Industry in Greece*, state that per capita meat consumption in Greece is at an unbelievable (at least to this vegetable lover) 183 pounds (83 kg) annually, or about ½ pound (225 g) per day. More than a third of that is pork, with poultry running second at about 21%, beef at 20%, and the traditional goat and lamb lumped together at 15% of total consumption.

What I have tried to do in this chapter on meats and the Ikarian table is to present a fairly wide gamut of the kinds of meat dishes Ikarians a generation and more ago did eat, typically when they sat down to a holiday, or, for a few more fortunate families, Sunday, meal. For many Ikarians up until the early 1970s, meat was affordable at best three to four times a year. Slaughtering a goat or lamb meant losing a source of milk; slaughtering a chicken meant losing a source of eggs. No one did this capriciously. The family pig was fattened up all year and slaughtered around the holiday; its meat provided sustenance to an extended family for almost half the year.

In the traditional diet of the island, what little meat people did consume was dictated by the season. Pork was the winter meat, roosters and chickens saved for various festive events, kid and lamb savored in the spring. Game—mainly partridges and hares—was also seasonal, and is now regulated. Cattle were never really raised on the island. There just isn't enough land.

As for seasonings and pairings, most meat dishes were and still are stews that are married with other vegetables or herbs, everything from fennel to taro root. Oregano, garlic, and warm spices like cinnamon and allspice flavor meat dishes that are cooked in tomato sauce. Avgolemono, the egg-lemon liaison that is such an iconic Greek sauce, goes into more than a few meat stews, too.

BABY GOAT BRAISED WITH FENNEL

Katsikaki sto Tsikali me Maratho

Everywhere you look on Ikaria you see goats. Sometimes they are in people's yards, tied to a tree or penned; mostly they roam free and you see them along mountain roads, in forests, even near the sea. They are the basic meat on almost all Aegean islands, and Ikaria is no exception. I've always found it a little ironic that Greek cuisine outside of Greece is known mainly for perfectly roasted lamb. Greeks eat goat at least as often, if not more often, than lamb. Goat meat is leaner than lamb.

The combination of goat and fennel is a springtime classic, evincing yet again how much the seasons come into play on the Ikarian and wider Greek table. The meat should be beautifully seared and crusty, to counter the billowy softness of everything else in the pot. It is also cooked bone-in, which is more flavorful than filleted cuts and how Greeks generally tend to eat both goat and lamb. You may easily substitute lamb for goat in this and any other recipe.

MAKES 4 TO 6 SERVINGS

⅓ cup Greek extra virgin olive oil

2 pounds (900 g) bone-in goat, preferably shoulder, cut into serving pieces

10 scallions or spring onions, finely chopped

2 fresh green garlics or 3 garlic cloves, finely chopped

⅔ cup dry white wine

Salt and freshly ground black pepper

Pinch of sugar

2 cups chopped wild fennel*

Juice of 1½ lemons, strained

In a large pot, heat the olive oil over medium heat. Add the meat and sear, turning it to brown on all sides. Remove the meat to a plate and tent with foil to keep warm.

Add the scallions (or spring onions) and garlic to the pot and stir for a few minutes until soft. Return the meat to the pot. Pour in the wine and as soon as the alcohol steams off, add enough water to cover the meat. Season with salt and pepper. Cover, bring to a boil over medium heat, reduce the heat to low, and simmer until the meat is so tender it falls off the bone, 1 hour 30 minutes to 2 hours. Check the liquid content every so often and add water as needed. About halfway through the cooking time, add the wild fennel to the pot. Pour in the lemon juice, stir, and resume cooking until the meat is done. Cool slightly before serving.

*Substitute 2 medium fennel bulbs with fronds, finely chopped, and 1 bunch dill, finely chopped. Cook the chopped fennel along with the scallions and garlic. Add the dill when you would have added the wild fennel.

OREGANO-ROASTED GOAT

Katsikaki Riganato sto Fourno

Roasted goat with oregano is as iconic a dish as the better-known roasted lamb with garlic and oregano. On Ikaria, goat prevails over lamb as the meat of choice, although they are interchangeable in recipes. There is nothing bashful about the flavors in this dish. With 10 cloves of garlic and heaps of fresh and dried oregano, it is robust and vibrant. Ikarians pick oregano twice a year, once in the spring before it flowers, then again in midsummer when it erupts with tiny white blossoms. There are several varieties that grow wild on Ikaria, and they are all very aromatic.

MAKES 4 TO 6 SERVINGS

- 1 whole goat or bone-in lamb leg about 5 pounds (2.5 kg)
- 10 garlic cloves, finely chopped
- Leaves from 10 sprigs fresh oregano, finely chopped
- Grated zest of 1 lemon
- ⅔ cup Greek extra virgin olive oil
- Salt and cracked black pepper

- 3 pounds Yukon Gold potatoes, skin on, quartered
- 2 tablespoons dried Greek oregano (see resources on page 299)
- 2 sprigs fresh rosemary, cut into 1-inch pieces
- 1 cup white wine
- Juice of 1 to 2 lemons (to taste), strained

(continued)

OREGANO RULES

It's not by accident that Ikarians flavor almost all their meat dishes and many vegetable dishes with oregano. Four to five different varieties grow wild all over the island. A professor of pharmacology at the University of Athens has studied Ikarian oregano, compared it to oregano from other parts of Greece, and found it to be three times more aromatic and nutrient-dense.

Oregano is a rich source of vitamin K, antibacterial compounds, and antioxidants. It is high in iron, manganese, potassium, calcium, magnesium, and omega-3 fatty acids. But oregano's special simpatico relationship with meat dishes on the island and around Greece touches on something at once intangible and scientifically proven. Empirically, local cooks use it profusely in meat recipes, especially but not exclusively with goat. It helps digestion by increasing the secretion of bile, and it is great for heartburn and bloating.

Oregano, *rigani* in Greek, means "mountain joy" . . . exactly the sentiment I feel when savoring wild goat perfumed with this amazing herb.

Trim the fat from around the goat or lamb leg and, using a sharp paring knife make incisions about 1 inch (2.5 cm) deep all around the meat.

Preheat the oven to 375°F (190°C).

Using a mortar and pestle, pound the garlic, fresh oregano, lemon zest, 1 tablespoon of the olive oil, and pepper until the mixture becomes a paste. Season with salt.

Push a little of this mixture into each of the incisions around the meat.

Toss the potatoes in a large bowl with ½ cup of the olive oil, the dried oregano, rosemary, and salt and freshly ground black pepper.

Rub the outside of the meat with the remaining olive oil and season generously with salt and pepper. Place in the middle of a large roasting pan and spread the potatoes evenly around the pan. Pour in the wine.

Cover the pan with a lid (or with parchment paper, then a layer of foil to seal) and roast the meat and potatoes until tender, about 2 hours 30 minutes. Check occasionally for liquid content and turn the potatoes in the pan juices. Add water to the pan if the potatoes are very dry. Remove the lid (or parchment and foil) 15 to 20 minutes before the meat and potatoes are done, for them to brown nicely. Pour in the lemon juice and toss it with the potatoes.

Remove it from the oven and let it stand for 20 minutes before carving.

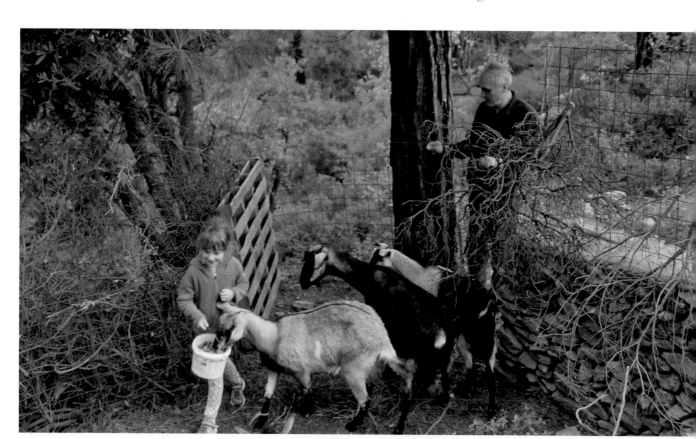

GOAT BANE

The preferred meat on Ikaria is, no doubt, goat, which is healthier than lamb, and better for you than beef or chicken. In fact, goat meat is more than 50% lower in fat than American beef and about 40% lower in saturated fat than chicken, even chicken cooked with the skin off, according to the USDA.

But on Ikaria it is indelibly linked to both survival and destruction.

To see goats in Ikaria is to see not only the animal, but the ancient instrument called a *tsambouna*, made from the skin, a primitive bagpipe for cavorting Ikarians during their wildest *panygyria*. It is to see the *filaki*, the most unusual of satchels, none other than a whole, intact goatskin, legs and hair and all, slung backpack style around the shoulders of Ikarian men of all ages. It's to see the bells dangling from Sideris Spanos's shop in Christos, Raches, to know how important it has always been for local shepherds to keep track of their animals. It's to know the "Invisible One," not God, but a goat rustler whose nickname has been passed down two generations!

But goats are also the bane of island life. The census says it all: There are about 8,000 permanent inhabitants on Ikaria and anywhere between 30,000 and 50,000 goats! (All those goats and there is no cheese facility or slaughterhouse.)

For most of their history, Greek islanders have herded goats for sustenance and minimal income. Then, in the name of progress, EU subsidies corrupted old, ecologically sound island ways. There was supposedly funding for a cheese facility, which would have helped island shepherds sell their milk, but it never materialized. Numbers became important. The more goats one had, the bigger one's subsidy. The policy has wreaked havoc on the island's ecosystem and, ultimately, on the quality of its treasured goat meat. Once, there were actually "wild" goats in the mountains, a limited number, which was ecologically unremarkable. They could feed at will on wild food. But today, the majority of shepherds don't herd their animals and instead let them roam free all over the island. When you drive on Ikaria's mountain roads you see gates seemingly in the middle of nowhere, where private land crosses public; private citizens put up the gates to keep the goats away.

All those free-roaming goats survive on a diet of cotton meal and wild, foraged food; the cotton makes them thirsty, so they seek out any source of moisture they can chew on. It becomes a vicious cycle. As a result, they have desiccated trees, shrubs, and just about anything else that grows within reach in many parts of the island.

But shepherds are stubborn and resist returning to old, sounder habits, because the money is easy. The meat doesn't taste as good as it once did and parts of the island have lost valuable flora to uncontrolled grazing. As of this writing, not much seems poised to change.

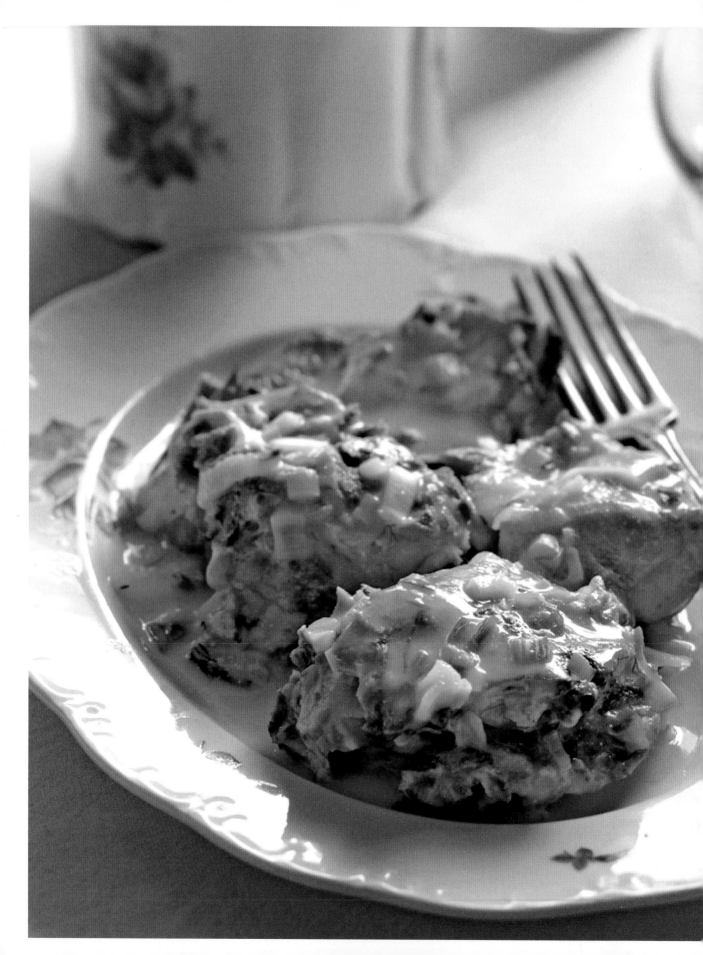

BABY GOAT WITH YOGURT AVGOLEMONO

Katsikaki me Yiaourtato Avgolemono

The Greek yogurt craze affected me one Easter a few years ago, as I was preparing the family feast and decided, on a lark, to add some yogurt to an otherwise classic dish of goat with egg-lemon sauce. I've since experimented with this dish for the menu at Molyvos, too, the Greek restaurant in New York City where I am collaborating chef. This is not a traditional Ikarian recipe. I do use ingredients that I've always used on Ikaria, however, including fennel.

MAKES 6 SERVINGS

½ to 1 cup Greek extra virgin olive oil

3 pounds bone-in baby goat or lamb shoulder, cut into serving portions

8 scallions, chopped

2 to 3 fresh green garlics or 3 garlic cloves, finely chopped

1 fennel bulb, finely chopped

2 bay leaves

6 or 7 sprigs fresh thyme

1 cinnamon stick

1 cup Samos muscat or other sweet white wine

1 cup white wine

3 cups chicken stock or water

Salt and freshly ground black pepper

1 cup snipped fresh dill

AVGOLEMONO

3 egg yolks

3 tablespoons fresh lemon juice

4 tablespoons plain Greek yogurt

1 teaspoon cornstarch

In a large, wide pot, heat ½ cup of olive oil over medium-high heat. Add the meat and brown on all sides, turning with kitchen tongs. Do this in batches if necessary, then return the browned meat to the pot.

Add the scallions, garlic, and chopped fennel bulb. Reduce the heat to medium and stir occasionally until wilted, about 10 minutes. Add the bay leaves, thyme, and cinnamon stick. Pour in the wines. As soon as they steam up, add the stock (or water). Season to taste with salt and pepper. Cover and simmer until the meat is falling off the bone, 1 hour 30 minutes to 2 hours. Ten minutes before removing from the heat, add the dill.

For the avgolemono: In a bowl, whisk the egg yolks until frothy, 6 to 8 minutes. Slowly add the lemon juice and continue whisking until creamy. Whisk in the yogurt and cornstarch.

Remove a ladleful of hot pan juices and, whisking all the while, very slowly drizzle it into the egg-lemon mixture. Repeat 2 more times, whisking all the while. Pour this mixture back into the pot and tilt the pot back and forth for the avgolemono to go all over. Serve immediately.

EASTER: SOLIDARITY, VIOLINS, AND FEASTS

The Easter trip is our first family jaunt to the island after months in Athens. At Easter, my husband, Vassili, usually plants the garden. In the spring, the island is lush and green and quiet, with nothing of the frenzy that overtakes it in July and August.

During Holy Week, rhythms of life are palpable. Much revolves around the table and its preparations. The butcher shops buzz with orders. In the beginning of the week, women get together at each other's houses to make *koulourakia*, the twisted and braided cookies. Easter Thursday is the bread-baking bonanza and it all happens around the village baker's cavernous oven. Dozens of women are inside and outside the bakery, a tight-squeeze of a place, where, weighing their *tsoureki* (Easter bread) dough on ancient scales, twisting and braiding and coiling loaf after loaf, then inserting in each a deep-red dyed egg. Stacks of coal-black baking pans crowd the bakery, and Yianni, our local baker, sweats his way through them all day. The sweet, fruity smell of *mahlepi*, a cherry kernel boiled as a spice for the bread, and the musky smell of *mastiha*, or gum mastic, a crystal resin spice, as well as the sticky perfume of orange, permeate the air. We dye eggs on Thursday, too, the old Ikarian way, with onion skins for color.

Good Friday is solemn and people generally observe it as such. But on Saturday, almost everyone is busy making *mageiritsa*, the Greek Easter soup of offal, lettuce, wild herbs, spring onions, and egg-and-lemon that we eat after the Saturday midnight liturgy to break the fast.

The highlight of Easter on Ikaria is a social phenomenon, one that speaks of the underlying solidarity and sense of common fate that binds people together here and provides an emotional as well as material welfare net: the *mnymosyno*. The word means "memorial" but it refers now to a communal meal organized on all the major holidays, but especially Easter, in which everyone who can donate meat to the village. Volunteers cook it and anyone who wants to come may, whether he or she contributes meat or not, whether Ikarian or not. The tradition was a way to ensure that everyone ate a little meat at least two or three times a year, but it has morphed into a communal feast. Almost no one celebrates Easter Sunday privately at home on Ikaria. Instead, everyone congregates at the village center, where long tables are laid. They bring their own wine and any other side dishes they want, from salads to savory phyllo pies to *tzatziki* and more. The meat, spit-roasted and boiled goat, is free. People generally start to head over after 3 or 4 in the afternoon. Kids run about.

When everyone is sufficiently sated and soused, the music starts. The first violin riffs of the *kariotiko* sound. It takes at least an hour or so for people to feel sufficiently inspired to get up for that first round, but once they do the party begins to roar and doesn't stop until 9 or 10 the next morning. Even then, people continue the feast. The day after Easter is usually marked by a late-afternoon lunch (after enough time to catch some sleep) for family and close friends.

The week or two each Easter we are lucky enough to spend here gives me a sense of renewal and of reassurance that even as the island's ways are exposed, its traditions are still alive.

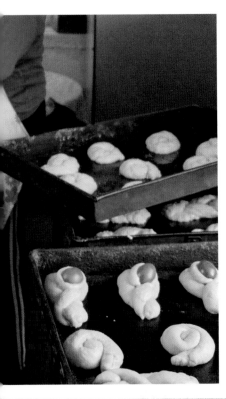
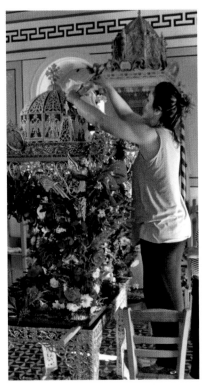
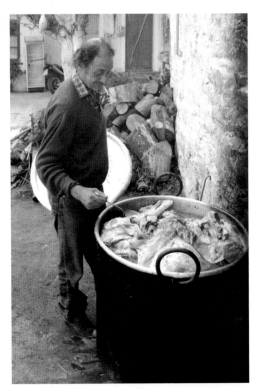
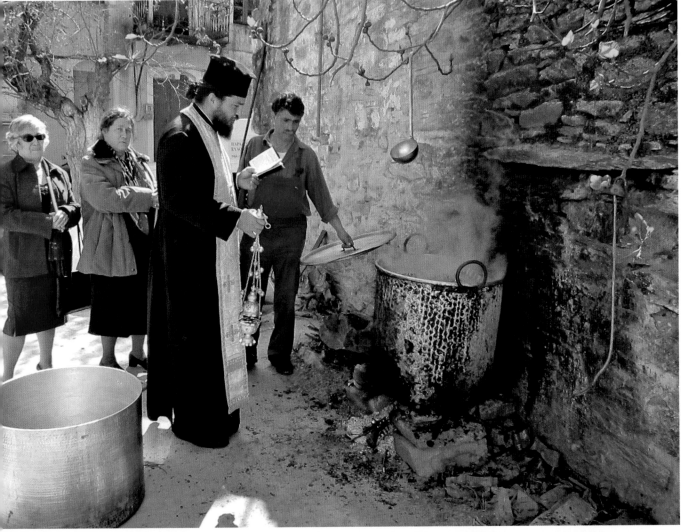

OVEN-ROASTED EASTER GOAT

Ofto

The cliché image of lamb and goat on a spit at Easter time is one that belongs more to the mainland than to the Greek islands. On Ikaria, as on most Aegean islands, the Easter tradition is for an oven-roasted whole goat, stuffed with rice or bulgur and herbs, and usually brought to the village baker's wood-burning oven, which imparts its own flavorful addition to the final dish. This dish is a showstopper. It's as though all the herbs of an island spring are stuffed into the meat. The rice filling could easily stand on its own as a pilaf. The flavor palette is complex: herbaceous thanks to all the herbs, but earthy, too. You don't have to add the organ meats if you're not a fan of such things. If you can't find lemon balm you can add a little lemon verbena or the grated peel of 1 large lemon into the rice mixture. You can substitute lamb for the goat.

MAKES 12 TO 16 SERVINGS

1 cup Greek extra virgin olive oil

15 scallions, chopped

Liver and other organ meats from a baby goat or lamb, rinsed well and trimmed

1½ cups short-grain rice

1¾ cups water

Salt and freshly ground black pepper

1 bunch flat-leaf parsley, finely chopped

1 bunch dill or wild fennel, finely chopped

1 cup finely chopped lemon balm (if available)

1 whole baby goat or lamb, about 10 pounds (4 to 5 kg)

1 cup strained fresh lemon juice

2 to 3 tablespoons dried Greek oregano

8 garlic cloves, very finely chopped

White wine (optional)

Preheat the oven to 375°F (190°C).

In a large, deep skillet, heat 2 tablespoons of the olive oil over medium heat. Add the scallions, reduce the heat to low, and cook slowly, stirring occasionally, until softened, about 10 minutes.

Meanwhile, chop the liver and any other organ meats.

Add the chopped liver mixture to the scallions, increase the heat to medium, and brown on all sides. Add the rice to the skillet and toss to coat in the oil. Add ¾ cup of the water and cook until it is absorbed. Season with salt and pepper. Add the chopped herbs and remove from the heat to let cool. Add 1 cup of water to the rice mixture.

Place the goat in a large shallow oiled baking pan. Season the outside and inside of the goat generously with salt and pepper. Stuff the goat's cavity loosely with the rice mixture and secure it closed, either by sewing or with metal skewers.

In a bowl, whisk or puree the remaining ¾ cup plus 2 tablespoons olive oil, the lemon juice, oregano, and garlic. Brush the goat with about half of the mixture. Roast, turning once, until the goat turns golden brown, about 1 hour 30 minutes, then reduce the temperature to 350°F (175°C) and continue roasting until the meat is tender, about 3 hours, basting with the pan juices, additional marinade, and white wine (if using) every so often.

Let rest for at least 20 minutes before carving.

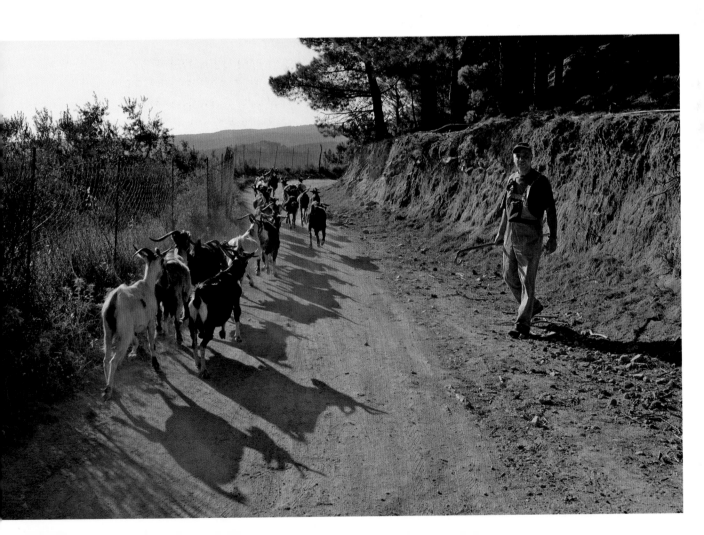

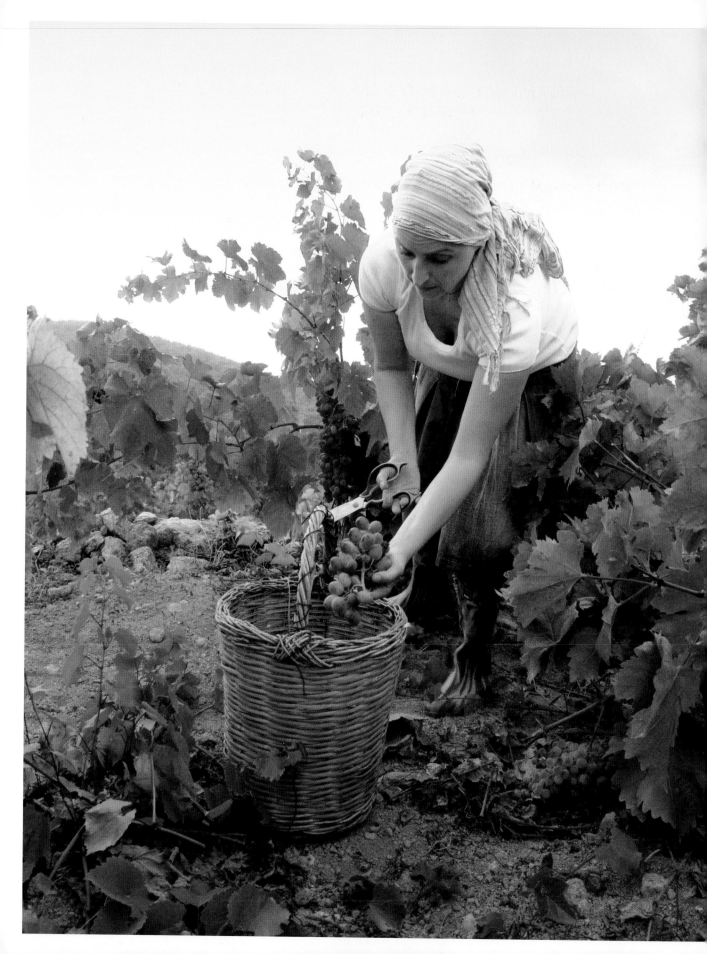

ELENI'S GOAT OR LAMB STEW WITH GRAPE MOLASSES

Katsikaki tis Elenis me Petimezi

I sing the praises of my friend Eleni Karimali throughout this book. She is a great cook and the meals I have enjoyed over the years at her country winery in Pygi have always left me deeply satisfied because her food, almost all of it produced on the estate, tastes so fresh, so real, so delicious.

Eleni produces *petimezi* (grape molasses) from the grapes on her farm and estate. She uses it in many different ways, from an addition to salad dressings to a flavor enhancer in meat dishes like this one, to a sweetener—one of the world's oldest—in various desserts. *Petimezi* is available in Greek and Middle Eastern food shops. If you can't find it, substitute sweet red wine, such as port or Mavrodafni and reduce 1½ cups of the wine to about ¾ cup to get a more intense sweetness, akin to *petimezi*.

MAKES 4 TO 6 SERVINGS

- ⅔ cup Greek extra virgin olive oil
- 3 pounds (1.5 kg) bone-in goat or lamb shoulder, trimmed, washed, and patted dry
- 2 red onions, finely chopped (about 2 cups)
- 2 large carrots, chopped (about 1½ cups)
- 5 garlic cloves, finely chopped
- 2 to 3 cups dry red wine

- ⅔ cup *petimezi* (grape molasses)
- 3 bay leaves
- 4 allspice berries
- 1 cinnamon stick
- 5 or 6 sprigs fresh thyme
- 5 or 6 sprigs fresh oregano or savory
- Salt and freshly ground black pepper

In a large, wide pot, heat the olive oil over medium-high heat. Add the meat and brown, turning it to color on all sides. Do this in batches if necessary, then return the browned meat to the pot.

Reduce the heat to low, add the onions and carrots, and cook, stirring until wilted, 10 to 12 minutes. Add the garlic and turn it in the pan juices a few times.

Add the wine, *petimezi*, spices, herbs, and salt and pepper to taste. Add water, if there isn't enough liquid, so that the meat is just barely covered. Bring to a boil, reduce the heat to low, cover, and simmer until the meat is falling off the bone and the sauce thick, about 2 to 2 hours 30 minutes.

Let cool for 10 to 15 minutes, then serve.

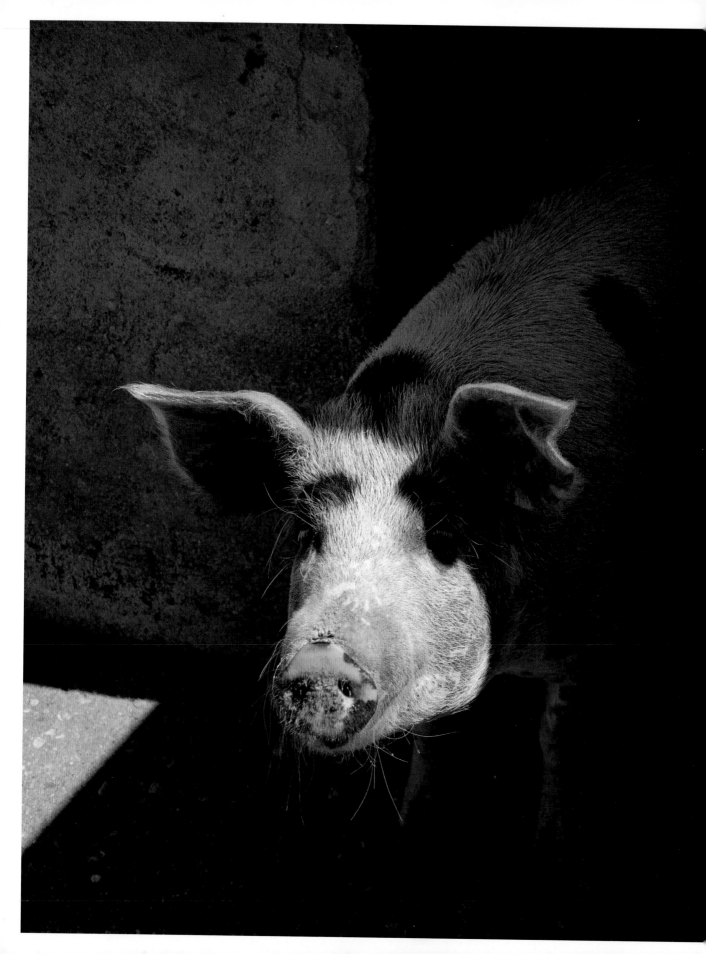

FAMILY HOGS AND CHRISTMAS

Christo Kouvdos, in his midtwenties, feeds the pigs he keeps acorns, table scraps, and whey left over from his mother's, Argyro's, cheese making. They seem happy! Around Christmastime or, more likely, around December 6 when his dad, Nikolas, celebrates his name day, one of his little piggies will become, well, food for an ongoing feast. The holiday pork slaughter, whether there is a Nikolas in the family or not, is still a living tradition on Ikaria and—pork is still the winter meat. It takes several men to help out with the slaughtering, shaving, evisceration, and butchering of the pig, and several women to handle all the culinary work that ensues: intestines, washed inside and out, become the casings for sausages; the lungs are made into a stew (*stifado*) with whole small onions, rosemary, bay leaf, and wine; the liver is sautéed with vinegar and olive oil, a meze par excellence; the head becomes *pikti*, headcheese, which takes hours to simmer, before the meat can be shredded and the gelatin set; bits of boneless meat become *kaourmas*, a kind of confit, in which the meat is preserved in its own fat. The belly—pancetta—is either cut into thick slabs and grilled or stewed with collard greens, a treat that Ikarians to this day still love. Thighs become Ikarian prosciutto, called *hoiromeri*, which is salted, pressed, and smoked. Over the mantle in Christos' parents' home, for example, the whole salted pork thigh is wrapped in muslin and hangs above the fireplace, where it is smoked for days over lemon wood and *schino*, lentiscus in English, the same tree that the spice *mastiha* is made from. Both woods are aromatic.

The fat itself is a whole chapter. Pork fat was a valuable source of energy and a beloved treat when rendered and spreadable—poor man's butter. Friends who are my age, in their 50s, still speak lovingly of the best finger-licking childhood treat: a piece of bread smeared with rendered pork fat and sprinkled with sugar. Remember, this was a generation that knew no television (which came to the island between the late 1960s and early 1970s, together with electricity), worked and played outside, and walked, sometimes 2 hours each way, to school and back. The best fat is the alabaster-white fat from the belly of the pig, what Ikarians call *kayias*.

The humble pig provides both nourishment and the reasons for a feast.

It might seem counterintuitive to write about the importance of pork in a book that aims to take a peek at the cooking traditions of a people known for their longevity. Pork is not, of course, the first food that comes to mind when one thinks of healthy eating. But it is a very important part of the local Ikarian diet, and, more so, an integral part of the Mediterranean diet, so long as we understand it in context—it was eaten neither in quantities nor daily, but rather sparingly over the course of a few cold months, until the start of Lent, and, if there was any left, then after Easter, too.

PORK, WILD FENNEL, AND BARLEY RUSKS

Hoiromeri sto Tetzeri me Maratho kai Paximadi

What intrigued me about this dish when I came across it in a book about the traditional foods of Ikaria and also in older people's descriptions of it, was not only its simplicity but its unwitting elegance. It reminded me of a dish I had stumbled upon years ago, on the other side of Greece, a simple asparagus broth served over rusks, with a bit of olive oil and shaved cheese. It touched the chef in me. Originally, this recipe called for smoked *hoiromeri*, something akin to prosciutto cotto (cooked prosciutto), but saltier and not as refined in taste. You can use either cotto or smoked pancetta for this. Some Greek regional cured pork products such as *pasto* and *singlino* from the Peloponnese, are available in Greek specialty food shops and are also well suited to this dish. I just love the idea of a smoky broth, sweetened with onions and herbs, served over a barley rusk. Rusks, for anyone not familiar with them, are the hard twice-baked breads that come shaped like thick slices or small bite-size chunks. They are also available in Greek and Middle Eastern food shops.

MAKES 4 TO 6 SERVINGS

½ cup Greek extra virgin olive oil

1 pound (450 g) prosciutto cotto, cut into cubes (1 inch [2.5 cm]), or smoked pancetta, cut into half-moons (½ inch [1 cm] thick)

1 large red onion, chopped (about 1 cup)

2 garlic cloves, chopped

5 cups water

Sea salt and cracked black pepper

1 cup chopped wild fennel fronds

Juice of 1 to 2 lemons (to taste)

4 to 6 barley rusks

In a large, wide pot, heat 2 tablespoons of the olive oil over medium heat. Add the prosciutto (or pancetta) and lightly brown. Add the onion and garlic and cook, stirring, until soft, 8 to 10 minutes.

Pour in the water and season to taste with salt and pepper. Simmer, covered, until the meat and vegetables are tender, about 45 minutes. About 10 minutes before removing from the heat, add the fennel. Season with some of the lemon juice.

To serve, place a barley rusk in the bottoms of 4 to 6 individual soup bowls. Pour the pork-and-fennel broth on top. Drizzle in the remaining 6 tablespoons olive oil and additional lemon juice to taste.

PORK AND COLLARD GREEN STEW

Hoirino Mageiremeno me Lahanides

Pork and cabbage is a globally loved combination of flavors, and this dish is essentially a version of that, since collards are in the cabbage family. This lemony pork and collard stew is probably the most popular winter recipe on Ikaria, a Sunday and Christmas treat that calls for strong wine and company. There are at least three versions of this dish. The first, below, is with fresh pork, preferably bone-in (for more flavor). But the more traditional versions, if you have a family pig and a fireplace over which to smoke it once you slaughter it, are for smoked pork. The leg is usually smoked, but I've also come across this recipe made with smoked pancetta (see Variations, on page 255), which you can find in Italian markets.

In the recipe below the pork and collards are finished with a thick, lemony sauce, which helps balance the richness of the pork and the almost musky, cabbagy flavor of the collards. If you can't find collards, you can use bok choy (Chinese cabbage). This dish is usually served with roasted potatoes.

MAKES 4 TO 6 SERVINGS

²/₃ cup Greek extra virgin olive oil

2¼ pounds (1 kg) bone-in pork shoulder or leg, cut into serving-size pieces

Salt and freshly ground black pepper

2 large red onions, chopped (about 2 cups)

2 tablespoons all-purpose flour

1 cup dry white wine

1 to 2 cups water or stock

3 pounds (1.5 kg) collard greens, trimmed and cut into ribbons 1½ inches (4 cm) wide

Juice of 1 to 2 lemons (to taste)

In a large wide pot, heat the olive oil over medium-high heat. Add the pork, in batches if necessary, and sear, turning with kitchen tongs to brown on all sides. Season with salt and pepper.

Push the pork to one side of the pot and add the onions. Reduce the heat to medium and cook, stirring the onions occasionally, until soft and translucent, 8 to 10 minutes. Sprinkle the flour into the pot. Mix gently to combine with the onions and pork. Cook for 2 to 3 minutes.

Pour in the wine. When the alcohol sizzles off, add enough water (or stock) to come about halfway up the height of the meat. Cover, reduce the heat to low, and simmer until the meat is tender but not completely done, 1 hour to 1 hour 15 minutes.

Add the collards to the pot. Mix in gently. Season again with salt and pepper. Cover and cook until the greens and meat are both very tender and the meat is falling off the bone, another 35 to 40 minutes. About 5 minutes before removing from the heat, pour in half the lemon juice, taste it, and pour in the rest if desired. Remove from the heat and serve.

(continued)

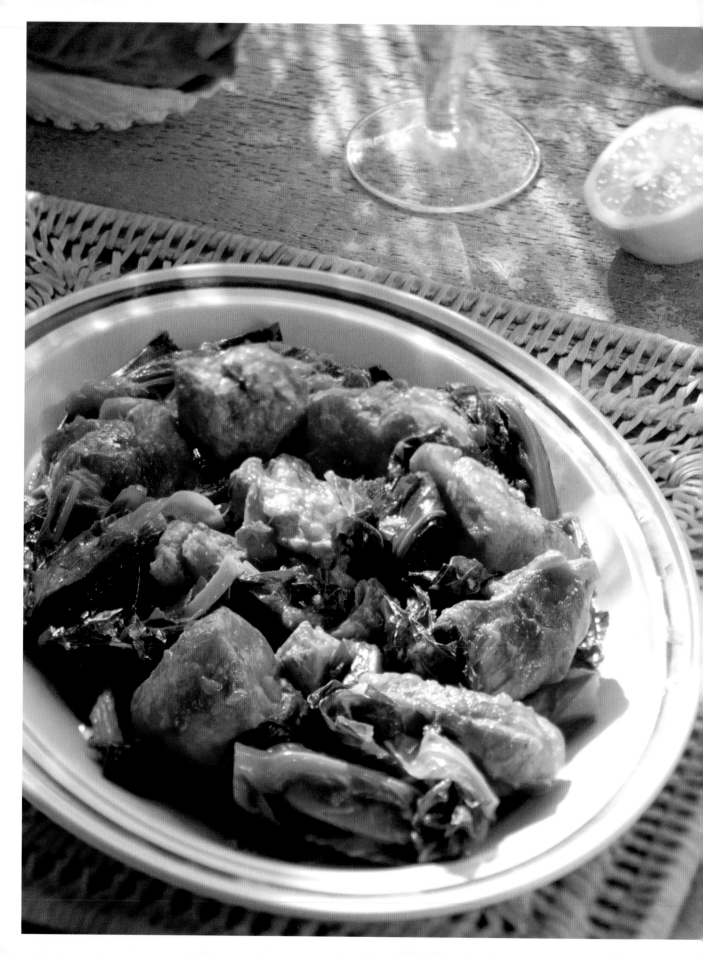

Collards and Pancetta Stew: Look for either smoked or fresh pancetta or whole slab bacon, preferably smoked, either of which needs to be cut into 2-inch (5 cm) chunks. Lightly brown 2 pounds of cubed pancetta or slab bacon in ½ cup olive oil over medium heat in a large, wide pot. Add the onions, a pinch of flour, then the collards. As soon as they wilt, add enough wine, water, and/or stock to come about halfway up the contents of the pot. Season to taste with salt and pepper. Simmer, covered, until the greens and pancetta are tender, 45 minutes to 1 hour. Add lemon juice, or bind with avgolemono, as in the variation below.

Pork and Collards Avgolemono: Instead of plain lemon juice, you can finish the dish with avgolemono, the egg-lemon liaison that is used to thicken and flavor so many Greek dishes, especially those in which greens and meat or fish are cooked together. To add avgolemono, whisk 3 egg yolks until frothy and slowly drizzle in 1 cup lemon juice, whisking all the while, until the mixture is thick and creamy. Take a ladleful of the pot juices and very slowly drizzle them into the egg-lemon mixture, whisking vigorously while you do this. Repeat 2 to 3 more times. Pour the whole mixture back into the hot pot, tilt the pot from side to side so that the avgolemono is evenly distributed, and serve.

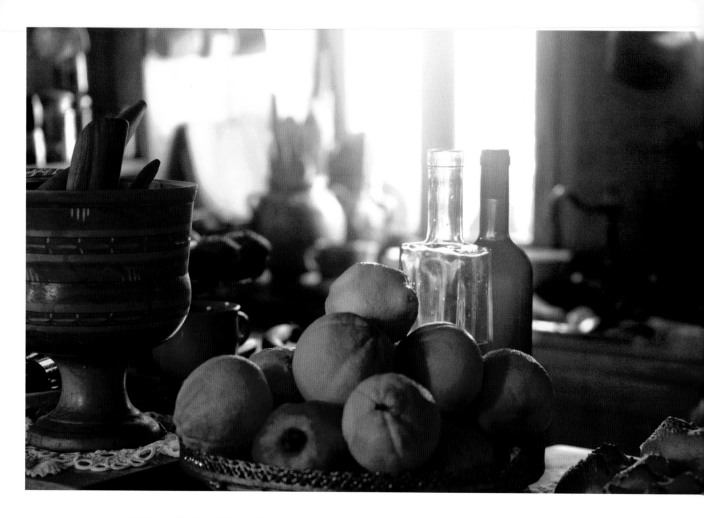

SIPHONING OFF THE WINE

We are at our friend Kollia's for a meal, one of so many over the years. Wine waits on the table for the food to arrive, but we have no issue pouring some in anticipation. His wife, Argyro, is a great cook and the table is already laden with her cheese, her olives, boiled greens, and her bread. The wine, dark red and strong, edges slowly toward the bottom of a carafe and Kollia swings out of his chair, takes the bottle, and heads outside to the cellar to siphon off some more.

This is an old habit among wine-making Ikarians—the siphoning—that dates to the days, within my own living memory, when people kept their homemade wine in amphorae in the ground and served it from dried-out, swan-necked squashes. To transfer it required literally sucking it up through a small cut-off hose or straw only to then release it into the container. Now, wine is served in glass pitchers or bottles, but the trip to the siphon room, aka cellar, is still something men like to do. Needless to say, the more siphoners the merrier. There is no dearth of excuses for having to run to the cellar with a buddy or two to test and transfer the vino.

AUNT ATHINA'S IKARIAN HEADCHEESE

Pikti tis Theias Athinas

"You have to put Ikarian *pikti* [headcheese] in your book," my friend Aneza insists, scooping up a lump of it and spooning it onto my plate. We're at her Aunt Athina's house in Athens and the woman has prepared a post-holiday feast, right after New Year's but before the Epiphany and the name day of St. John the Theologian, which families in Greece celebrate, John being a common name.

I wince. The last time I had *pikti* I was at another Ikarian home, across the Atlantic, one New Year's Day about 25 years ago. His mother Mary's *pikti* was there on the table, abandoned to some outer ridge until one of us, with the help of a little Johnny Walker, dared the other to taste it.

It took a score and some years for me to reassess *pikti*, and that only after tasting Aunt Athina's version, which is light, and very lemony. She never uses the head but boils trotters and shoulder instead.

MAKES 12 TO 15 SERVINGS

3 whole pork trotters

6 pounds (2.75 kg) boneless pork shoulder, in large chunks

10 allspice berries

6 whole cloves

6 bay leaves

Salt and freshly ground black pepper

2½ cups fresh lemon juice (from about 15 lemons)

Place the trotters and meat in 2 separate pots and pour in enough water to cover by 2 inches (5 cm). Divide up the herbs and spices and add them to each pot. Season with salt and pepper.

Boil the trotters until all their gelatin has been released and the meat is falling off the bone, 2 to 2 hours 30 minutes. Boil the boneless meat, simmering until it is so tender it shreds. While both pots are simmering, skim off any foam that accumulates on the surface.

Remove the pork shoulder with a slotted spoon and let it cool slightly. Shred or cut it into bite-size pieces. Discard the cooking liquid.

Remove the trotters and let cool. Reserve their boiling liquid. Shred the meat off the trotters. Discard the spices from both pots.

Place the shredded meats in a large bowl. Strain the cooking liquid from the trotters into the meat mixture and add the lemon juice. Mix.

Pour the mixture into a deep serving dish, glass bowl, or Bundt pan. Cover with plastic wrap and refrigerate for 4 to 6 hours, until set. Serve cold.

ONE-POT PORK AND TARO

Hoirino me Kolokasi

This is one of the most traditional ways to stew pork and use taro on the island. Greeks consider pork a winter meat and taro is also generally harvested in the damp cold months between November and February. Together they make for extremely hearty fare. Taro is rich in complex carbohydrates and dietary fiber but very low in fat and protein. It is used in this dish the way potatoes would be, to provide even more substance and stretch the meal. Pork is high in protein. If you add a salad to this dish, you've got a nutritionally complete meal.

MAKES 4 TO 6 SERVINGS

2¼ pounds (1 kg) bone-in pork shoulder, cut into serving pieces

⅓ cup Greek extra virgin olive oil

2 large red onions, chopped (about 2 cups)

2 leeks, cleaned and chopped

2 large carrots, cut into ½-inch (1 cm) rounds

1 cup dry white wine

1 cup chopped canned tomatoes

3 bay leaves

5 or 6 allspice berries

2 or 3 dried chile peppers (to taste)

Salt and freshly ground black pepper

2 pounds (1 kg) taro root, peeled and cut into 1-inch (2.5-cm) rounds (keep in acidulated water to prevent browning)

Rinse and pat dry the meat.

In a large flameproof casserole or Dutch oven, heat the olive oil over medium-high heat and brown the meat, turning with kitchen tongs to sear on all sides.

Remove the meat with a slotted spoon. Drain off all but 3 tablespoons of the fat. Add the onions, leeks, and carrots and cook over medium heat, stirring occasionally, until slightly softened, 8 to 10 minutes.

Return the meat to the pot. Pour in the wine. As soon as the alcohol steams off, add the tomatoes, bay leaves, allspice, chile peppers, and salt and black pepper to taste. Cover and simmer until the meat is very tender and falling off the bone, 1 hour 30 minutes to 2 hours. About 45 minutes before removing from the heat, add the taro pieces and gently stir. When they, too, are tender, remove the stew from the heat and serve.

MY CHICKEN STIFADO WITH AN URBAN TOUCH

Kotopoulo Stifado me Astiki Pinelia

The door to my kitchen on Ikaria opens up onto our little stone terrace and a few years ago my husband, Vassilis, planted an herb bed in a dirt patch he left unpaved right in the middle, under a trellis of grapes and between a few very old almond trees. We've planted rosemary, sage, mints, lavender, oregano, thyme, and, every spring, replenish with all the annuals: different varieties of basil, parsley, cilantro, chives, lemon balm, and more. All of these find their way into my cooking. I get inspired by the absolute freshness and immediacy of ingredients on Ikaria, the fresh-cut herbs, the chicken that strutted in my neighbor Titika's coop until she brought some of it over for me to cook for the kids, by the onions we pick out of the ground that are so peppery and sharp you want to cry before you even peel them. This is real food, the ultimate locavore diet.

The urban touch in this recipe comes from the addition of almonds, which is not something one finds in the savory cooking on the island, even though so many people have their own almond trees. Note: Potatoes fried in olive oil are the dish to serve with this as an accompaniment.

MAKES 4 SERVINGS

½ cup plus 2 tablespoons Greek extra virgin olive oil

4 bone-in, skinless chicken thighs

1 large red onion, finely chopped (about 1 cup)

2 garlic cloves, finely chopped

Sea salt and freshly ground black pepper

1½ cups semisweet white or rosé wine

2 bay leaves

1 sprig fresh rosemary

4 or 5 sprigs fresh thyme

2 or 3 fresh sage leaves

4 or 5 sprigs fresh marjoram, oregano, or savory

3 or 4 allspice berries

6 or 7 black peppercorns

1 cinnamon stick

1 tablespoon tomato paste, preferably from sun-dried tomatoes

1 to 2 tablespoons water

12 boiling onions, peeled

1 cup fresh green almonds (if available) or blanched almonds

2 to 3 tablespoons red wine, sherry, or balsamic vinegar (to taste)

In a large, wide pot or Dutch oven, heat ½ cup of the olive oil over medium heat. Place the chicken in the pot, top side down, and brown. Using kitchen tongs, carefully turn to brown on the other side, too, for a total of 10 to 15 minutes. Transfer the chicken to a plate and drain off all but 2 tablespoons of fat from the pot.

Add the chopped onion and cook until wilted, about 10 minutes. Stir in the garlic.

(continued)

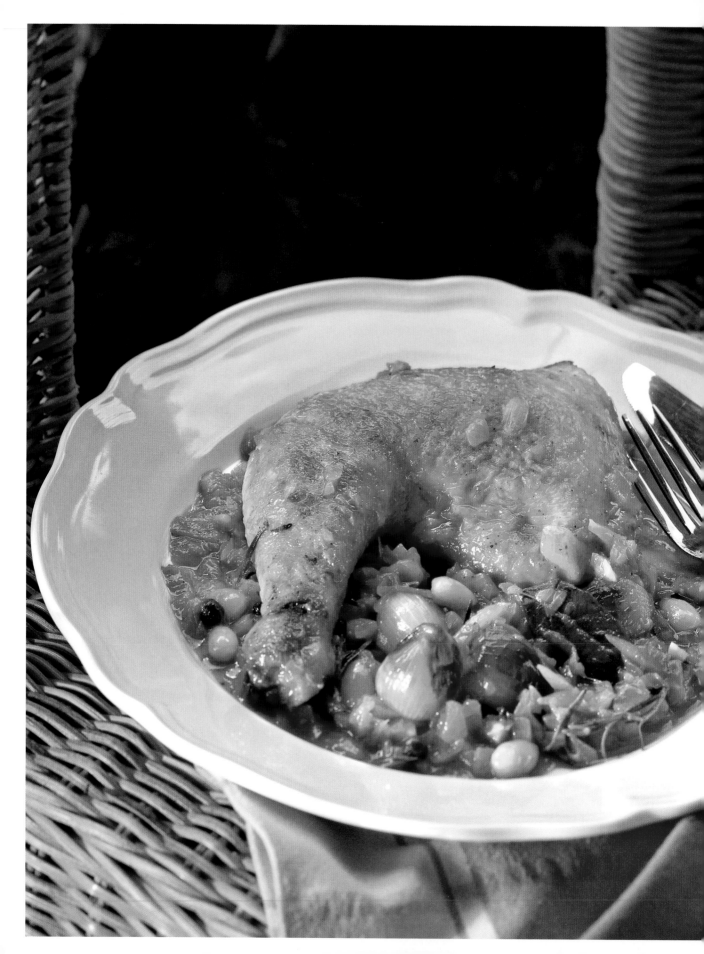

Season the chicken with salt and pepper and return to the pot. Pour in the wine. Add the herbs and spices. Dilute the tomato paste with the water and add to the pot. Add enough additional water to come about halfway up the chicken pieces (there might already be enough liquid in the pot, so this may not be necessary). Season with salt and pepper. Cover the pot, reduce the heat, and simmer the chicken until falling-off-the-bone tender, 50 minutes to 1 hour.

While the chicken is simmering, in a large, heavy skillet, heat the remaining 2 tablespoons olive oil. Add the whole onions and cook, covered, over low heat until they caramelize lightly, 20 to 25 minutes.

Twenty minutes before removing the chicken from the heat, gently stir in the whole onions, the almonds, and the vinegar.

VARIATION

This same recipe, with or without the almonds, which are my addition, may also be made with rabbit, cut like the chicken, into serving pieces (minus the head). Cooking times are the same.

WINE-COOKED ROOSTER AND ROOSTER BROTH WITH RICE

Kokoras Krasatos kai Soupa me Ryzi

Ikarians still cook rooster for a holiday or other special occasion, literally making the most of it. In the following recipe, the rooster is first cooked in a soup pot then removed and finished with a wine-based tomato sauce; its broth becomes a soup. Both are served together. Rooster meat is tough and sometimes sinewy, so needs much more cooking time than chicken does. Boiling it first creates the broth for a soup; then the meat is repurposed, so to speak, by continuing to cook it in an aromatic tomato-wine sauce. The end result is meat that is literally falling off the bone; its natural gelatin over such long hours of cooking is released and helps thicken both the soup broth and the tomato-wine sauce. This is ultimate comfort food, made for good bread and strong country wine.

MAKES 6 TO 8 SERVINGS

1 large rooster or free-range chicken, about 5 pounds (2.25 kg)

2 large red onions, 1 whole and 1 chopped

3 carrots, cut into 3 or 4 large pieces each

½ cup Greek extra virgin olive oil

Salt and freshly ground black pepper

2 cups chopped plum tomatoes (canned if fresh are out of season)

1 cinnamon stick

4 or 5 sprigs fresh basil

2 sprigs fresh sage

2 bay leaves

1 cup dry red wine

1 chicken liver, finely chopped (optional)

¾ cup short-grain white or brown rice

Juice of 2 lemons (optional)

Place the rooster or whole chicken in a large soup pot together with the whole onion, the carrots, ¼ cup of the olive oil, and a little salt and pepper. Pour in enough water to cover the bird by about 2 inches (5 cm). Bring to a boil, reduce the heat, and simmer until the meat is almost cooked, about 1 hour. As the broth simmers, skim the foam off the surface and discard.

Reserving the broth, remove the bird with a slotted spoon. Place in a bowl and when it is cool enough to handle cut into large serving pieces, bones and all.

In a shallow, wide pot, deep skillet, or Dutch oven, heat the remaining ¼ cup olive oil over medium heat. Add the chopped onion and cook until soft. Add the rooster or chicken pieces and season with salt and pepper. Add the tomatoes, cinnamon, and herbs. Pour in the red wine. Cook until the bird is very tender and falling off the bone, 20 to 30 more minutes.

Meanwhile, bring the broth to a boil and add the liver (if using). Simmer until the liver is halfway cooked, about 10 minutes, skimming the foam off the surface of the soup as it forms. Add the rice. Season to taste with salt and pepper. Simmer, partially covered, until the rice is tender and adjust the seasoning with salt and pepper, about 20 to 25 minutes. The soup should be thick and dense. Season it, if desired, with lemon juice.

Serve the chicken on a platter and the soup separately, in bowls.

POULTRY IN THE DIET

When I am on Ikaria in the summers, nothing seems more rural to me than the cock-a-doodle-do alarm clock we wake up to at sunrise as roosters sing in the new day from every which direction.

Almost every family keeps a chicken coop, but hens and roosters weren't the stuff of everyday meals. To this day, rooster is a special-occasion meat or major holiday fare. Roosters, for example, are scarce and have always been esteemed for their dark, flavorful meat. Rooster continues to be the traditional Christmas and New Year's main course.

Hens were more valuable for their eggs than for their meat.

Most of the dishes for either are simple. Roasted chicken and a lot of stewed chicken dishes, often with vegetables, such as Chicken in a Pot with Okra (page 264), are still a part of the island recipe repertoire. Stews are mainly simmered in tomato-based sauces. Sometimes old hens are boiled for soup, which is thickened with rice or bulgur and finished with avgolemono, the egg-lemon liaison that defines much of Greek cuisine.

Roosters, on the other hand, have tough meat that requires slow, wet cooking and so are typically simmered for hours. The most common way to cook a rooster on Ikaria is in an hours'-long wine sauce (opposite).

Today, of course, chicken is a much more frequent part of the dinner table and there is at least one commercial producer of chickens on the island. You can find the bird at local supermarkets. There is no comparison, as anyone with a chicken coop will say, between the commercial bird and its garden-strutting cousin.

CHICKEN IN A POT WITH OKRA

Kotopoulo Yiahni me Bamiyes

Throughout the book, there are recipes called *yiahni*, which is the term for an oniony tomato sauce. Almost any protein or vegetable can be cooked *yiahni*. These dishes are rich and pleasingly unctuous, with an unabashed quantity of olive oil, the kind of dishes that were cooked for hours until every ingredient melded and all that was left in the pot was "a little olive oil," which was actually a cooking instruction a generation ago. I've toned down the quantity of olive oil. This is a summer dish, when okra is in season. You can also make it with green beans.

Saucy dishes like this one are usually served with thickly cut potatoes pan-fried in olive oil. A nice big green salad or village salad would almost surely be on the table, too.

MAKES 6 SERVINGS

½ cup Greek extra virgin olive oil

1 large chicken, about 4 pounds (2 kg), cut into serving pieces

2 large red onions, chopped (about 2 cups)

2 garlic cloves, chopped

1 pound okra, trimmed and soaked in vinegar (see Note)

2 cups chopped canned plum tomatoes or grated fresh tomatoes

2 bay leaves

2 or 3 sprigs fresh oregano

Salt and freshly ground black pepper

In a large stewing pot or Dutch oven, heat half the olive oil over medium heat. Working in batches if necessary, brown the chicken, turning with kitchen tongs to brown on all sides.

Transfer the chicken to a plate, and drain off all but 3 tablespoons of fat. Add the onions and garlic. Stir until soft, 8 to 10 minutes. Place the chicken back in the pot.

Add the okra, tomatoes, herbs, and salt and pepper to taste. Add enough water so that the liquid in the pot comes about halfway up its contents. Bring to a boil, cover, reduce the heat to low, and simmer until the chicken and okra are tender, 50 minutes to 1 hour.

Let cool slightly before serving. Drizzle with remaining olive oil and serve.

NOTE: *To trim okra, take a small paring knife and cut around the circumference of the stem, discarding the tough, thin stem piece. Rinse the okra and drain, then place in a bowl and sprinkle with red wine vinegar. Let stand for 1 hour. Rinse and use as needed. Soaking the okra in vinegar helps rid it of its mucilaginous texture.*

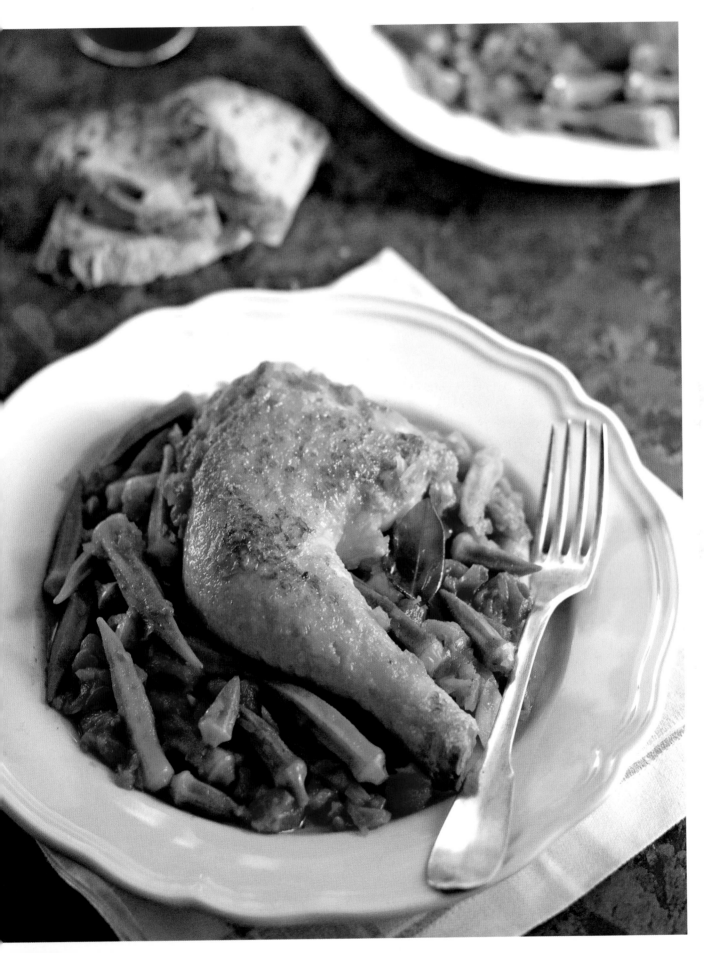

RABBIT STEW

Kouneli Stifado

Hares and partridges are the two main game meats on the island. Both are cooked in the most traditional ways—hares and rabbits are cooked stifado-style, in an aromatic tomato sauce with plenty of onions and partridges are typically roasted with olive oil and oregano.

In this dish, you'll notice a lot of the same flavor components that run through many of the stews and casseroles in this book, the warm spices like allspice and cinnamon, the red wine, and an overabundance of onions, all of which cook together slowly to help make this dish comfortingly sweet. Hare, which is tough, certainly benefits from a lengthy marinade, but so does rabbit, with its lean, mild flesh. The most popular way to serve this is with a mountain of potatoes fried in olive oil or with mashed potatoes.

MAKES 4 TO 6 SERVINGS

1 medium rabbit, about 3 pounds (1.4 kg), cut into serving pieces

4 cups dry red wine

4 bay leaves

6 to 10 allspice berries

2 cinnamon sticks

Flour, for dredging

¾ cup Greek extra virgin olive oil

Salt and freshly ground black pepper

1 large onion, finely chopped (about 1 cup)

2 garlic cloves, finely chopped

1 cup chopped tomatoes

2 pounds (900 g) small boiling onions, peeled and whole

1 tablespoon tomato paste diluted in 1 tablespoon water

Place the rabbit in a large bowl and cover with 2 cups of the red wine, 2 of the bay leaves, the allspice berries, and 1 of the cinnamon sticks. Marinate for 2 to 8 hours (you can do this overnight). Remove the rabbit from the marinade and pat dry.

Dredge the rabbit lightly in flour.

In a large, wide pot or Dutch oven, heat ¼ cup of the olive oil over medium heat. Working in 2 batches, add half the rabbit and brown on one side. Turn with kitchen tongs to brown on the other side. Season with salt and pepper. Replenish the pot with another ¼ cup olive oil to brown the second batch. Remove and set aside.

Add the chopped onion to the pot. Cook, stirring, until wilted, 8 to 10 minutes. Stir in the garlic. Add the rabbit pieces back in.

Add the remaining 2 cups of wine, 2 bay leaves, cinnamon stick, and the tomatoes. Bring to a boil, reduce the heat to low, cover, and simmer until the rabbit is tender and falling off the bone, 1 hour 30 minutes to 2 hours.

Meanwhile, in a large skillet, heat the remaining ¼ cup olive oil over medium heat. Add the whole onions and cook until lightly browned, shaking or turning in the pan so that they are evenly colored.

Thirty minutes before the rabbit is done, add the onions. Add the diluted tomato paste and stir gently. Season to taste with salt and pepper. When the rabbit is cooked and tender, remove and serve.

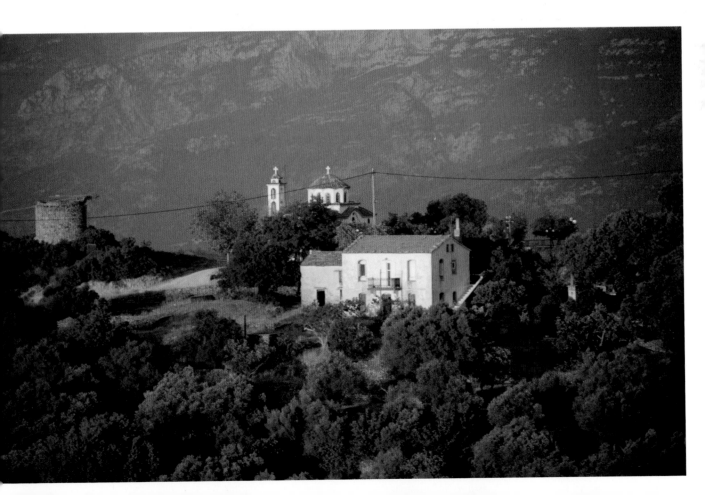

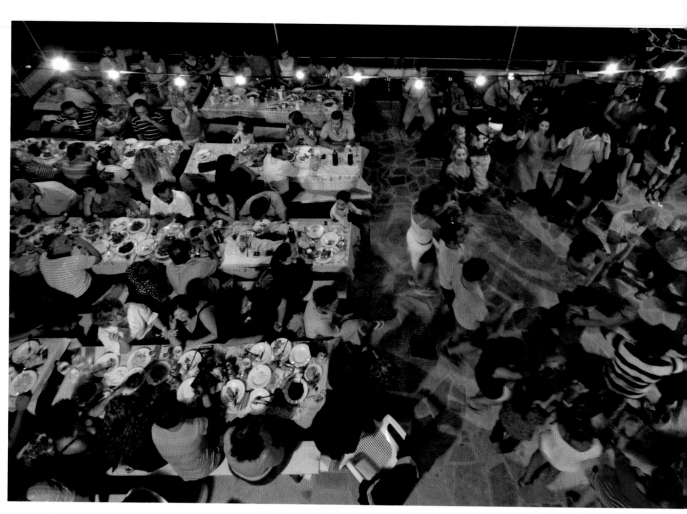

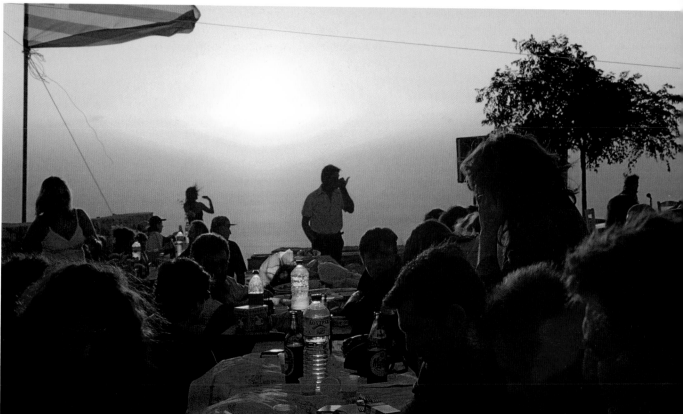

PANYGYRIA: FEASTS OF LIFE

August 15 is the height of Greek summer and the Ascension, one of the holiest days of the year. In the villages around Raches, most people head to morning liturgy at Moundé, a 17th-century monastery. By late morning, the day's other character starts to take shape. August 15, despite its sobriety, is also a time of unbridled revelry at one of about half a dozen *panygyria* all over Ikaria. The largest and by far most infamous is in Langada, one of the earliest settlements on the island, nestled in a valley on the north side. Literally thousands of people, the great majority young, descend on Langada for what one Greek newspaper a few years ago described as the biggest rave party in the Aegean. The only difference is that the music is traditional demotic Greek. To get there you park a good kilometer or more away and walk down a dusty road into the heart of the valley. The crowd here starts to gather early. By midafternoon the searing sound of a traditional *tsambouna*, bagpipe, wailing out the rhythm of a *kariotiko*, the local song and dance, has most people locked shoulder-to-shoulder in circles, dancing the dance.

Panygyria are festivals, replete with food and dancing, traditionally held to commemorate a saint's name day. Over the last three decades they have morphed into almost nightly affairs all over the island in summer. Ikaria is famous throughout Greece for her *panygyria*.

To the uninitiated it is hard to explain the pleasure of a *panygyri*. To an outsider, it might simply appear as a ragtag congregation with hundreds, sometimes thousands, of fellow islanders who squeeze onto highly uncomfortable, rough-hewn wooden benches, wait in line for food that largely consists of boiled goat, Greek salad, and cold fries; drink local wine that is sometimes a little rough around the edges; and then dance. And dance. And dance. If you have the stamina, you can literally dance 'til dawn since most *panygyria* wind down in the midmorning hours after a good 10 hours of revelry.

All in all, between May and September, there are more than 100 *panygyria* all over the island, the vast majority of them in July and August, when the island is most populated. Money from the sale of food and wine goes toward some charitable cause related to the host village. Many a road and community hall have been built with the money collected at *panygyria*.

Locals know to avoid the feasts that have gotten so huge they no longer have any real character. (Langada is an exception because the venue holds a certain place in the island's history, as its earliest settlement.)

At most *panygyria*, the festivities don't really get underway until around midnight. Some start early in the day and last until the next morning.

For us on the island, the *panygyria* are the means by which we embrace our Ikarian identity. They are one more expression of the solidarity that runs through the heart of this place and its people. To this day, they are a unifying force, bringing people together to express, in the most uninhibited ways, their common culture. They are also a lot of fun.

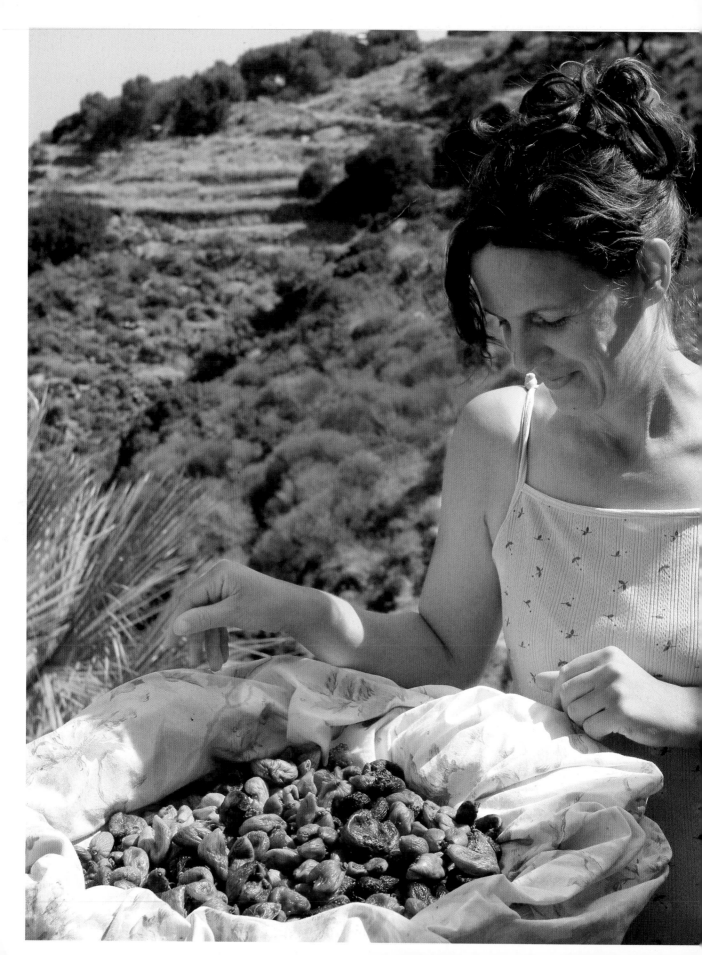

IKARIA'S
ICONIC SWEETS

THERE ARE A FEW SWEETS THAT FOR ME SPELL Ikaria, mainly because I remember them in the fondest way from the very first time I set foot on the island, in 1972.

My Aunt Mary was the arbiter of taste for me then. As old and eccentric an aunt as any 12-year-old could have, she had spent a lifetime away from Ikaria, mainly in Argentina, but returned to the island to live out the remainder of her life, which proved to be long and robust. She passed away 35 years later, at the ripe age of 95, and until almost the very end she tended her garden, knew the status of every tree in it, and worked hard to put their fruits to good use. Her *vyssino* (the classic sour-cherry preserve that is made in many parts of Greece but is a specialty of Ikaria, especially the north side, with its cooler, damper climate, perfect for cherry trees) is a flavor etched in my memory, smoky from her simmering the mix inside a blackened old pot in her fireplace. Her walnut spoon sweet, one of the most difficult of the Greek preserves, subtly spiced with clove, was laced with that same smokiness.

Other sweets remind me of other friends, like the *pasta flora*, a Greek jam tart that my lovely neighbor Titika makes several times a summer; or the spice cake for St. Fanourios, which I tasted for the first time at our friend Dafni's house, which is in the heart of the village and always filled with people and good things to eat.

The sweets on Ikaria are not unlike the sweets that are made elsewhere in Greece, but some things stand out because of what is on hand naturally: cherries and sour cherries, walnuts, apricots, peaches, young green (male) figs. These are all commonly made into spoon sweets, which are essentially preserves of fruits, young nuts, and certain vegetables that are put up in sugar syrup (or, in days gone by, grape molasses).

Honeyed sweets, made with Ikaria's excellent pine, heather, blossom, and thyme honey are also popular, with the best among them the *loukoumades*—dough puffs that are deep-fried and drenched in local honey. The best place to have them is at the Theoktisti Monastery in Pygi.

Walnuts and almonds also grow well on the island, but the former are more popular in sweets. One confection that is somewhat unique to the island are the Lenten *kaltsounia*, olive-oil-based cookies filled with nuts, grated orange, and raisins, and sprinkled with sugar. Another are the *xerotygana*, strips of fried dough drizzled with honey, the de rigueur Christmas, New Year's, and wedding confection.

Most of the confections in the Greek repertoire, and by default on the local Ikarian table, too, are pretty healthy so far as desserts go. That is, olive oil plays a role in cakes and cookies, and fruits and nuts are the main ingredients in many traditional sweets. Very few desserts call for cream or dairy, so very few contain saturated fat.

That said, I have not made a point of presenting specifically "healthy" desserts, but rather am showcasing some of my own favorites, culled from indulgent experiences on the island, in friends' homes, in local cafes, etc. When it comes to dessert, in my book, there is always room for a little sinfulness, so long as one is guided by sense. Abide by those ancient Greek words of wisdom, *Pan metron ariston*, or "nothing in excess," and enjoy!

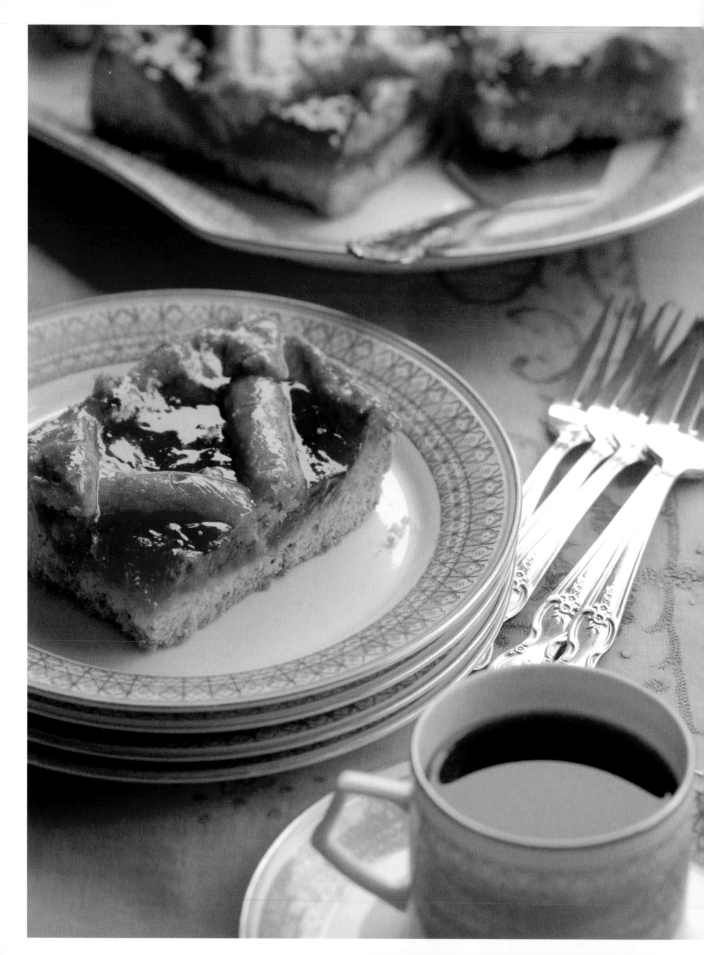

GREEK JAM LATTICE-TOP TART

Pasta Flora

We usually arrive in Ikaria at the end of apricot season, the one tree in our garden bent with the weight of hundreds of beautiful ripe fruits. Apricots are something of a specialty fruit on Ikaria, and the island has long been known for one variety, the small, sweet kaisia.

Almost every summer, as if on cue, Titika comes over with one of her jam tarts, called *pasta flora*. Elsewhere in Greece *pasta flora* is made with berry or cherry jams, but on Ikaria this lattice-topped tart is almost always made with local apricot jam. It should not be cloyingly sweet but rather be imbued with the refreshing tartness of apricots and have a crisp, crumbly pastry.

MAKES 6 TO 8 SERVINGS

3 cups all-purpose flour

1 teaspoon baking powder

1 tablespoon finely grated lemon zest

9 ounces (250 g) unsalted butter, at room temperature, plus more for greasing the tart pan

2 tablespoons sugar

1 egg

3 tablespoons brandy or fruit liqueur, preferably orange or apricot

1 teaspoon vanilla extract

1½ cups good-quality apricot jam, or any other good-quality fruit jam of choice

1 egg yolk, lightly whisked with 1 tablespoon water

In a bowl, combine the flour, baking powder, and lemon peel.

In a stand mixer fitted with the whisk attachment, beat the butter and sugar until fluffy. Add the egg and continue mixing until blended. Beat in the brandy (or liqueur) and vanilla.

Change the whisk attachment to a dough hook and slowly add the flour mixture, in ½-cup increments, until a dough forms. Knead for a few minutes, but don't overwork it. Remove the dough and let it rest at room temperature for 20 minutes.

Divide the dough into 2 balls, one slightly larger than the other. Break off a golf ball–size piece from the larger ball and set it aside.

Position a rack in the center of the oven and preheat it to 350°F (175°F). Lightly butter a 10-inch tart pan.

Spread a sheet of parchment paper or wax paper on a work surface and flour it lightly. Roll out the larger ball of dough to a round slightly larger than the circumference of the pan. Lift the paper

(continued)

carefully, place with dough side down over the tart pan, and carefully peel away the paper on the back side of the dough so that it folds gently and evenly into the tart pan. Press the edges slightly. Take a knife and skirt the edge of the pan to cut away any excess dough.

Collect the scraps and combine them with the smallest ball of dough. Roll it out to a round about ⅛ inch thick. Cut out 4 to 6 strips, each ½ inch wide. Position these around the rim of the tart pan, going all around the circumference of the pan, to form a ledge that you can attach the lattice strips to after the tart is filled with jam. Press lightly to anchor in place.

On a floured piece of parchment or work surface, roll out the remaining pastry ball to a sheet about 10 inches (25 cm) square. Cut ½-inch strips of dough to form the lattice.

Spread the jam evenly inside the tart shell.

Take the lattice strips one at a time and place them over the tart, first in one direction and then in the other, to form a decorative latticed top. Secure the lattice strips to the pieces you've already pressed around the rim. Trim any excess dough with kitchen shears or a small sharp knife.

Brush the lattice top with the egg yolk. Bake until the pastry is set and golden, 30 to 35 minutes. Let cool for at least 30 to 40 minutes for the jam to set before serving.

OLIVE OIL AND DESSERT

Olive oil has long been used in many Greek desserts, especially the sweets made during periods of fasting, when butter and dairy are prohibited. Over the years, I've learned to bake almost every imaginable cake with olive oil instead of butter.

Olive oil dramatically cuts back on the cholesterol and saturated fat content of desserts. It allows the flavor of the other ingredients to come forth. Because olive oil contains vitamin E, it helps to naturally maintain the freshness of baked goods and creates moist cakes, biscuits, and muffins. Every recipe in this chapter—save for Titika's Greek Jam Lattice-Top Tart (page 275), Diamando's Messy Orange Phyllo Pie (page 285), and the spoon sweets—contains olive oil.

SPICE CAKE FOR THE REVEALING SAINT

Fanouropita

One of my favorite things to do on August 27 is to go to the early morning liturgy at one of the little churches in various nearby villages named for St. Fanourios, the patron saint of lost things and the saint to whom one prays for help in finding misplaced possessions or, more metaphorically, for revealing everything from one's future spouse to the path toward faith. He is celebrated in a sprightly manner on Ikaria, and in the evening there is one of the most-beloved local *panygyria* (festivals) in the inland village of Maratho.

But the church tradition involves baking a cake, called *Fanouropita*, and at the service in the morning almost everyone there has brought a rendition of this spiced, raisin- and nut-filled sweet, which the priest blesses then distributes to parishioners right after the ceremony is over.

MAKES ONE 10- OR 12-INCH CAKE

4½ cups self-rising flour

1 teaspoon ground cinnamon

1 teaspoon ground cloves

1 teaspoon freshly grated nutmeg

Grated peel of 2 oranges

¾ cup Greek extra virgin olive oil

¾ cup granulated sugar

1 scant teaspoon baking soda

2 cups fresh orange juice

3 tablespoons brandy or orange liqueur

1 cup raisins

1 cup coarsely ground walnuts

Powdered sugar, for garnish

Preheat the oven to 350°F (175°C). Lightly oil a 10- or 12-inch round cake pan. In a bowl, combine the flour, cinnamon, cloves, nutmeg, and orange peel.

In a stand mixer fitted with the whisk attachment, beat together the olive oil and granulated sugar at medium speed until creamy.

Dissolve the baking soda in the orange juice. Reduce the mixer speed and add the orange juice mixture and brandy or liqueur. Whisk until smooth.

Replace the whisk attachment with the paddle attachment and mix in the flour mixture, raisins, and walnuts. Or, alternatively, do so with a spatula or wooden spoon. Transfer the batter (it will be dense) to the baking pan and spread evenly. Bake until a toothpick inserted in the center comes away clean, 35 to 40 minutes.

Let the cake cool in the pan for 15 minutes and then transfer to a rack to cool completely. Dust with powdered sugar and serve.

HONEYED DOUGH PUFFS

Loukoumades

Loukoumades are a special-occasion dessert and we enjoy them most at the monasteries of Theoktisti in Pygi and Mounte in Raches after the liturgy on several saints' name days during the summer.

MAKES 8 TO 10 SERVINGS

4 to 6 cups all-purpose flour, or more as needed

1 scant teaspoon salt

1 tablespoon instant dry yeast

1 tablespoon honey

2 cups warm water, or more as needed

Olive or other oil, for deep-frying

1 to 2 cups Ikarian pine honey or Greek thyme honey, for drizzling

Ground cinnamon

Coarsely ground walnuts

In a large stainless steel bowl, mix 4½ cups of the flour and the salt. Dissolve the yeast, honey, and 1 tablespoon of flour in ½ cup warm water.

Make a well in the center of the bowl of flour and pour in the yeast mixture. Add the remaining 1½ cups water. Either by hand (wear thin rubber gloves because the dough is very sticky) or with a large wooden spoon, gradually work enough flour into the liquid to form a thick, viscous, sticky, loose mass. Add more water in ¼-cup increments if necessary to achieve this texture. Cover the bowl with plastic wrap and place a large kitchen towel over it. Let stand in a warm, draft-free place for about 2 hours, or until doubled in bulk.

Fill a large, deep pot halfway with olive or other oil and heat to 375°F (180°C).

To shape the *loukoumades* traditionally: Lightly oil your hands with olive oil. Take up a handful of the dough about the size of a tennis ball; the dough will be loose, elastic, stringy, and yeasty. Clench your fist around it loosely. Have a cup of olive oil nearby to dip a tablespoon in. Squeeze out a knob of the batter between your curled-up index finger and thumb, scoop it up with the oiled tablespoon, then drop it carefully in the hot oil. Repeat with several more.

To shape the *loukoumades* with 2 tablespoons: Oil 2 spoons. Lift a little bit of dough up on one and push it off the spoon and into the hot oil with the other oiled spoon. Drop several balls at a time into the oil. Don't overcrowd.

As soon as the dough puffs rise to the top and are light golden brown, remove with a slotted spoon and drain on paper towels. Repeat until all the dough is fried. Replenish the oil if necessary.

Plate about 10 *loukoumades* and drizzle with honey. Sprinkle with cinnamon and walnuts. Serve.

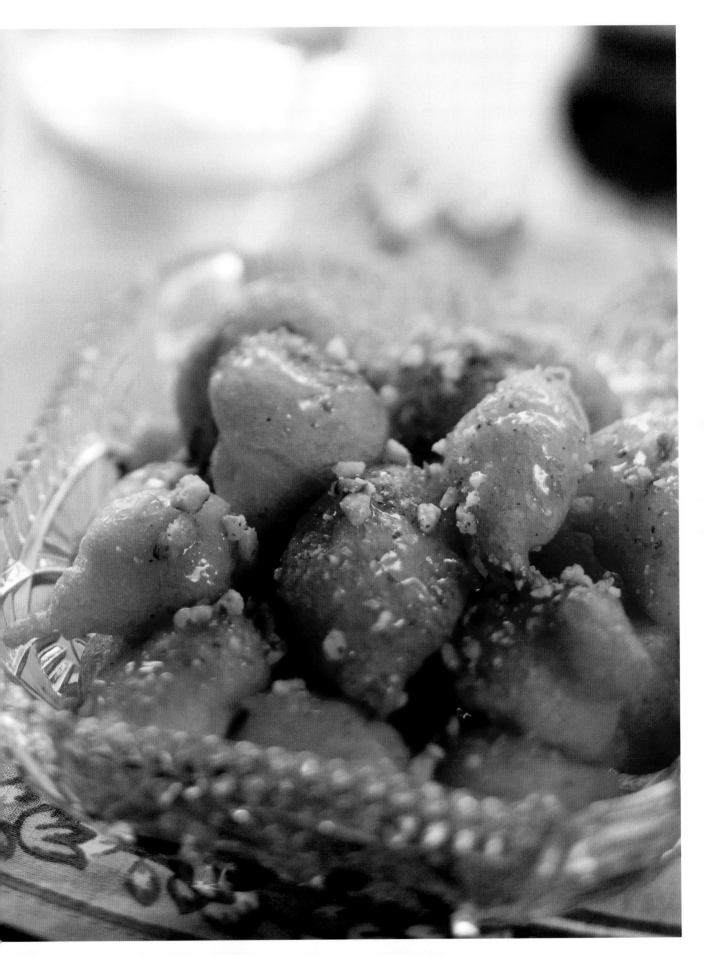

IKARIA'S AMAZINGLY PURE HONEY

"*Pharmaco*," says our friend Yiorgos Stenos, as he runs a heated knife across a framed honeycomb to scrape the last bits of *anamatomelo*, the unique, thick-as-peanut-butter honey drawn from bees that have fed on the tiny purple flowers of fall heather. "*Pharmaco* [medicine]. Every morning, I eat a tablespoon of this. When we were kids this was our breakfast—a cup of *fliskouni* [pennyroyal tea], a clove of garlic, and a spoonful of honey all mixed together. It's nature's antibiotic. And more," he adds as a wry smile opens across his face. Yiorgos is a very young, very robust 83. He is the most sought-after dancer on the north side of Ikaria, and at community gatherings, where he is a most frequent and welcome guest, he gladly whirls a waiting list of women eager to partner with him for an island waltz, or tango, or for the allure of a lyrical *ballo*, the "flirting dance." He is also one of Ikaria's most knowledgeable beekeepers and certainly one of its most generous, having taught many younger men and women the art and mystery of working with bees.

We have visited him on many dewy, early summer mornings, following his old white van up dusty roads to the places where he keeps his apiary: the pine forests in Carres or the coast along the south side, near Aghios Kyrikos, where the drier climate provides perfect growing conditions for thyme, which grows wild in the late spring.

Ikaria's honey, like almost all honey in Greece, comes from bees that feed on different plants throughout the year, thereby producing varietal types like pine honey, thyme honey, heather honey, etc. But what is arguably very different on the island is, first, the diversity and richness of the local wild flora and, second, the fact that it still really is wild; there are virtually no open fields or plains on the island that could make commercial farming viable, which means in turn that there is very little use of pesticides. So, too, chemical-free is the pollen and nectar collected by the local species of honeybees, which are themselves unique. From what Yiorgos has told me, the bee subspecies on Ikaria is more closely related to the more aggressive African bee than to the laid-back Greek, Macedonian, and Cretan honeybee species found in other parts of the country. For all of the Ikarians' own relaxed lifestyle, their bees are a cantankerous lot that happen to produce some of the purest, most delicious honey on earth!

Most of Yiorgos's activity as a beekeeper takes place from the early spring to the late fall. In the winter, bees hibernate, feeding off the honey they've stored. "You always have to leave enough for them," he says, fingering one of the frames he's opened to show us a swarm. "We're taking their food, remember!"

(continued)

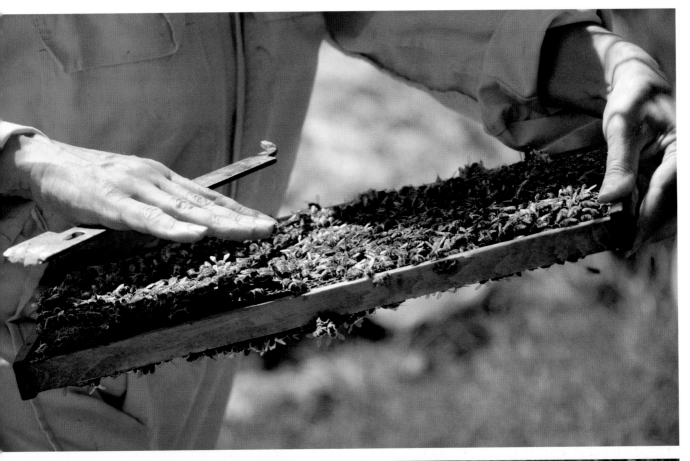

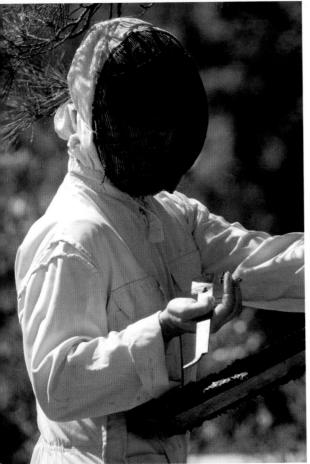

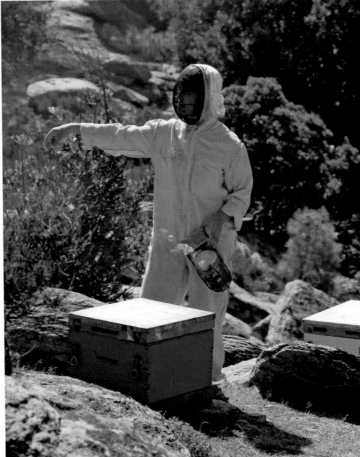

Honey Seasons, Varieties, and Medicinal Qualities

Honey varieties are distinguished by the plants that bees feed from, but that does not mean, for example, that for "thyme honey" the bees have fed exclusively on thyme. Honey types are an indication of the majority of plants from which the bees have collected pollen and nectar; but, of course, bees are peripatetic, traveling in a range of 6 miles (8 km) from their hives, and so sucking nectar and scooping up pollen with their fine hind legs from myriad different plants. It's the beekeeper who knows where to take them so that they can collect the highest percentage of whatever pollen it is he or she wants them to collect. The categories are regulated by Greek law, so that each type of honey has to contain a legal minimum of whatever plant is listed on the label as the variety.

Early spring is the time that beekeepers take their hives to the spots around the island where the most wildflowers are in bloom. The honey produced by blossom-feeding bees is light in color, aromatic, and relatively thin, especially compared to the dark, minerally, viscous pine honey and the almost-solid heather honey.

Blossom Honey

In spring, white heather, which grows all over the island, from shoreline to mountain crest, blossoms. It's a resilient plant, reviving itself even after fires that do, unfortunately, sometimes sweep the island, especially when the weather is dry, hot, and windy—a nationwide bane.

The madrone—*koumara* to the islanders and arbutus to botanists—provides white pollen and rich nectar that bees are drawn to. But the honey produced from the arbutus berry, although said by many beekeepers to be most therapeutic, is decidedly bitter. It's a strange feeling to eat something at once sweet and bitter, but it's delicious in its own right.

Wild lavender, which blankets Ikaria with its long, billowing purple flowers and green-gray stems, provides some of the most aromatic nectar—no pollen—and also some of the most perfumed honey.

Thyme Honey

Then, later in the spring and early summer, around June, the thyme bushes blossom. Their tiny purple-pink flowers are delicious fodder for bees, and Yiorgos, like most beekeepers, takes his hives to the south side of Ikaria, where the terrain is bone-dry and dusty—not unlike the Cyclades—the only place on the island where thyme flourishes. Thyme honey is one of the most sought after of all Greek honeys because it has one of the most distinct aromas and flavors, but also because less honey is actually produced by bees when they feed from its blossoms. Demand drives its price higher than that of other honeys. As a folk remedy, it is said to be antiseptic, heal wounds, and boost the immune system.

Pine Honey

Summer is the time for pine honey, and it is mostly in the pine forests on Ikaria's north side that we've seen Yiorgos and other beekeepers in action. Of all honeys produced on the island and in Greece in general, the most nutrient rich is pine. It is dark, mahogany brown, thick as the finest silks, delicious and easy to enjoy on its own or in syrups, desserts, and even savory dishes.

Pine honey is rich with proteins, amino acids, and minerals and also has somewhat fewer calories than other honeys produced from pollen.

What I find most fascinating about pine honey is that it is actually drawn not from the tree, which doesn't flower, but from the honeydew secreted by a parasite, *Marchalina hellenica, Pinus sp.*, commonly known as the aphid, which feeds off the branches and bark of Aegean pine species. The insect feeds off the trees' sap, sucking out more than it can process, then filters it into the sugary secretion that bees love. They collect the sugary secretion (it's about 20% protein, 80% carbohydrate) and convert it to honey. Ikarian kids also love the sticky drops on the barks of pine trees and scrape them off with their fingers as a kind of snack—the forests are kids' playgrounds even today; my son has spent many a childhood summer day playing hide and seek, cops and robbers, and whatever other adventure games boys like to play. Most pine honey is produced in July and August and collected in mid to late August.

Fall Heather

Beekeepers keep a keen eye on the weather at all times, but perhaps more than ever in the midfall, after the first rains. If it gets too cold, the season's purple heather won't flower. But if the conditions are right, and they often are, *anama* (heather) explodes all over the northern side of Ikaria. It is from this bush that Ikarian beekeepers produce what they will say is the island's rarest, best, most therapeutic and delicious honey. *Anamatomelo* or *riki* as it is called is thick and spreadable. It has a beautiful, rich reddish caramel color. Folk wisdom says it is a tonic and the best thing to consume for bronchitis and chest colds.

How Honey Is Used on the Island

Honey is often taken as medicine or as preventive medicine, especially among older people on the island. But it is also used to make many of the syrups served with traditional desserts and as a sweetener for the dozens of different wild mountain herbal teas that Ikarians drink, themselves an important component of the folk pharmacopeia.

Honey as Medicine and Nutrition

The belief that honey is medicine is founded in truth. Indeed, honey has a long medicinal history.

All honey, for example, is antibacterial. It contains hydrogen peroxide, which the bees create from glucose with the aid of an enzyme, glucose oxidase, which is deadly to microbes such as salmonella, *E.coli*, *Helicobacter pylori* (thought to cause stomach ulcers), and even certain strains of staphylococcus.

Even though honey contains simple sugars, it is *not* the same as white sugar or artificial sweeteners. Its exact combination of fructose and glucose actually helps the body regulate blood sugar levels. Ancient Olympic athletes would eat honey and dried figs to enhance their performance. This has now been verified with modern studies, showing that it is superior in maintaining glycogen levels and improving recovery time compared to other sweeteners.

Honey is also rich in flavonoids and antioxidants, which help fight against certain cancers and heart disease.

And, as at least one dancing beekeeper claims . . . honey is nature's very own Viagra!

CORNMEAL PIE WITH GREEK YOGURT, DRIED FRUIT, AND HONEY

Bobota

Cornmeal, *bobota* in Greek, was the stuff of poor man's porridges and desserts in Greece until the early 1960s. Like many "poor man's" foods, it is a nutritional treasure trove of thiamin, niacin, and folate. It is rich in carbs and fiber, so satisfies an empty belly easily. Cornmeal is rich in iron, which helps our red blood cells transport oxygen throughout the body and drives our metabolism by activating enzymes required for energy production. It's a great source of phosphorous and also contains magnesium, potassium, zinc, copper, manganese, and selenium. As for vitamins, it contains a few from the B group, as well as vitamins E and K.

This simple cake was traditionally made with goat's milk, which I have replaced with Greek yogurt which is easier to find stateside; I've added orange peel and the result is a hearty dessert that also doubles as a great breakfast treat.

MAKES 6 TO 8 SERVINGS

Oil or butter, for greasing the pan

2 cups coarse cornmeal or polenta

¼ cup sugar

1 tablespoon baking powder

½ teaspoon baking soda

½ teaspoon salt

¾ cup fresh orange juice, strained

½ cup Greek extra virgin olive oil

½ cup plain Greek yogurt

Grated peel of 1 orange

½ cup golden or dark raisins

½ cup chopped dried figs (optional)

½ cup Greek or Ikarian pine honey

1 cup hot water

1 strip orange peel

Position a rack in the center of the oven and preheat it to 375°F (190°C). Grease an 8 x 8-inch square baking dish. In a medium bowl, combine the cornmeal (or polenta), sugar, baking powder, baking soda, and salt. In a large bowl, whisk together the orange juice, oil, and yogurt.

Slowly add the cornmeal mixture to the orange juice mixture, stirring by hand with a wire whisk until smooth. Using a spatula or wooden spoon, mix in the orange peel, raisins, and figs, if using. Pour the batter into the baking dish. Bake in the center of the oven until light golden and set, about 40 minutes.

Meanwhile, in a small saucepan, combine the honey, hot water, and orange peel and bring to a boil. Simmer over low heat for 8 to 10 minutes to make a viscous syrup.

Remove the cake from the oven, prick the surface all over with a toothpick, and pour the hot syrup over the warm cake. Let it cool. Cut into squares and serve.

DIAMANDO'S MESSY ORANGE PHYLLO PIE

Patsavouropita y Portokaloglyko

This is a favorite Greek dessert. The pie is made by tearing up pieces of commercial phyllo into a "mess," and mixing them with a tangy yogurt-orange custard. Anyone who remembers a Creamsicle will understand the flavor combination I am talking about! After the pie is baked and the top crisp and golden, it is drizzled with orange syrup. This isn't health food as dessert, but it's delicious.

MAKES 10 TO 12 SERVINGS

SYRUP

1½ cups sugar

2 cups water

1 cinnamon stick

1 strip (1 inch [2.5 cm wide]) orange zest

PIE

Butter, for the baking dish (or ramekins)

1 cup plain Greek yogurt

¾ cup sugar

3 large eggs

½ cup fresh orange juice

1 teaspoon vanilla extract

2 sticks (8 ounces [224 g]) unsalted butter, melted

Grated peel of 2 large oranges

½ pound thin phyllo (#4 or #7), 9 to 12 sheets

Greek yogurt, Greek honey, and orange slices, for garnish

For the syrup: In a medium saucepan, bring the sugar and water to a simmer and stir until the sugar is dissolved. Add the cinnamon stick and orange peel. Simmer for 8 to 10 minutes to form a thin syrup.

For the pie: Preheat the oven to 375°F (190°C). Butter a 13 x 9 inch (33 x 23 cm) glass baking dish or 10 to 12 individual ramekins 2½ inches (6 cm) wide. Using a stand mixer fitted with a large bowl and whisk attachment, whisk together the yogurt, sugar, eggs, and orange juice at medium-high speed until creamy. Add the vanilla, melted butter, and orange peel and whisk until smooth.

Tear the phyllo into irregular pieces about 2 inches (5 cm) long and ½ inch (1 cm) wide. Add them to the yogurt mixture combining well by hand and separating any pieces that might be stuck together.

Spread the mixture evenly in the baking dish or the individual ramekins. Place the baking dish or ramekins inside another, larger, pan and fill it one-third of the way up with water. Bake until puffed and golden, 35 to 40 minutes. Let cool slightly before serving.

To serve: if using ramekins, invert and flip again so that the golden-brown side is on the top. For the larger pie, cut into serving pieces. Serve with a dollop of the yogurt, honey, and orange slices, if desired.

WALNUT-OLIVE OIL COOKIES
DIPPED IN HONEY

Finikia

Finikia are walnut cookies made with an olive oil dough, a specialty of Christmas.

Because the dough contains no butter or dairy, these delicious cookies are also transformed into a larger nut-stuffed Lenten pastry called *skaltsounia* (page 289).

These cookies are dark, damp, and crumbly, yet substantial and surprisingly filling. They make excellent breakfast fare and go perfectly with a steaming cup of coffee, Greek or otherwise.

MAKES 40 TO 50

SYRUP

3 cups honey, preferably Ikarian pine honey

1 cup water

1 tablespoon lemon juice

2/3 cup sugar

Juice of 2 oranges, strained

2 teaspoons ground cinnamon

1/2 teaspoon freshly grated nutmeg

Heaping 1/4 teaspoon ground cloves

COOKIES

6 to 8 cups all-purpose flour

1 teaspoon baking powder

1/2 teaspoon baking soda

2 cups Greek extra virgin olive oil

FILLING

3 1/2 cups finely chopped or ground walnuts

4 teaspoons ground cinnamon

Preheat the oven to 350°F (175°C). Line a baking sheet with parchment paper or a silicone baking mat.

For the syrup: In a medium saucepan, bring the honey, water, and lemon juice to a boil. Reduce the heat and simmer for 10 minutes. Set aside.

For the cookies: In a large bowl, sift together 6 cups of the flour, baking powder, and baking soda.

In a stand mixer fitted with the whisk attachment, whisk together the olive oil and sugar until fluffy. Add the orange juice, cinnamon, nutmeg, and cloves and beat to combine.

Add 2 cups of the flour mixture to the batter and whisk to combine. Remove the whisk attachment. Using a spatula or wooden spoon, slowly add as much of the remaining flour as you can in 1/2-cup increments to form a smooth, soft, but dense dough, kneading as you add.

For the filling: Combine the walnuts and cinnamon. Set aside 1 cup for the garnish.

Break off a nugget of dough and shape it into an oblong piece about 2½ inches (6 cm) long, 1¼ inches (3 cm) wide, and 1 inch (2.5 cm) high. Using your thumb, make an indentation in the center. Add ½ teaspoon of the walnut-cinnamon mixture and pinch the top of the biscuit closed. Place the cookies 2 inches (5 cm) apart on the lined baking sheet. Continue with the remaining dough. Bake in batches, until set, 20 to 25 minutes. Cool on a rack.

Reheat the syrup. Immerse the cooled cookies in the hot syrup, remove with a slotted spoon, and transfer to a platter. Sprinkle with the reserved nut mixture.

NUTS MAKE GREEK PASTRIES HEALTHY

Nuts are a basic ingredient in countless Greek sweets. A few, like the *Finikia* (opposite), *skaltsounia* (Stuffed Lenten Cookies, page 289), and the Spice Cake for a Revealing Saint (page 277) are represented here. That's not to say, of course, that baklava, *kataifi* (nut-filled shredded wheat pastry), and other classics aren't made on the island; I've just chosen a few favorites and the most prevalent.

Nut trees grow in Greece and flourish on Ikaria, too, which is one reason why they appear in certain foods and in a bevy of sweets. But there is a nutritional reason, too, once more evincing the innate wisdom in eating like an Ikarian, or more generally like a Greek!

Nuts are protein- and fat-based foods. Sweets contain carbohydrates. The protein in nuts counteracts the effects of the carbohydrates, which in turn reduces the burden on our pancreas to produce high amounts of insulin. Many of the Greek nut-filled sweets may actually be consumed by people who are insulin resistant. Nuts basically keep the balance of glucose levels in the blood more stable.

They are, of course, filled with good nutrition, too. Some nuts, especially walnuts, which are prevalent in Greece and in Ikaria—there is even a village named for them, Karidiyes, on the north side of the island—provide some rare anti-inflammatory and antioxidant phytonutrients that help reduce the risk of prostrate and breast cancer. They contain a high amount of vitamin E, which is heart healthy. The skin is actually the healthiest part of the walnut, where almost 90% of its health-inducing phenols are found.

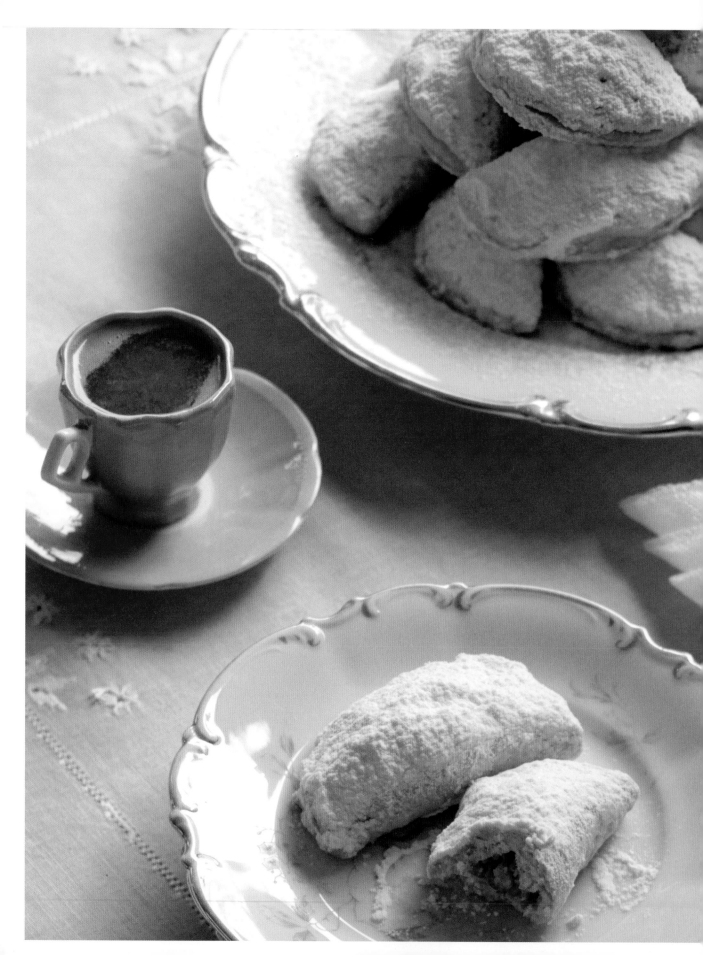

STUFFED LENTEN COOKIES

Skaltsounia Nystisima

These delicious nut- and raisin-stuffed traditional Lenten cookies are totally vegan. They are one of the few simple sweets people traditionally ate during Lent. Home cooks still make them. Redolent of spices and filled with nuts, they are both wholesome and filling. I often bake these to have on hand all throughout the year.

MAKES 25 TO 30

Finikia dough (page 286), without the syrup or filling

2 cups ground walnuts

1½ teaspoons ground cinnamon

½ teaspoon ground cloves

½ cup raisins (optional)

Grated peel of 1 orange

2 tablespoons Ikarian pine or other honey

Powdered sugar or granulated sugar (see Note), for garnish

Preheat the oven to 350F° (175°F).

Prepare the *finikia* dough and divide it into 3 balls.

In a bowl, combine the walnuts, cinnamon, cloves, raisins (if using), orange peel, and honey.

Roll out a ball of dough to a round about 15 inches in diameter. Take a 3-inch (8 cm) glass or cookie cutter and cut rounds out of the dough. Place 1 tablespoon of the filling in the center of each circle and fold over to form a half-moon. Wet the inside edges with a little water and press closed with your fingers or with the tines of a fork. Continue until the dough and filling are used up. Gather up any excess dough and roll it out and fill it, to finish off the cookies.

Bake until lightly golden, about 25 minutes. Remove the *skaltsounia* from the oven and cool slightly on a rack. Sift a generous amount of powdered sugar over them.

NOTE: *Instead of sprinkling powdered sugar on the cookies after baking, you can sprinkle them with a generous amount (about 2 teaspoons per cookie) of granulated sugar before baking.*

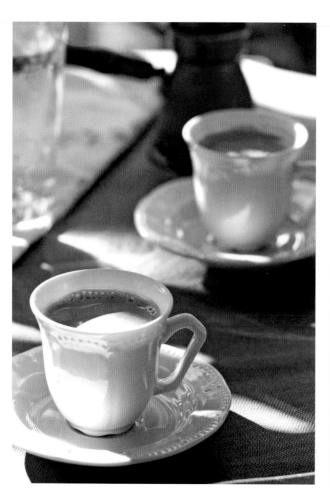
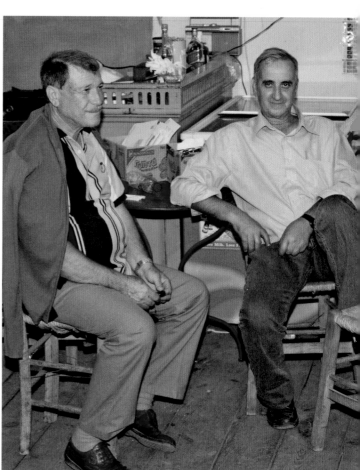
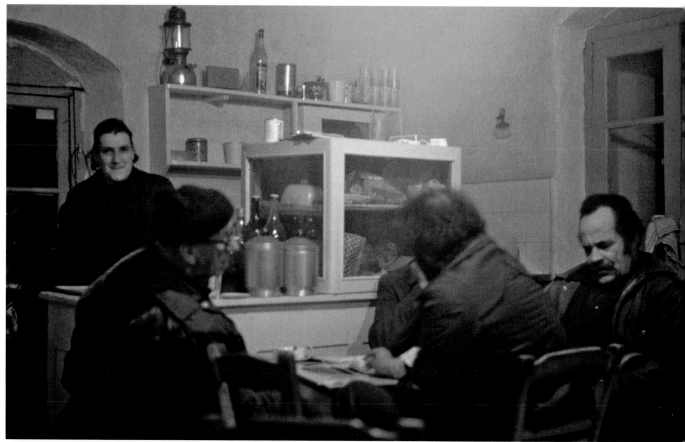

GREEK COFFEE, HEART DISEASE, AND LONGEVITY

Coffee and dessert go hand in hand. Greek coffee made headlines in 2013 as the elixir of life, the secret to longevity among the inhabitants of Ikaria, all thanks to a study conducted by Dr. Gerasimos Siasos, MD, and professor at the University of Athens Medical School, and published in *Vascular Medicine* in March 2013. It essentially found that drinking a daily cup of Greek coffee may be good for our hearts and one more in the long list of food and lifestyle clues behind these islanders' enduring life spans.

Moderate coffee consumption in general is thought to have a beneficial effect on cardiovascular health. Dr. Siasos and his team researched the link between coffee-drinking habits and endothelial function. The endothelium is a layer of cells that lines blood vessels and is affected by aging and lifestyle habits, such as smoking.

Siasos's team randomly selected 71 men and 71 women over the age of 65 on the island. They were tested for high blood pressure and diabetes and asked to fill out questionnaires about their medical history, lifestyles, and coffee-drinking habits. The team tested the endothelial function of the 142 people who participated in the study. More than 87% of those tested said they drank Greek coffee daily. The subjects, even those with high blood pressure, had better endothelial function than those who drank other kinds of coffee.

The reason might lie in the nature of Greek coffee itself. Greek coffee is lightly roasted and finely ground, almost powdery. It is prepared by boiling, usually with a little sugar, in a tapered small pot called a *briki*. Boiling helps extract more of the healthy compounds, such as polyphenols and antioxidants, than are found in, say, brewed or filtered coffee.

A Few Empirical Observations, and How to Make Greek Coffee

I can add my own observational two cents here, too: Making Greek coffee is something of a ritual. First you have to measure out a demitasse cup of water and pour it into the *briki*. Then you measure out a heaping teaspoon of coffee and as much sugar as desired, typically 1 teaspoon for a *metrio*, or medium-sweet cup, and add these to the water. With a long-stemmed spoon or miniature whisk you then proceed to stir the coffee over a light flame until it begins to swell and rise in the *briki*. The best Greek coffee is lifted two or three times over the flame as it swells, which helps create a creamy surface, called *kaimaki*. To make Greek coffee requires mindfulness and presence; it's not just a matter of pressing the button on an automated espresso maker or turning on the coffeemaker for a cup of filtered coffee. It is something you have to do slowly and deliberately. A typical cup of Greek coffee is not more than a demitasse full, or 2 to 4 ounces, compared to 8 ounces in a regular cup of filtered coffee.

FRIED DOUGH STRIPS WITH HONEY
Xerotygana

Xerotygana literally means "dry," as in crunchy and fried. This confection, essentially dough strips fried in olive or other oil and drizzled generously with honey and nuts, is one of the classic Christmas sweets on the island. My dad made mountains of them every Christmas in our New York home, perhaps waxing nostalgic, if in private, about his love of the island where he grew up. Some cooks pinch the strips together in the center to form little bows. The pastry should be crisp and lightly redolent of eggs. These may be made a day in advance, but not drizzled with honey until just before serving, to prevent them from softening.

MAKES 4 TO 5 DOZEN

1 teaspoon baking powder

¼ teaspoon baking soda

2½ to 3 cups all-purpose flour

5 egg yolks

1 egg white

2 tablespoons butter, at room temperature

¼ cup powdered sugar

2 tablespoons brandy

Grated peel of 1 orange

½ teaspoon vanilla extract

Olive or other vegetable oil, for deep-frying

Honey, preferably Ikarian pine honey, warmed slightly

Ground cinnamon

Finely chopped walnuts

In a medium bowl, sift together the baking powder, baking soda, and 2½ cups of the flour.

Using an electric mixer, beat the egg yolks and egg white at medium-high speed until fluffy. Slowly add the butter, powdered sugar, brandy, orange peel, and vanilla, beating well after each addition.

Remove the bowl from the mixer and gradually add the flour mixture by hand, in ½-cup increments, mixing it in with a spatula. Knead until the dough is elastic and smooth, then divide into 3 balls.

Lightly flour a work surface. Using a rolling pin, roll out each ball, one at a time, until as thin as a dime. As you roll, rotate the dough and sprinkle lightly with flour, so that it opens up evenly on all sides and becomes elastic and silky. You can also do this using a pasta maker, passing the balls through it in ever-narrowing sequence, until you have long, thin strips.

There are many shapes for *xerotygana*, but on Ikaria the preferred shape is the simplest: a strip about 2 inches wide and 4 inches long. Cut the strips and set them aside, covered, until you finish and until you have heated the oil.

In a large, deep pot, heat 4 inches (10 cm) of oil to 350°F (175°C). Using tongs or a slotted spoon, place several dough strips at a time in the oil, being careful not to overcrowd them. Fry for a few seconds, until the *xerotygana* turn light golden and bubble and float to the surface. Remove with a spider or slotted spoon and drain on paper towels. Repeat until all the dough is used up.

Place the *xerotygana* on a large platter or platters and drizzle generously with warm honey. Sprinkle with cinnamon and walnuts. Serve.

PETIMEZI: A VITAMIN-RICH SYRUP FROM GRAPES

I love to be in Ikaria in September, when the light starts to change, the air goes crisp, and the sweet, sticky smell of pressed grapes is on every breeze. On the island almost everyone we know makes wine. Most people make wine for their own consumption; a few families produce it commercially, either to sell locally or, bottled, to export to Athens and beyond. One Ikarian winemaker, at the Afianes estate in Raches, has succeeded in getting a few bottles of his Begleri, wine made from the local, eponymous grape, onto New York menus.

Being on the island during wine season has another advantage: access to a seemingly unlimited supply of *petimezi*, the syrup made by clarifying grape must (the juice of pressed grapes before it ferments), then boiling it until it is sufficiently reduced. On Ikaria, most people who make wine also make *petimezi* and they use it as a sweetener in specific, seasonal confections like *moustalevria* (a *petimezi* and flour pudding), *moustokouloura* (spiced cookies sweetened with *petimezi*), and, finally, *petimezopita*, a cake (see Grape Molasses–Chocolate Cake, page 294).

Petimezi contains all the nutrients and healthful characteristics of grapes, including disease-fighting antioxidants, vitamins, and minerals. The juicy part of the grape, which is used to make molasses, contains vitamins A, C, and B$_6$, along with minerals such as potassium, calcium, iron, and magnesium. *Petimezi* is a great source of iron and a delicious way to help restore the body's iron if you are anemic. Our bodies can easily metabolize the natural sugars in *petimezi*, too.

GRAPE MOLASSES–CHOCOLATE CAKE

Petimezopita me Sokolata

It's funny how recipes travel. *Petimezopita* is a cake I've been making for years, waiting anxiously every September for a supply of *petimezi* (grape molasses) from friends on Ikaria who make wine and go to the trouble to take the must, clarify it, and boil it down to syrup. One afternoon while I was visiting my friend Eleni, whose husband makes wine on a large and gorgeous estate in Pygi in the center of the island, she served us chocolate *petimezopita* cupcakes, of all things, and said, "You know, I used your recipe!" So, here is my recipe, reworked with Eleni's twist, to make something modern out of something utterly traditional and old-world.

The *petimezi* has a subtle sweetness, nowhere near as cloying as either honey or sugar. The result is a dense, dark cake that is moist and faintly reminiscent of the smell of grapes as they ferment.

MAKES 6 TO 8 CAKE SERVINGS OR 12 CUPCAKES

- 1 cup water
- 1 cinnamon stick
- 5 whole cloves
- 1 cup Greek extra virgin olive oil
- 6 tablespoons brown sugar
- 1½ cups *petimezi* (grape molasses)
- Grated peel and juice of 2 large oranges

- ¼ cup Greek *tsipouro*, ouzo, or grappa
- 1 teaspoon baking soda
- 5 to 6 cups all-purpose flour
- 1 cup dark chocolate chips
- 2 tablespoons granulated sugar
- ½ cup sesame seeds

Preheat the oven to 350°F (175°C). Lightly oil a 12-inch (30-cm) springform pan or 12 cups of a muffin tin.

In a small pot, combine the water, cinnamon stick, and cloves and bring to a boil over medium heat. Turn off the heat and let the spices steep for 15 minutes. Strain.

In a stand mixer fitted with the whisk attachment, whip the olive oil and brown sugar together until fluffy. Add the spice water, *petimezi*, orange peel, and tsipouro (or ouzo or grappa). Mix well.

Dissolve the baking soda in the orange juice and stir into the *petimezi* mixture.

Sift 5 cups of the flour into a medium bowl.

Gently whisk the flour into the *petimezi* mixture. If the batter is loose, add a little more flour. Stir in the chocolate chips, if using.

Scrape the batter into the springform or muffin cups. Toss the granulated sugar and sesame seeds together and sprinkle over the cake. Bake until a toothpick inserted in the center comes out clean, 50 minutes for the cake, 40 to 45 minutes for the cupcakes.

Serve the cake as is, or with a bit of *petimezi* or chocolate syrup drizzled over or around it. Serve the cupcakes, if making, the same way. *Petimezopita* is delicious with vanilla ice cream, too.

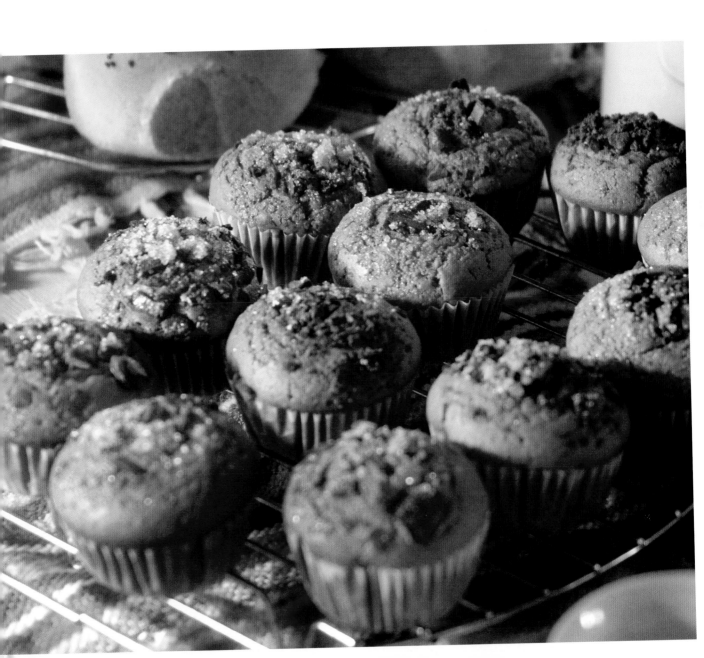

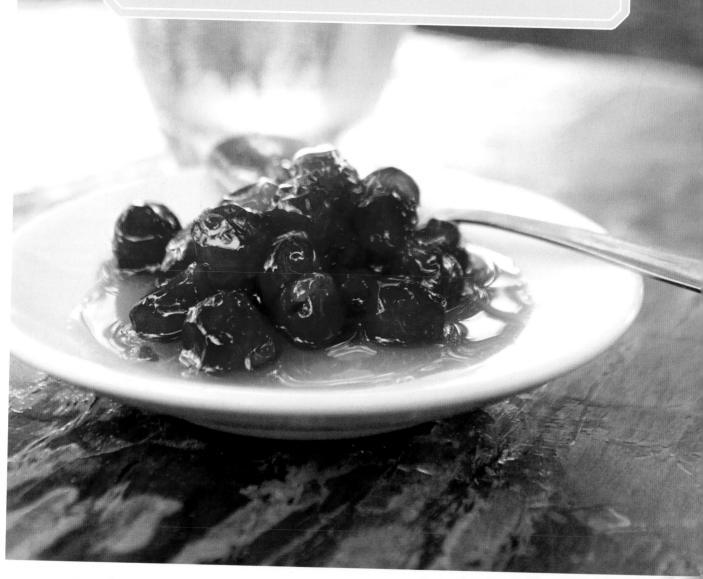

A WORD ABOUT SPOON SWEETS

No other sweet calls to mind the traditions of hospitality and seasonality better than the *glyka tou koutaliou*, sweets on a spoon. These are basically preserves of fruits, unripened nuts, and some vegetables put up either in sugar syrup, *petimezi* (page 293) or, sometimes, honey.

Today, *glyka tou koutaliou* are made all over Greece and the range of nature's bounty put up in syrup is enormous. But every region has certain specialties. On Ikaria, they are: sour cherries, called *vyssino*, which both grow wild and are cultivated all over the northern, mountainous part of the island; sweet cherries, *kerasia* in Greek; walnuts, which are picked green and soft in early June, then debittered in a lengthy process of soaking and changing the water over weeks; and green figs, made into a spoon sweet from hard, unripe wild figs when they are in season in early June. That's not to say local cooks don't make other spoon sweets. These are simply the most prevalent.

SOUR CHERRY SPOON SWEET

Cherries and sour cherries abound on the north side of Ikaria and we pick them in June by the kilo to make this delicious spoon sweet. The flavor of sour cherry spoon sweet is both, well, sweet and tart. The cherries taste a little like dried cranberries. They are small, with tiny pits that require patience to remove. The syrup ends up being very dark, almost black, and it takes extra care to make it. If you are inattentive at the final few minutes of simmering, you can easily burn the whole batch and end up with a caramelized sweet that tastes more like burnt sugar than fruit.

MAKES 6 PINTS

2¼ pounds (1 kg) fresh sour cherries

2¼ pounds (1 kg) sugar

1 cup water

2 tablespoons lemon juice, strained

Wash the cherries. Remove their stems. Using a cherry pitter or the loop end of a hairpin, push out the pits.

Place ½ pound (225 g) (about a fifth) of the cherries on the bottom of a large, wide pot. Sprinkle with a fifth of the sugar. Repeat, layering cherries and sugar. Let the cherries stand for 8 hours or overnight, refrigerated.

The next day, bring the cherry-sugar mixture up to room temperature by letting them stand unrefrigerated for about 2 hours.

Place the pot over low heat and pour in the water. As soon as the mixture comes to a simmer, add the lemon juice. Simmer carefully over low heat, without stirring much but skimming the foam off the surface, until the syrup is thick enough to coat the back of a spoon, 30 to 40 minutes. As soon as it's done, remove from the heat. *Vyssino* is one of the easiest of the spoon sweets to master, but the secret to making it well is in the timing and in those pivotal few minutes between knowing when the syrup is right and burning it. Let the mixture cool to room temperature.

Ladle the spoon sweet into 6 clean 1-pint (0.5-l) canning jars, filling each to about ¾ inch (2 cm) from the top. Loosely screw the lids on the jars. Place in a clean pot with enough water to come about two-thirds of the way up the height of the jars. Cover and bring to a boil. Reduce the heat and simmer for 5 minutes. Using kitchen tongs, carefully remove each jar and with a pot holder or towel screw on the lids very well. Immediately flip the jars upside down to create an air vacuum. Let stand until cool. Store, well sealed, in a cool, dark place. The *vyssino* spoon sweet will last for months, even years, if stored properly.

ACKNOWLEDGMENTS

All of us who belong to the island of Ikaria feel blessed to have her in our lives. We touch ground there whenever possible. With this book I hope to give something back to the island that has given me and my family so much joy, so many friendships, the fondest memories, and an enduring perspective on life.

My first encounter with the island would never have happened if my sister Athena and her husband, Paul, hadn't taken me there in the summer of 1972. Thanks to them, I fell in love at first sight with Ikaria. I met my husband, Vassilis Stenos, there. His larger-than-life personality, encyclopedic knowledge of the island and just about everything else, and telling pictures grace this book. Thanks to all my family, always, for an endless store of unconditional love and support: Kyveli and Yiorgo, Koko, Trif, George, Tom, Kristy, and Katharine.

I would never have gotten to know the island if it weren't for lifelong friends and fellow villagers whose homes are always open, and from whom I've learned so much about the local food, lore, and ethos. Among them: Argyro and Nikos Kouvdou; Argyro and Christos Malahias; Eleni and Yiorgos Karimalis; Aneza, Popi, Olga, and Captain Yiannis Manoli; Aris and Anna Tsapaliaris; our wonderful neighbors, Titika Karimali and Stefanos Tsantiris; the inimitable Yiorgos Stenos, beekeper, friend, and philosopher; and so many others too numerous to name. The Safos clan has always figured prominently in my experience of Ikaria, both stateside and on the island. Thanks to all for so many great times around the table.

Five other friends also helped with their knowledge and aesthetics: Dietician Maria Byron Panayidou provided all the nutritional information and Dr. Tassos Kyriakides, a research scientist at the Yale School of Public Health, helped me make sense of the Ikaria study and other related scientific information. My good friend Lizana Mitropoulou ran the kitchen and helped style the food when we shot the book. Another great friend, Despina Velonia, took over the lion's share of the food styling. I owe a debt of gratitude to Lefteris Trikiriotis, who was always there generously sharing his knowledge of the island's flora, history, and more.

I owe a big hug and special thanks to Peter Poulos, who once again let me strip his cupboards bare of antique Greek plates to use as props in many of the photographs. An old friend, Katya Mavroyiorgou, provided a mountain of beautiful plateware, too.

I am grateful to my agent, Angela Miller, who saw the potential in a cookbook about remote Ikaria, island of longevity and a Blue Zone. Thank you Dervla Kelly for seeing the book to fruition with a keen eye and gentle spirit, and thanks Elissa Altman for beginning that process. The designer, Kara Plikaitis, has taken our raw material and turned it into a most visually stunning portrait of the island.

Thanks, too, to Molyvos restaurant in New York City, where I am collaborating chef and where many of the recipes I have collected from Ikaria are slowly finding their way onto the menu.

RESOURCES

For Mastiha and other gourmet and
regional Greek food products:
mastihashop.com

For specialty produce and greens:
melissas.com

For Ikarian products and honey:
dianekochilas.com
ikariamag.gr/ikariastore

For general Greek food products:
demeterspantry.com
greekshops.com
titanfoods.net

For acorn flour:
iloveacorns.com

SELECTED BIBLIOGRAPHY

In Greek

Bauman, Helmut. *Greek Flora*. Athens: Elliniki
Etaireia Prostasia tis Fyseos, 1993.

Diamandis, Stefanos. *Ta Manitaria tis Ellados*.
Athens: Ekdoseis Ion, 1992.

Dimitrakis, K. L. *Agria Fagosima Horta*. Athens:
Kalliergitis, undated.

Heldrech, Theodore. *Lexico ton Dimodon Onomaton
ton Fyton tis Ellados*. Athens: Adelfoi Tolidi, 1980.

Jovanovic, Ana, and Laura Mandleberg. *Ta Farmakeftika
Votana tis Ikarias*. self-published, 2004.

Kerpis, Ioulios. "Laikes Trofes tis Ikarias." *Laografia*
Magazine 34 (1988): 416–20.

Milingou-Markantoni, M. "Heirografes Sylloges
Protogenous Laografikis Ylis tou Spoudastiriou
Laografias toy Panep. Athinon." *Parousia* 5
(1987): 539–50.

*Oula Einai Fadia tis Koilias—H Kouzina tis Ikarias
kai Oi Syntages tis Zois Mas*. Syllogos Kavos-
Papas, 2007.

Paschari-Kouloulia, Argentoula. "Painemata ki
aitimata sta Katiotika Kalanta." *Ikariaka*, 1992.

———. "To krasi stin Laiki Paradosi tis Ikarias." In
Pramnios Oinos—"Ethos, Istoria, Laografia."
Athens: Syllogos Kavos-Papas, 1999.

Poulianos, Alexis. *Laografika Ikarias*. Vols. 1, 2, and
3. Athens: Etaireia Laografikon kai Istorikon
Meleton Ikarias, 1976.

Samara-Gaitlich, Natalia. *Oi Syntages tis Katohis*.
Athens: Marathia, undated.

Yannetou Louvari Vasilia. *Paradosiaka Stoiheia kai
Gefseis tou Vorioanatolikou Aigaiou*. Athens:
Papazisi, undated.

In English

Bhanoo, Sindya N. "The Secret May Be in the
Coffee," *New York Times*, March 25, 2013.

Brill, Steve, with Evelyn Dean. *Edible and Medicinal
Plants in Wild (and Not So Wild) Places*. New
York: Harper, 1994.

Buettner, Dan. *The Blue Zones*. Washington, DC:
National Geographic Society, 2008.

Chrysochoos, John. *Ikaria—Paradise in Peril*.
Pittsburgh: RoseDog Books, 2010.

Davidson, Alan. *Mediterranean Seafood*. Baton
Rouge: Louisiana State University, 1981.

Kallas, John. *Edible Wild Plants: Wild Foods from
Dirt to Plate*. Layton, UT: Gibbs Smith, 2010.

Kochilas, Diane. *The Glorious Foods of Greece*. New
York: William Morrow, 2001.

Panagiotakos, D. B., C. Chrysohoou, G. Gerasimos
Siasos, et al. "Sociodemographic and Lifestyle
Statistics of Oldest Old People (>80 Years)
Living in Ikaria Island: The Ikaria Study."
Cardiology Research and Practice (2011), Article
ID 679187, 7 pages, doi:10.4061/2011/679187.

Papalas, Anthony J., *Ancient Icaria*, Wauconda, IL.:
Bolchazy-Carducci, 1992.

———, *Rebels and Radicals*, Wauconda, IL.: 2005.

Thayer, Samuel. *The Forager's Harvest—A Guide to
Identifying, Harvesting, and Preparing Edible
Wild Plants*. Birchwood, WI: Forager's Harvest
Press, 2006.

Weed Research & Information Center. *Weed
Control in Natural Areas in the Western United
States*. Davis, CA: University of California,
Davis, 2013.

INDEX

Boldface page numbers indicate photographs. Underscored references indicate boxed text.

CONVERSION CHART

These equivalents have been slightly rounded to make measuring easier.

VOLUME MEASUREMENTS

U.S.	Imperial	Metric
¼ tsp	–	1 ml
½ tsp	–	2 ml
1 tsp	–	5 ml
1 Tbsp	–	15 ml
2 Tbsp (1 oz)	1 fl oz	30 ml
¼ cup (2 oz)	2 fl oz	60 ml
⅓ cup (3 oz)	3 fl oz	80 ml
½ cup (4 oz)	4 fl oz	120 ml
⅔ cup (5 oz)	5 fl oz	160 ml
¾ cup (6 oz)	6 fl oz	180 ml
1 cup (8 oz)	8 fl oz	240 ml

WEIGHT MEASUREMENTS

U.S.	Metric
1 oz	30 g
2 oz	60 g
4 oz (¼ lb)	115 g
5 oz (⅓ lb)	145 g
6 oz	170 g
7 oz	200 g
8 oz (½ lb)	230 g
10 oz	285 g
12 oz (¾ lb)	340 g
14 oz	400 g
16 oz (1 lb)	455 g
2.2 lb	1 kg

LENGTH MEASUREMENTS

U.S.	Metric
¼"	0.6 cm
½"	1.25 cm
1"	2.5 cm
2"	5 cm
4"	11 cm
6"	15 cm
8"	20 cm
10"	25 cm
12" (1')	30 cm

PAN SIZES

U.S.	Metric
8" cake pan	20 × 4 cm sandwich or cake tin
9" cake pan	23 × 3.5 cm sandwich or cake tin
11" × 7" baking pan	28 × 18 cm baking tin
13" × 9" baking pan	32.5 × 23 cm baking tin
15" × 10" baking pan	38 × 25.5 cm baking tin (Swiss roll tin)
1½ qt baking dish	1.5 liter baking dish
2 qt baking dish	2 liter baking dish 325°
2 qt rectangular baking dish	30 × 19 cm baking dish
9" pie plate	22 × 4 or 23 × 4 cm pie plate
7" or 8" springform pan	18 or 20 cm springform or loose-bottom cake tin
9" × 5" loaf pan	23 × 13 cm or 2 lb narrow loaf tin or pâté tin

TEMPERATURES

Fahrenheit	Centigrade	Gas
140°	60°	–
160°	70°	–
180°	80°	–
225°	105°	¼
250°	120°	½
275°	135°	1
300°	150°	2
160°	3	
350°	180°	4
375°	190°	5
400°	200°	6
425°	220°	7
450°	230°	8
475°	245°	9
500°	260°	–

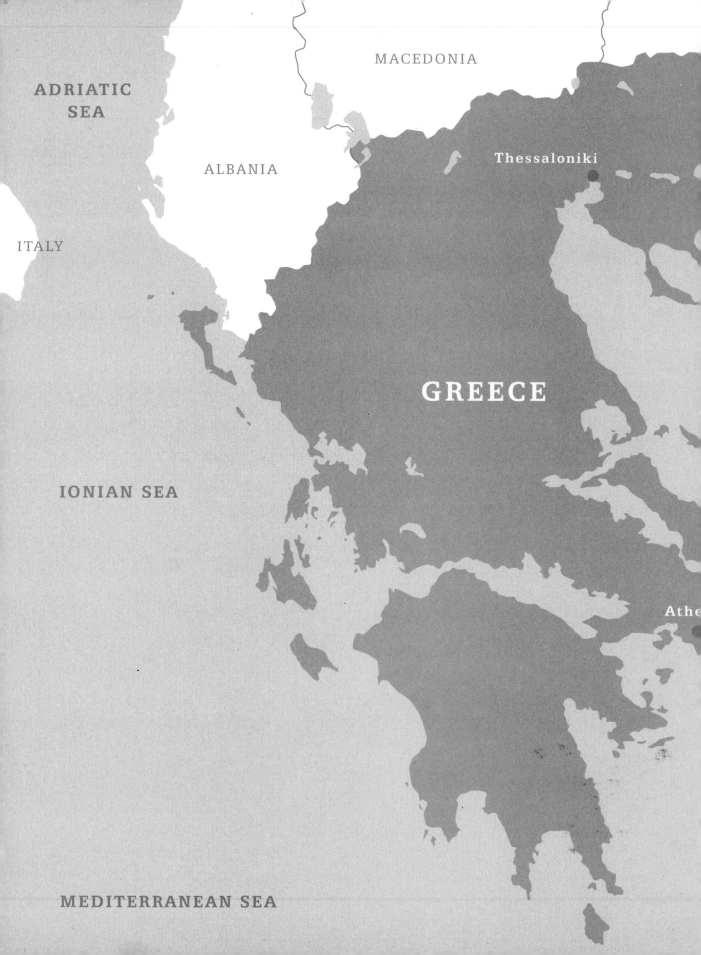